CLINICAL
FORENSIC
MEDICINE

CLINICAL FORENSIC MEDICINE

SECOND EDITION

Edited by

WDS McLay OBE

$\langle\!\langle$ G $\backslash$ M $\backslash$ M $\rangle\!\rangle$

© 1996

Greenwich Medical Media
507 The Linen Hall
162-168 Regent Street
London
W1R 5TB

First Edition 1990
Second Edition 1996 © GMM

ISBN: 1 900151 200

A catalogue record for this book is available
from the British Library

Designed and produced by
Derek Virtue, DataNet

Printed in Hong Kong

CONTENTS

PREFACE xi

CONTRIBUTING AUTHORS xiii

1 – CONTEMPORARY CLINICAL FORENSIC MEDICINE 1

2 – LEGAL SYSTEMS AND THE POLICE

    PART I: English Legal System 7

        The courts 7
        Appeals to the Court of Appeal 8
        Civil and criminal procedure 9
        The nature of evidence 9
        The law of evidence 10
        Admissibility of evidence 10
        Types of evidence 10
        Standard and burden of proof 11
        Presumptions 12
        Competence and compellability 12
        Spouses 12
        Children 12
        The mentally ill and handicapped 13
        The order of trial 13
        The right of silence 15
        Hearsay 17
        Confessions 19
        Opinion and expert evidence 21
        Similar fact evidence 22
        Corroboration 22
        Professional privilege and disclosure 23

    PART II: Scottish Legal System 25

        History 25
        Criminal jurisdiction 26
        Procurator fiscal 27
        The Crown Office 28
        Solemn cases 28
        Criminal procedure 30
        Civil jurisdiction 31
        Children's hearings 31

PART III: The Police in the United Kingdom 33

The duties and structure of the police service 33
The investigation of crime, and prosecutions 36
Other operational matters 36
Police personnel 37
Complaints against police officers 37
Other forces 38

3 – THE PRACTITIONER'S OBLIGATIONS 39

Introduction 39
The legal framework 42
Consent 43
Intimate samples 46
Capacity 50
Confidentiality 51
Disclosure 56

**4 – CLINICAL EXAMINATIONS IN
THE POLICE CONTEXT** 59

General considerations 59
Facilities for examination 60
Doctor/patient relationship 61
Beginning the investigation 62
Specific forensic examination 66
Summary 72

5 – THE DOCTOR IN COURT 75

Statements 76
Attendance at court 79
Defence experts 87
Fees 88

6 – CARE OF DETAINEES 91

Introduction 91
Clinical notes 92
Some general considerations 92
Treatment plans 93
Specific conditions 94
Head injury and altered consciousness 99
Intoxication and drug abuse 102
Fitness to be interviewed 103
General aspects 103
Clinical assessment of interviewee 104

Responsibilities of forensic clinician 108
Annex C 108

7 – CHILDREN 111

Non-accidental injury 111
Child sexual abuse 119
The Children Act 1989 135
Child protection procedures in Scotland 137

8 – INJURY 143

Describing wounds 143
Types of injury 146
Defence wounds 153
Self-mutilation 154
Firearm wounds 155
Torture 160
Investigation of suspicious death 161

9 – SUBSTANCE MISUSE 163

Introduction 163
Criminality and drug use 163
Drug laws 164
Definitions 164
General principles 165
Specific drugs 166
Treatment of opiate withdrawal 169
Harm minimisation 170
Overdose 171
Mental Health Act 171
Concealment 172
Notification 172
Alcohol 173
Alcohol and crime 176
Alcohol withdrawal 177

10 – PSYCHIATRIC DISORDER 181

Introduction 181
Examination of the mental state 182
Clinical syndromes 183
Assessment of suicide risk 185
The Mental Health Act 1983 186
Arrangements in Scotland 189
Mens rea, the M'Naghten rules
    and diminished responsibility 191

11 – ADULT SEXUAL OFFENCES AND RELATED MATTERS 193

Introduction 193
Definitions 193
Examination facilities 196
History of the allegation 196
Forensic exhibits 196
Consent 201
Medical and sexual history 201
Physical examination 201
Female genitalia 203
Male genitalia 205
Anal area 206
Special techniques 206
General injuries 207
Genital and anal findings 208
Subsequent to the examination 210
The psychological consequences of sexual assault 211
Sexually transmitted diseases. 213
Defendant (alleged suspect) examinations 214
The medico-legal implications of pregnancy 215
Premenstrual syndrome 216
Sexual variations 217

12 – ACCIDENTAL INJURY AND TRAFFIC MEDICINE 219

Introduction 219
Accidents on the road 220
Role of the forensic medical examiner in traffic accidents 224
Legal aspects of traffic medicine 225
Accidents in the home 242
Accidents at work 244

13 – THE SCENE OF CRIME AND TRACE EVIDENCE 247

Preservation of the scene 247
Techniques used at the scene 249
Documents 254
The doctor at the scene 254
The role of the forensic scientist 255
DNA profiling 258
Physical examinations 261
Drugs and toxicological examinations 263

The medical examination –
  the requirements of the forensic scientist 264
Forensic science in the UK 270

14 – DEATH AND ITS INVESTIGATION 271

Confirmation of death 271
Examination of the body and
  estimation of the time of death 272
Historical aspects 275
Death certification 277
Natural deaths 279
Unnatural deaths and inquests 280
Disposal arrangements 282
Death certification in Northern Ireland 283
Death certification in Scotland 284

15 – FORENSIC ODONTOLOGY 287

Marks which should raise the police surgeon's
  suspicions that an odontologist is required 287
Differential diagnosis of bite mark injuries 290
Action taken by the forensic physician 291
Action taken by the forensic odontologist 293
Odontology's place in identification 293
Age determination from the teeth 294

16 – DEALING WITH A MAJOR DISASTER 297

Police objectives in the aftermath of
  a major incident 297
Planning for disasters 301
The ambulance service 301
The clinical foresnsic examiner 302
Mortuary phase 303
Identification 304
Special instances 307
Operational debriefing 307

17 – OCCUPATIONAL HEALTH OF
POLICE OFFICERS 309

Conditions of service of police officers 310
Conditions of work 311
Recruits 311
Cadets, special constables and civilian employees 313
Specialists 313
Physical and chemical hazards 316

Biological hazards 317
Stress and alcohol 317
Sick leave 319
Maternity leave 320
Pensions 320

TABLE OF CASES 323

TABLE OF STATUTES 324

INDEX 326

PREFACE

A fresh reading of the preface (does anyone other than the editor read the preface?) to the first edition of *Clinical Forensic Medicine* published in 1990 shows many of the ideas expressed there to still be valid. Greater emphasis is placed now upon the care of those in police custody, but this simply puts into context the need for clinical acumen in a wide sense. Since 1990, the service provided by police surgeons has become more written about in general medical journals, a healthy development, although much of the comment is hostile. The trial of two doctors whose lamentable standard of care towards a prisoner led to his death was described by Brahams (*Lancet* 1993; **341**:428), then in a *Lancet* editorial (1993; **341**:1425). Rix discussed the same case and related matters in the *British Medical Journal* (1993; **341**:861), with an answer from Davis (15 May 1993). Moon and his colleagues argued for better legal and forensic training (*BMJ* 1995; **311**:1587). That, and the refrain by Patel on deaths in police custody (*BMJ* 1996; **312**:56) were answered in the issue of 6 April by members of the Association of Police Surgeons. Forensic medical examiners are now assumed to have a valid contribution, for example in debating the topic "Should doctors be more proactive as advocates for victims of violence?" Knight put the police surgeon's point of view ("Medical paternalism is unacceptable") in the *BMJ* of 16 December 1995.

The journal for long published by the Association of Police Surgeons has become the *Journal of Clinical Forensic Medicine*, attracting relevant and significant articles from around the world. The Association itself is likely to adopt an altered title, but this must not detract from the major task of assisting the police and the prosecuting authorities in the investigation of crimes and offences by use of medical techniques.

Assiduous attention to the whole text will reveal some discrepancies, some variation in emphasis or practice between authors when they refer to the same topics. This is both realistic and inevitable, for consensus has still to be reached. In similar vein, police surgeons are strongly recommended to familiarise themselves with local procedures and the sometimes subtle differences in law between jurisdictions.

Readers will also appreciate that political and legal ideas change and develop. For the forensic clinician, this imposes a duty to keep abreast of events. As an example, the General Medical Council published *Duties of a Doctor* at the end of 1995 as an up to date statement of the ethics of practice by which doctors would be judged. Portions of this publication are referred to repeatedly in the pages that follow. The British Medical Association and the Association of Police Surgeons issued guidelines on such matters as consent and confidentiality based upon the GMC view, but the foundation for that view must inevitably change when impending statutory provisions on disclosure come into force. In turn, the stance taken by police surgeons as they deal with prisoners will be affected.

This edition of *Clinical Forensic Medicine* is designed, as was the last, primarily to be of value to the many practitioners who are concerned with people whose medical condition is of interest to the courts, be they witness, accused, victim, or party to civil litigation. We know how often the previous edition is referred to in court. In this edition authorship of each chapter is clearly identified; an unforeseen outcome of the decision in 1989 not to do this has been to saddle the editor with both undeserved praise and blame! Once again, I have depended upon the accumulated knowledge of many colleagues in writing the text and in reviewing contributions. To those who are not members of the Association of Police Surgeons a special debt is owed.

In a more technical sense, I am pleased to acknowledge the assistance of Mr John Meyer, Advocate, who has kindly taken time and trouble to guide me around many legal pitfalls. Officers of Strathclyde Police have given me sound information over the years. The book has been designed by Mr Derek Virtue, of DataNet, who has both set the text and enhanced many of the illustrations. Geoffrey Nuttall and Jason Payne-James, directors of Greenwich Medical Media, and their assistant Justine Santer, have contributed their publishing expertise, not to mention patience in time of trouble. Finally, wifely forbearance has been both precious and necessary over many months.

W.D.S.M
MAY 1996

CONTRIBUTING AUTHORS

1: CONTEMPORARY CLINICAL FORENSIC MEDICINE

DAVIS Neville
FRCGP FFOM LMSSA(Lond)

Senior Forensic Medical Examiner Metropolitan Police, Lecturer Detective Training School, Senior Honorary Secretary Royal Society of Medicine, Vice President Section of Clinical Forensic Medicine Royal Society of Medicine, Honorary Medical Secretary Medico-Legal Society, Member Editorial Board *Forensic Science International,* First President Section of Clinical Forensic Medicine Royal Society of Medicine, Formerly Member of Executive Council British Academy of Forensic Sciences, Formerly Honorary Secretary Association of Police Surgeons, Consultant Occupational Physician National Intitute for Medical Research (MRC), Member of Medical Survival Committee Royal National Lifeboat Institution.

2: LEGAL SYSTEMS AND THE POLICE
PART I: ENGLISH LEGAL SYSTEM

WALL Ian
MB BS BA DCH DRCOG MRCGP

Barrister at Law, Forensic Physician, Forensic Medical Examiner Metropolitan Police, Forensic Medical Examiner City of London Police, Approved Medical Practitioner Mental Health Act.

PART II: SCOTTISH LEGAL SYSTEM

Mc LAY WDS
OBE MB ChB LLB FRCS

Chief Medical Officer Strathclyde Police, Honorary Clinical Senior Lecturer in Forensic Medicine Glasgow University, Lectures in forensic medicine and science to law classes at Strathclyde University, Past President Association of Police Surgeons.

PART III: THE POLICE IN THE UNITED KINGDOM

STRACHAN Crispian
QPM MA MIMgt

Assistant Chief Constable Community Services Strathclyde Police, Formerly Metropolitan Police Service London.

3: THE PRACTITIONER'S OBLIGATIONS

KNIGHT Michael A
MB BS LLM DA DMJ(Clin)

> Principal Police Surgeon and Force Medical Adviser Suffolk Constabulary, Honorary Secretary Association of Police Surgeons.

WILKS Michael
MB BS DRCOG

> Forensic Medical Examiner, Executive Member Metropolitan and City Group, Member BMA Medical Ethics Committee, Chairman APS/BMA Working Group on Disclosure, Member BMA/APS Working Group on Healthcare of Detainees.

4: CLINICAL EXAMINATIONS IN THE POLICE CONTEXT

BUNTING Reginald
MB ChB DMJ DObstCOG

> Force Medical Officer and Principal Police Surgeon Avon and Somerset, President Association of Police Surgeons, Police Surgeon Training Officer.

5: THE DOCTOR IN COURT

CLARKE Myles DB
MB ChB MRCS LRCP MRCGP DMJ

> Consultant Forensic Physician, Former Divisional Police Surgeon Merseyside, Former Deputy Police Surgeon Cheshire, Late Honorary Lecturer Department of Forensic Medicine University of Liverpool, Late Visiting Lecturer Merseyside Police Training School, Visiting Consultant in Clinical Forensic Medicine to the Department of Health, Government of Singapore, Visiting Lecturer Netherlands School of Public Health Utrecht, Tutor and Lecturer to the FAGIN (Forensic Academic Group in the North) Manchester, Member of the Examining Board for the Diploma in Medical Jurisprudence Society of Apothecaries London, Past Editor of "Police Surgeon Supplement"

6: CARE OF DETAINEES

ROBINSON Stephen P
MB ChB DMJ

> Senior Police Surgeon to Greater Manchester Police. Honorary Lecturer in Clinical Forensic Medicine to the University of Manchester. Co-ordinating director of the Forensic Academic Group in the North (FAGIN). Listed in the Law Society's Directory of Expert Witnesses, member of the Acadamy of Experts, in the Register of Experts. Specialist knowledge for treatment and reporting of patients with mental disease approved under section 12 of the Mental Health Act. Examiner for Diploma in Medical Jurisprudence. Member of the Association of Police Surgeons, the Clinical Forensic section of the Royal Society of Medicine. Member of the British Acadamy of Forensic Sciences, the Forensic Science Society and the Manchester and District Medico-legal Society

7: CHILDREN

ROBERTS Raine
MBE MB ChB FRCGP DCH DMJ(Clin)

Clinical Director (Honorary Consultant) Sexual Assault Referral Centre Manchester, Forensic Physician Greater Manchester Police, Convener Panel of Examiners for Diploma in Medical Jurisprudence Society of Apothecaries London.

8: INJURY

CRANE Jack
MB BCh FRCPath DMJ(Clin et Path) FFPathRCPI

State Pathologist for Northern Ireland, Professor of Forensic Medicine Queen's University Belfast, Consultant in Pathology Northern Ireland Health and Social Services Boards, Member Home Office Policy Advisory Board on Forensic Pathology.

9: SUBSTANCE MISUSE

NORFOLK Guy A
MB ChB LLM MRCGP DMJ

General Practitioner and Police Surgeon Bristol, Honorary Assistant Secretary Association of Police Surgeons, Member of Education and Research Sub-Committee, Association of Police Surgeons, Member of the International Editorial Board *Journal of Clinical Forensic Medicine,* Lecturer on Alcohol Drugs and the Law.

STARK Margaret M
MB BS LLM MFFP DGM DMJ(Clin) DAB

Forensic Medical Examiner, Metropolitan Police, Chairman Education and Research Sub-Committee Association of Police Surgeons, Council Member Section of Clinical Forensic Medicine Royal Society of Medicine, Member Medical Working Group on Substance Misuse Detainees in Police Custody, Lecturer on Substance Misuse Basic Training Course Metropolitan Police, National Development Training Programme, and SEAL (South East and London Legal Medicine Study Group)

10: PSYCHIATRIC DISORDER

BAIRD JA
MD FRCPsych DObst DCH

Consultant Forensic Psychiatrist Leverndale Hospital and Douglas Inch Clinic Glasgow, Visiting Psychiatrist Barlinnie Prison and Greenock Prison.

EVANS J Victoria
MB BS MRCGP DFFP DMJ(Clin)

Police Surgeon Greater Manchester Police, Hospital Practitioner Paediatric Forensic Medicine, Clinical Assistant Drugs North West, Visiting Specialist Substance Abuse HMP Manchester.

11: ADULT SEXUAL OFFENCES AND RELATED MATTERS

HOWITT Josephine Burnell
MB BS MRCS LRCP DMJ(Clin)

Forensic Medical Examiner Metropolitan Police Service, Council Member Section of Clinical Forensic Medicine Royal Society of Medicine

ROGERS Deborah
MB BS DCH DRCOG MRCGP DMJ(Clin) DFFP

Forensic Medical Examiner, Honorary Secretary Section of Clinical Forensic Medicine Royal Society of Medicine, Member of Education and Research Subcommittee Association of Police Surgeons, Lecturer and Tutor South East and London Legal Medicine Study Group.

12: ACCIDENTAL INJURY AND TRAFFIC MEDICINE

MARSDEN Andrew K
MB ChB FRSCEd FFAEM DiplMRCSEd

Consultant Medical Director Scottish Ambulance Service, Former Consultant in Accident and Emergency Medicine Wakefield, Force Surgeon West Yorkshire Police, Former Chairman Rescucitation Council UK.

13: THE SCENE OF CRIME AND TRACE EVIDENCE

HOGG Ian

Chief Inspector, Head of Identification Bureau, CID Support, Strathclyde Police.

RANKIN Brian WJ
BSc MSc CChem FRSC

Forensic Scientist Forensic Science Service.

SHAW Ian C
BSc

Forensic Scientist Forensic Science Service.

14: DEATH AND ITS INVESTIGATION

DEAN Peter
MB BS BDS(Hons) LLM DRCOG DFFP

HM Coroner for the County of Essex, Forensic Medical Examiner London, Formerly Secretary Section of Clinical Forensic Medicine Royal Society of Medicine, President-Elect Section of Clinical Forensic Medicine Royal Society of Medicine, Member of the Journal Committee of the *Journal of Clinical Forensic Medicine*, Member of the Council of the Medico-Legal Society, Member of the Steering Group of the National Confidential Enquiry into Perioperative Deaths.

15: FORENSIC ODONTOLOGY

CLARK Derek
CStJ BDS PhD LDSRCS DFO CAvMED SRN

Scientific Director Kenyon International Emergency Services UK, Lecturer Civil Emergency Management Centre University of Hertfordshire, Consultant Physicians for Human Rights.

16: DEALING WITH A MAJOR DISASTER

BUSUTTIL Anthony
MD FRCPath DMJ(Path) FRCPE FRCPG

Police Surgeon Lothian & Borders, Regius Professor Forensic Medicine University of Edinburgh, Chairman European Council for Legal Medicine.

17: OCCUPATIONAL HEALTH OF POLICE OFFICERS

McLAY WDS
OBE MB ChB LLB FRCS

Chief Medical Officer Strathclyde Police, Honorary Clinical Senior Lecturer in Forensic Medicine Glasgow University, Lectures in forensic medicine and science to law classes at Strathclyde University, Past President Association of Police Surgeons.

1

CONTEMPORARY CLINICAL FORENSIC MEDICINE

N Davis

In his foreword to the first edition of this textbook published in 1990, the Lord Chancellor, the Rt. Hon. Lord Mackay of Clashfern, wrote "I know from my own experience just how important the quality of expert evidence is; and in no area is it more vital than where medical matters are in issue." Clinical forensic evidence, when given by a forensic physician relating to an individual whom he or she has examined, is the product of a chain of events. It begins with an understanding of the terms of reference, and progressively links the clinical examination, the writing of a report or statement, and the appearance in court. This is the "professional" witness – a witness as to fact. The witness box is the place where findings and opinions will be tested out. Where such evidence is subjected to scrutiny by an independent "expert" witness, the basic quality of the original evidence is the foundation on which the expert can build – or a house of cards waiting to be demolished.

If the evidence is to be of the desired quality, the clinical ability, the impartiality, the ethics and the judgement of the practitioner must all be of a high standard. Do these high standards generally prevail today?

The academic world in the United Kingdom does not recognise clinical forensic medicine (CFM) as a specialty or even as a subspecialty. On the forms which doctors complete for the Medical Directory (an informative list of doctors on the Medical Register) CFM does not appear in the catalogue of specialties, unlike forensic pathology and forensic psychiatry. The undergraduate medical curricula, with few exceptions, pay scant attention even to the basics of CFM, so newly qualified doctors find themselves hard put to describe injuries accurately – and even harder put to draw any reasonable conclusions as to their causation. Raw young doctors, working in accident and emergency departments, are called upon to treat a considerable proportion of the victims of criminal injury and the police rely on their evidence. Given the current academic attitude to CFM, it is not surprising that such evidence may be unsafe and misleading. Similar criticism applies to general practitioners, who also suffer from this educational deprivation. As general practitioners see most of the results of domestic violence, this is again of some importance. So, regrettably, much is left to be desired in the knowledge and practice of CFM in the various disciplines of our profession as we approach the end of the twentieth century.

Calls made on the services of doctors assisting police have increased in number, in complexity and in variation over the years. Such services have traditionally been given by general practitioners, working part-time and paid on a retainer plus item of service fee basis. Historically, such services were initially confined to attendance at cases of sudden or unexpected death, the health care of detainees and of police officers and their families. With the advent of the National Health Service (NHS) in 1948, responsibility for the primary health care of the latter shifted to the local general practices. The duties of doctors assisting the police had already broadened out to include the provision of evidence from victims and perpetrators of criminal injury, the multitude of alcohol related offences, adult sexual crime, and the rest of the catalogue of "crimes against the person". Later activities which came to the fore included drug misuse, non-accidental injury to children and child sexual abuse.

In the United Kingdom, many mental hospitals have been closed as a result of government policy. Their inmates have been released into the community, which in these early days has not always provided that concentration of assistance which the move from a protected environment into our current, often traumatic, society necessitates (Bluglass 1990; Davis 1990). Many of these unfortunates find their way into police stations on account of bizarre, antisocial or otherwise abnormal behaviour. Forensic Medical Examiners (FMEs) are called upon to make an initial assessment and offer advice about subsequent management.

In 1984, the Police and Criminal Evidence Act (PACE) was passed, a statute unmatched anywhere else in the world. This is fully discussed in later chapters, but is mentioned here as it markedly impinges on the work of FMEs. Numerous safeguards for detained persons are written into this legislation, of direct relevance to the responsibilities of the FME. Recent judgements by the Court of Appeal (for example, R v Ward [1993] 2 All ER, 577 CA) in which confessions made during police interviews were regarded as unsafe, years after conviction, have further heightened the need for psychiatric skill. It has become good practice to show that detainees who are going to be interviewed are seen to be fit for this purpose. From time to time it is also desirable to show that the interviewee has not suffered as a result of the questioning. These assessments are now a major responsibility of the FME. On these accounts it is necessary for FMEs to be more proficient in psychiatry than the average general practitioner.

The next element which is influencing standards is a high degree of public exposure. Cases have occurred where doctors employed by the constabularies have patently failed in their duty of care towards detainees or prisoners (Brahams 1992) and it is clear that in some instances the doctors concerned had no specific training in CFM or even in primary health care in a custodial setting. The Crown Prosecution Service, established in 1986 to instigate and conduct prosecutions and thereby separate the investigation of crime from the prosecution of its perpetrators by the constabularies, is showing little reluctance to lay charges against doctors whose breach of their duty of care falls into the category of "gross negligence" (R v Prentice and anor; R v Adomako [1993] 4 All ER 935). Doctors in general are thus increasingly vulnerable, and perhaps this vulnerability is one factor involved in increasing attendances at medico-legal meetings. In the winter of 1994, the Royal Society of Medicine put on a seminar for medical students on the legal aspects of medicine. It was a cold, wet Saturday, yet more than forty students attended, many from provincial medical schools. Their interest, shown in the busy question and answer sessions, vividly demonstrated their need.

Another aspect of the development of CFM is the increasing use of its practitioners by defence lawyers in criminal cases. As it became obvious that the evidence of FMEs was very influential, defence lawyers had to seek out doctors who could assess and, if possible, rebut their evidence, and for this they had to look to other FMEs who were the only ones with experience enough to do the job. The constabularies initially frowned upon their doctors accepting defence work, but since this deprived the defence of legitimate assistance, the situation had to alter. But before it did, many FMEs, finding themselves very much in demand by defence lawyers, resigned from their constabularies and succeeded in establishing themselves in new careers as expert witnesses. The current situation is that it is generally accepted that FMEs should be free to act on behalf of the defence, but that this should be avoided in their own locality, for reasons which are not difficult to understand. The other side of the coin is that, where their FMEs are found to be inexperienced in serious cases, the constabularies are increasingly backing them up in court with more senior doctors in order to equate with a skilful ex-FME – or even a current FME – outside his own area assisting the defence.

In the UK, the fact that most FMEs are active general practitioners in the NHS poses a potential problem. New contracts offered to FMEs by the constabularies are likely to include a requirement similar to "...be immediately contactable if required and available to attend immediately on being requested to attend any Police Station or other place within the Area..." This requirement could conflict with the doctor's obligations to his patients in the NHS. It does mean that rotas have to be scrupulously organised and maintained. Even so, several FMEs have given up general practice and are concentrating successfully on medico-legal work. This trend is likely to increase. Provided that it does not compromise the impartiality of the doctor, it is perhaps to be welcomed, particularly if it means that the standard of CFM evidence will be raised on both sides of our adversarial system.

Looking back on the development of training for FMEs, it is clear that the Association of Police Surgeons was its initiator and that it continues to promote high standards in this discipline. The development of in-house training by the constabularies is a direct result of the activities of the Association. It would not have been possible without the expertise of its members.

So we need to look at two levels in which clinical forensic skills will be utilised. Basic skills, including at least the study of wounds and their causation, the recognition of factors which should give rise to suspicion in cases of sudden or unexpected death, and some understanding of the effects of alcohol and other recreational drugs, are needed by all clinicians; teaching these subjects should be mandatorily included in undergraduate curricula. Alongside this should be training in note-taking and report writing, together with information about the legal system and what is required of a professional witness in court. This should go a long way towards meeting the needs of junior hospital staff, in particular accident and emergency doctors, and general practitioners.

More advanced skills would be needed in various disciplines. For example, paediatricians would need in-depth knowledge of non-accidental injury and child sexual abuse; doctors working in prison health care need to know a great deal about suicide awareness, drug misuse and sexually transmitted diseases as well as mental subnormality (Report of the Working Party of Three Medical Royal Colleges 1992). FMEs need to be proficient through the whole range of CFM, because they are at the sharpest end of the medico-legal interface. Because of the present training deficiency, there is already a tendency towards a two-tier FME service, with 'generalists' who cope with daily 'run-of-the-mill' cases, and 'specialists' who are also competent, for example, in adult and child sexual abuse, and who are called upon specifically in these cases, but this is undesirable. It is the highest common denominator that is required, not the lowest.

The next stage which, bearing in mind existing pressures, must follow in the development of CFM, will be mandatory training, assessment and accreditation of those doctors whose work takes them regularly to this interface. In the UK, the role of the expert witness in civil cases is already under scrutiny (Woolf 1995) and a similar exercise for criminal cases cannot be far off. In these cases, the expertise of doctors in CFM is appreciated both by prosecution and defence. Since independence is a valuable commodity, most doctors would prefer to be appointed by the courts rather than called by either prosecution or defence in our adversarial criminal justice system. The lawyers, on the other hand, for reasons which are fairly obvious, would prefer the status quo. A pertinent – or perhaps impertinent – question that has been asked elsewhere is, "What is it that the court is seeking, justice or the most powerful legal gladiator?" (Davis 1995). At a meeting of the Medico-Legal Society in November 1994, it was evident that the majority of doctors present would prefer an inquisitorial system in which they were agents of the courts, a prospect strenuously resisted by the lawyers.

A major difficulty that has to be faced is finding an academic body willing to approve training and give its backing to assessment and accreditation in CFM. The preferred solution would be to involve the medical Royal Colleges. Such a scheme is currently being developed for doctors in the Prison Health Care Service, involving the Royal Colleges of Physicians, General Practitioners and Psychiatrists. It would not be too difficult to adapt it for use in the present context. The Royal College of Pathologists would also have a legitimate interest in such a venture. So would have the Royal College of Surgeons in respect of accident and emergency medicine. However, postgraduate diplomas already exist, in particular the Diploma in Medical Jurisprudence of the Society of Apothecaries of London, the DMJ(Clin.). This has been more widely taken up by doctors practising overseas than by UK doctors, but the diploma is experiencing something of a renaissance as more and more UK practitioners are finding that their services are in demand, which makes a career possible in CFM. Their need for recognition is leading to a considerable increase in the numbers of UK diplomates. The Society of Apothecaries has recently established the qualification of Master in Medical Jurisprudence (MMJ) which may meet the needs of those who wish to proceed further. However, many senior forensic clinicians and lawyers are convinced that a Medico-Legal Institute, backed by the medical Royal Colleges, the Law Society and the Bar Council, would meet both present and future needs. Efforts to found such an organisation have so far fallen on deaf ears. In the meanwhile, training for forensic medical examiners will continue to be given in-house by a number of constabularies and by specific courses, such as SEAL (South East And London) and FAGIN (Forensic Academic Group in the North) in Manchester. But, of course, this is just one facet, albeit a major one, of the medico-legal interface.

The effects of harmonisation of training in CFM in the UK resulting from European initiatives have yet to be assessed. It is already clear that our European colleagues are looking to a wider and more intense curriculum than is currently envisaged here. The deficiencies of UK forensic medicine relative to the situation in Germany, for example, were demonstrated by Dr David Wells from Melbourne, Australia, in his wide-ranging report to the Winston Churchill Memorial Trust (Wells 1993). A valuable contribution to European harmonisation would be the setting up of an international student exchange scheme. Outside Europe, students from Australia and Kenya have already been able to participate in the CFM activities of the Metropolitan Police in London.

Some progress has been made. The activities of the Section of Clinical Forensic Medicine, established in 1987 at the Royal Society of Medicine in London's

Wimpole Street, have provided a forum in which doctors of the several disciplines which involve the medico-legal interface have met with practising solicitors, barristers and judges as well as their colleagues from overseas. There is little doubt that the Section has forged valuable links and has contributed greatly to mutual understanding between the two noble professions of medicine and the law. Whether or not such contacts will lead to productive cooperation in the spheres of education and training remains to be seen. The Royal Society of Medicine is anxious to broaden its international connections, and therein lies an opportunity for a contribution by the Section of Clinical Forensic Medicine, particularly in the realm of information technology and the super-highway.

So a considerable task lies ahead. Training should be mandatory, standardised and approved. Practitioners must be seen to be independent, impartial and professional, aware of the significant role which society has decreed they must play in the judicial system. Accreditation will follow and this should permit recognition of CFM – but as what? Is it not a collection of subspecialties rather than a separate entity? Perhaps therein lies its strength, for all the medical Royal Colleges must have an interest in it. It is necessary for them to be made aware of this obligation.

References

Bluglass RS 1990 Letter to *The Times* March 3.

Brahams D 1992 R v Salim and Saha. *Lancet* **340**: 1462.

Davis N 1990 Letter to *The Times*, March 13.

Davis N 1995 Medicine and the Law: Hand-in-hand or Hand-in-glove?: *Medico-Legal Journal* **62**(2) 44-61.

Report of the Working Party of Three Medical Royal Colleges 1992: The Education and Training of Doctors in the Health Care Service for Prisoners: RCP, RCGP and RCPsych.

Wells D 1993 Current Practices and Future Directions in Forensic Medicine: Winston Churchill Memorial Trust.

Woolf LJ 1995 Access to Justice: Interim Report to the Lord Chancellor on the Civil Justice System in England and Wales, ch 23.

2

LEGAL SYSTEMS AND THE POLICE

PART I: ENGLISH LEGAL SYSTEM

I Wall

The English legal system is based on the common law tradition, where most law results from prior decisions of the court in the form of judicial precedent, though some law is 'codified' in the form of statutory enactments. The laws of most other European jurisdictions are codified and based on the Roman tradition which is formed from principles reasoned by the jurists of the first and second centuries AD. The modern *mores* of these societies can be reflected in statutes or 'judge-made' law.

Most legal systems are further broadly divided into civil and criminal jurisdictions. Criminal law is the corpus of law which governs wrongs done by persons which are thought to harm society. Civil law governs disputes between private individuals, such as actions in negligence. The substantive laws, procedural rules and the courts which hear the cases often differ between civil and criminal jurisdictions, as for example in the United Kingdom.

Ultimate legislative power in the UK resides in Parliament at Westminster, and though historical and political forces have fashioned entirely separate legal systems in England and Wales, Scotland, and Northern Ireland, there exist many similarities in their laws.

THE COURTS

In England and Wales civil cases are heard in the civil courts, which are arranged in a hierarchical manner. The most inferior of the civil courts are the magistrates courts, which have a limited role. The County Courts and the High Court are above the magistrates court, and most civil disputes will be heard in these courts, which share jurisdiction. Appeals from these courts will be to the

Civil Division of the Court of Appeal and thence, if the case raises a question of law of public importance, to the ultimate appellate court in the UK, the House of Lords.

The criminal courts are similarly arranged in a hierarchical manner. Again, the magistrates court is the most inferior of the criminal courts, though it hears the vast majority of minor criminal cases, either for full trial for 'summary' offences, or by way of a preliminary hearing. The role of the preliminary hearing is to decide whether the defendant will be tried at the magistrates court or the Crown Court if the offence is 'triable either way', or whether the defendant has a case to answer in front of the Crown Court if the offence charged is 'indictable' (a committal proceeding).

Above the magistrates court is the Crown Court where the more serious criminal cases are heard along with appeals against conviction and/or sentence from the magistrates court. Appeals against sentence and conviction from the Crown Court in England and Wales are made to the Criminal Division of the Court of Appeal, and thence to the House of Lords.

As a general rule courts are bound to follow their own previous decisions as well as those of the higher courts, when presented with a similar factual situation. The House of Lords is, however, permitted to depart from its own previous ruling. These binding judicial decisions then become a source of law.

APPEALS TO THE COURT OF APPEAL

Appeals to the Court of Appeal are governed by the Criminal Appeal Act 1968 s1 and can be made as of right if the issue involves a question of law alone; issues of fact alone or mixed fact and law require leave[1]. The grounds of appeal are that conviction is unsafe or unsatisfactory, that the trial court had made an incorrect decision on a question of law, or that there was a material irregularity[2] during the course of the trial. If any of these grounds is established the appeal will be allowed unless the court considers that no miscarriage of justice has actually occurred[3].

---

1. Leave is the permission of the court, and in this context leave may be granted by the trial judge, or a single judge of the Court of Appeal.

2. Such as certain procedural irregularities with the jury, or prejudicial interventions or comments by the trial judge.

3. Criminal Appeal Act 1968 s2; so called 'applying the proviso'.

CIVIL AND CRIMINAL PROCEDURE

In the UK the police are the principal gatherers of evidence for criminal prosecutions. The decision to prosecute, and the subsequent handling of the prosecution is, in England and Wales, undertaken by a centralised body, independent of the police, and under the auspices of the Director of Public Prosecutions, known as the Crown Prosecution Service (CPS). The decision on whether to pursue a case is based both on the public interest in prosecuting, and whether there is a realistic prospect of securing a conviction.

Civil cases in contrast are initiated by the injured party. The rules of civil procedure have been criticised as being too complex and the process too time consuming, though Woolf LJ (1995) has recommended a more streamlined procedure, particularly with regard to personal injury cases.

THE NATURE OF EVIDENCE

Evidence is information which has persuasive force: it need not in fact persuade; it is no less evidence because one chooses not to believe it, what is enough is that it has the *tendency* to persuade. In the deductive scientific paradigm, factual information or 'evidence' is derived from empirical observations, and these form the basis of scientific theory. Though a court of law uses evidence it does not conduct a scientific fact-finding exercise. The interposition of the human element would provide too much in the way of confounding variables for a true scientific exposition. Primary factual evidence, filtered through witnesses, may become distorted by individual perceptions, or corrupted by those who may be unable to recall information accurately, or who may be actuated by emotions other than a desire to tell the truth.

The courts indeed do not claim to discover 'the truth'. Contingencies of time and money, and the adversarial systems in the United Kingdom, mean that courts will only adjudicate, at one point in time, on the matter brought before them by the parties[4], and then only on the facts presented to them by these parties.

Finally, a complex and highly integrated corpus of rules exists which govern what information the court is permitted to hear, and which have the ability to exclude even highly relevant facts. These rules form the *law of evidence*.

---

4. Other jurisdictions such as those in Continental Europe employ a more inquisitorial system whereby an 'examining magistrate' acts as both investigator and judge, rather than just arbitrator.

THE LAW OF EVIDENCE

The largely exclusionary nature of the law of evidence in England and Wales evolved during the last century in response to a perceived need to protect the interests of the accused, at a time when criminal trials were largely perfunctory. There was concern that unsophisticated jurors or lay justices would be unduly influenced by certain types of prejudicial evidence, such as an accused's bad character. Fear of manufactured evidence contributed to the maintenance of the rules on hearsay, and led in part both to the exclusion of classes of persons from testifying, and to the exclusion of confessional evidence.

During this century there has been a shift away from this protective attitude. Changes to the rules of civil procedure have meant that most civil courts are presided over by professional judges sitting alone. This in turn has resulted in a considerable relaxation of the exclusionary rules in the civil jurisdiction, causing a divergence of the law of evidence between civil and criminal jurisdictions.

ADMISSIBILITY OF EVIDENCE

Parties in dispute must advance sufficient evidence before the court to prove their case and/or disprove the other party's case. Only evidence of 'facts in issue', or evidence relevant to facts in issue (the *facta probanda*) are admissible. Facts in issue are those facts which are essential to a case, and which must be proved in order to succeed. Facts in issue are usually a matter of substantive law, so, for example, in the offence of rape the facts in issue are that an act of intercourse has taken place (the actus reus) under circumstances where the accused knew the complainant was not consenting or was *reckless* as to that matter (the mens rea).

Evidence of facts which are *relevant*[5] to facts in issue are also admissible, and is known as circumstantial evidence. Despite this broad principle that all relevant facts are admissible, the judge retains a discretion to exclude relevant evidence[6] if in his opinion such evidence would have a prejudicial effect on the accused's right to a fair trial. Furthermore, relevant evidence may be excluded by the operation of the exclusionary rules discussed below.

TYPES OF EVIDENCE

The term evidence is used to describe the form by which information is presented to the court; that is orally, by way of documents or by way of real objects (for example weapons).

---

5. Relevance is a somewhat fluid term and most judicial definitions of relevance relate it to the concept of 'probative value'.

6. Such a discretion exisits at common law *R v Sang* [1980] AC 402, and under s78 of the Police and Criminal Evidence Act 1984 (see below).

The term is used also in a more substantive juridical context where the evidence may be direct, circumstantial, or hearsay, on the existence or non-existence of a fact in issue. Direct evidence is evidence that requires no act of mental process by the tribunal of fact, it is evidence that speaks directly of a fact in issue, such as an eye witness account. Circumstantial evidence, on the other hand, requires the tribunal of fact to draw logical or reasonable inferences from the information presented.

Circumstantial evidence, though commonly regarded as somewhat inferior, may in the absence of an eye witness account be the only evidence. In fact, it may have irresistible probative force, particularly in combination with other circumstances. Circumstantial evidence is not easily categorised, but includes issues such as opportunity, motive and habitual behaviour. Fingerprints, body fluids or DNA evidence from the scene of a crime are also forms of circumstantial evidence, inviting the tribunal of fact to conclude that the accused was present. An accused's silence may similarly invite the conclusion that he is in fact guilty (see below).

STANDARD AND BURDEN OF PROOF

The standard of proof is the degree of cogency needed of the evidence in order to persuade the tribunal of fact; put simply, it is a measure of how good the evidence is. In criminal cases the prosecution must tender evidence of a sufficient quality to convince the tribunal of fact 'beyond reasonable doubt' that the accused is guilty[7]. Generally speaking the burden of proving the case rests on the accuser, which in a criminal case in England and Wales is the Crown. The accused is innocent until proved guilty, and can sit back and let the prosecution try to prove the case against him (*Woolmington v DPP* [1935] AC 462, HL). This 'golden thread' of English criminal law has a number of exceptions, principally in the form of express statutory enactments. For example, under s2.2 of the Homicide Act 1957 an accused who raises the defence of diminished responsibility on a charge of murder bears the burden of proving diminished responsibility[8].

---

7. In civil cases the standard is based on the balance of probabilities, so that the tribunal of fact needs to be more than 50 percent sure of the defendant's culpability. The standard required may however vary in civil cases, with the requirement of a higher degree of probability commensurate with the seriousness of the allegations *Hornal v Neuberger Productions* [1957] 1 QB 247.

8. This is also true of other defences, such as provocation, duress or self defence. Here the accused must advance sufficient evidence for the judge to conclude that the jury *may* find in favour of the accused (the so called 'evidential' burden). The prosecution then has the 'legal' burden of disproving this defence.

PRESUMPTIONS

These are facts the court will accept as being established in the absence of sufficient or even any evidence, often because proof is difficult or indeed impossible. Presumptions may be of fact or law, and presumptions of the latter may be rebuttable or irrebutable. An example of an irrebutable presumption is that children under the age of 10 years (in Scotland, 8 years) cannot be guilty of committing a criminal offence.

COMPETENCE AND COMPELLABILITY

Whether the court will hear the evidence of a particular witness depends on the court's belief in his or her competence to testify, and, if competent, whether the witness can be *compelled* to testify. These matters fall to be decided before the witness testifies, in a *voir dire*[9].

Generally speaking all persons are competent witnesses and all competent witnesses are compellable, that is they can be forced to give evidence with the penalty of contempt of court if they refuse. The accused, though competent, cannot be compelled to give evidence in his own defence[10].

SPOUSES

A spouse of the accused is competent to give evidence for the prosecution. The spouse can be compelled to give evidence on behalf of the accused and, if the offence charged is a sexual offence in respect of a person under the age of 16, or an assault against the spouse or a person under the age of 16 for the prosecution. If a husband and wife are jointly charged neither spouse is competent or compellable to give evidence at trial[11].

CHILDREN

The particular problems attached to child witnesses giving evidence in court have been partly addressed by recent legislation. Evidence in court must be on oath otherwise it is a nullity, though many children have conceptual difficulties in understanding the nature of the oath. The Criminal Justice Act 1988, s33(a)[12] now makes it a mandatory requirement that the evidence of child witnesses

---

9. Also known as a trial within a trial, where evidence of disputed admissibility will be decided on by the judge when it arises, after hearing submissions from respective counsel. This is often conducted in the absence of the jury.

10. Criminal Evidence Act 1898 s1.

11. Police and Criminal Evidence Act 1984 (PACE) s80.

12. As inserted by Criminal Justice Act 1991 s52 (1).

(which the Act defines as persons under 14 years of age) must now be given unsworn; a child, therefore, over 14 years of age should be considered competent to give sworn evidence. The court, however, retains a power to exclude the evidence of children who appear incapable of giving intelligible testimony[13].

Similarly it had long been appreciated that children were vulnerable to the rigours of the criminal justice system, and particularly court appearances. These concerns have been partly alleviated by the introduction of live evidence by video link, and the recording of interviews with child witnesses under s32 Criminal Justice Act 1988[14]. Furthermore, s53 of the Criminal Justice Act 1991 allows sexual offences cases involving children to be transferred to the Crown Court without being first heard at the magistrates court, forestalling additional interrogation at the committal stage. Section 54(7) of CJA 1991 raises the eligibility to give such evidence to 17 for sexual offences.

THE MENTALLY ILL AND HANDICAPPED

When the mentally ill or handicapped are required to give evidence the secular approach to the oath, which governs child witnesses in civil cases, has been adopted. This approach is based on whether the witness has a sufficient appreciation of the seriousness of the occasion and a realisation that the taking of the oath involves something more than a duty to tell the truth in day to day life. A witness not satisfying this test is not competent to testify[15].

THE ORDER OF TRIAL

The criminal system in England and Wales is essentially adversarial, and the formalities of the hearing and the substantive rules of evidence reflect this. The adversarial system is shared with other common law jurisdictions such as Commonwealth countries and the USA. Some jurisdictions have a more inquisitorial model, such as France, where an inquisitorial magistrate or *juge d'instruction* acting as both investigator and judge is permitted to question the accused and witnesses both in and outside the court[16].

---

13. Section 168 (1) Criminal Justice and Public Order Act 1994.

14. Section 32 does not apply to the magistrates courts, but see s53 CJA 1991, and s55(1) CJA 1991 which prevents children in relation to offences of a sexual nature from giving evidence in magistrates courts unless the case is to be heard there.

15. *R v Hayes* [1977] 1WLR 234; *cf.* if a child fails to satisfy this test his evidence may still be heard.

16. A Look at French Criminal Procedure, Helen Trouille [1994] *Criminal Law Review*, 735-744.

The trial will commence with the charge being read to the accused and a plea entered. The jury will be empanelled where appropriate, and the prosecution will begin by outlining its case in the *opening speech*, though this is often omitted in summary trials before magistrates. Following this, the prosecution will present its evidence, prosecution witnesses will be called and questioned in turn by the prosecuting counsel in the examination in chief. The prosecution witnesses will then be subject to cross-examination by defence counsel. The prosecution will then have the option to re-examine the witnesses on fresh matters which have been raised during cross-examination. This process is then repeated *mutatis mutandis* for defence witnesses.

Examination in chief

During the examination in chief the questioning will be directed to elicit a cogent, relevant and credible story and to advance the case of the party calling. Witnesses, however, must not be asked 'leading' questions which suggest a particular answer.

The trial may be some time after the events of which the witness has direct knowledge. Under these circumstances witnesses are permitted to refresh their memory in the witness box by reference to documents, such as notes or medical records, provided that the records were made contemporaneously with the events in question, are in the original, and are available for the court to inspect. Contemporaneity is not literal, and includes circumstances where the document is made when the evidence is still fresh in the mind of the maker.

This memory refreshing document may be inspected by the parties' legal representatives, and in certain circumstances by the jury. Questions may be asked upon the document, in cross-examination, provided that the questioning does not go beyond the parts that are used to refresh the memory. The entire document can be put in evidence (that is inspected by the jury) if the questioning goes beyond the parts used to refresh the memory, or if there is a suspicion that the document has been fabricated or altered subsequently. The effect of this in criminal cases is that any consistencies or inconsistencies in the whole document can be used respectively to bolster or challenge the credibility or consistency of the witness.

Cross-examination

The main purpose of cross-examination is to undermine the other party's case, but it is also used to elicit favourable evidence for one's own case. If a witness is not questioned on disputed facts, the party conducting the cross-examination will be taken to have accepted the witness's version.

Evidence of character

Cross-examination may be conducted in an attempt to impugn a witness's good character, thereby suggesting to the court that he or she should not be believed.

Questions directed at such an end will only be permitted by the judge, in exercise of his duty to restrain oppressive conduct by counsel, when the answers would indeed seriously impair the witness's credibility. If such questioning does seriously imperil the witness's character, but his evidence is, in proportion, only of minor importance to the issue to be decided, then it will not be allowed.

A party in cross-examination may further be asked questions on his bias or impartiality, his previous convictions, his reputation for untruthfulness and on any handicap he may have which would affect the reliability of his evidence.

Rape

The issue of the character of a complainant in the case of rape is complex. The Sexual Offences (Amendment) Act 1976 s2 (1) preserves the common law principle that the complainant may be cross-examined on, and evidence produced on, prior *sexual experience* with the accused, but not about sexual experience with persons other than the accused *without the leave* of the judge. Leave will only be forthcoming if it would be unfair to the defendant to refuse to allow the evidence to be adduced or the question asked, notwithstanding the emotional effects that this may have on the complainant[17].

Leave is unlikely to be granted if the questions go merely to the credit of the complainant, as in any attempt to blacken her name, because her reputation is a collateral issue. If such questioning goes to a fact in issue, such as consent, leave is likely to be granted, though separating these two issues can sometimes be problematic.

THE RIGHT OF SILENCE

The common law in England and Wales, along with most advanced judicial systems, has traditionally protected the individual's right of silence[18], the benefit of which was that there was both no legal obligation for individuals to give evidence against themselves, and that no assumption of guilt should be inferred from an accused's silence. This was based on the understanding that there may be an innocent explanation for silence, such as fear or the desire to protect another. This privilege against self incrimination, linked to the right of silence, is an

17. The effect of s7(2) is to include the offences of attempt and aiding and abetting within s2, but does not include, for example, offences of sexual intercourse with minors.

18. Ths USA and Japan have rights to silence guaranteed by their constitutions.

implicit element of the right to a fair trial guaranteed under Article 6 (1) of the European Convention, to which the UK is a signatory. In contrast, there has always been support for the Benthamite proposition that 'guilt invokes the privilege of silence', based on concerns that terrorists, professional criminals and sophisticated fraudsters were exploiting the evidential machinery of the right to silence to obtain unjust acquittals.

This in turn resulted in an agenda for reform designed to curtail the right of silence. A succession of reports and statutes in the UK[19] culminated in the introduction of the Criminal Justice and Public Order Act 1994. Its intention was, *inter alia*, to exert pressure on suspects to co-operate with police, and on the accused to give evidence in their own trials in order to avoid any adverse inferences of guilt resulting from silence.

Pretrial silence

Silence prior to the police caution or charge will usually provide no basis for judicial comment, or adverse inferences, particularly in the absence of legal representation. Section 34 of the CJPO 1994 seeks to address the situation where the accused produces exculpatory evidence, or raises a defence in the subsequent court case, which he had not mentioned to the police under caution during the pretrial investigation, and under circumstances where it would have been reasonable for him to do so (so called ambush defences)[20]. Section 34 of the CJPO 1994, by reversing the common law, permits the prosecution to invite the jury to infer that the defence was in fact a sham.

Silence at trial

Section 35 CJPO 1994 allows the court to draw adverse inferences as appear proper on the accused's refusal to be sworn, or to answer questions after being sworn. In order to benefit from the provisions of s35 to bolster their case, the prosecution has to have presented a 'clear prima facie case' against the accused, as silence would not in itself be sufficient to surmount the required standard of proof of guilt. Section 38 (4) prevents a person from being convicted solely on inferences drawn from silence.

---

19. This began with the eleventh report of the Criminal Law Revision Committee 1972 whose agenda for reform can be seen in PACE 1984, CJA 1988 and the Criminal Evidence Act (N I) Order 1988 (which was the forerunner of the CJPO Act 1994) all of which represent an attempt to liberate the judge and jury from the complex rules of evidence, so enabling the guilty to be convicted. See The Criminal Justice and Public Order Act 1994; Ian Dennis, *Criminal Law Review* [1995] 4.

20. A principle reflected in the new caution that the police in England and Wales must use on arrest.

The nature and extent of these inferences are based on the application of common sense to each particular case[21]. Applying common sense to a failure by the accused to advance an innocent explanation when circumstances demand would imply that there was none, and that in fact he is guilty[22].

HEARSAY

Hearsay is the most pervasive of the exclusionary rules in the English law of evidence. Hearsay is any statement made by any person other than the witness giving evidence from the witness box (that is any out of court statement) which is presented before the court in order to assert that the facts contained in the statement are true. Suppose A gives evidence in the witness box stating that B had informed him that he, B, had seen C commit a crime. If A's assertion is adduced as evidence of the fact that C had truly committed a crime, then it is hearsay, and as such is inadmissible in court. B would thus need to give direct evidence to the court that he had witnessed C's wrong doing.

The rule against hearsay is seen as providing a measure of protection against manufactured evidence, by ensuring that the jury has the benefit of both observing a witness's demeanour first hand, and of assessing his truthfulness under challenge. Nevertheless, hearsay evidence may have considerable probative force because it may have passed through an unimpeachable source.

The rule against hearsay is also one aspect of an individual's right to a fair trial, where the accused's opportunity to examine all witnesses giving evidence against him in open court is of central importance. The common law in England and Wales has traditionally respected this right, and Article 6(3)(d) of the European Convention guarantees it, thereby imposing a strict rule against hearsay, though the European Court's handling of hearsay under article 6 has been somewhat conflicting[23].

---

21. Interpretations of the provisions in the CJPO are likely to be influenced by rulings under identical provisions in operation in Northern Ireland since Criminal Evidence (NI) Order 1988 and see Interpreting Silence Provisions; JD Jackson [1995] *Criminal Law Review* 587-601.

22. As is the case under the doctrine of recent possession in the law of theft *R v Aves* [1950] 2 All ER 330 (CA).

23. In *Unterpertinger v Austria* (case 1985/87/134) the European Court held that convictions based on the evidence of witnesses not present and not testifying at court were in breach of Art 6, while in the subsequent cases of *Asch v Austria* (1990) case 30/1990/221/283, the European Court declined to find a breach of the Article despite almost identical facts as *Unterpertinger*. In general see Hearsay and the European Court of Human Rights, [1993]*Criminal Law Review* 257.

Changes in civil procedure and successive statutory enactments[24] have led to the result that hearsay evidence is more likely to be admitted in civil than in criminal proceedings. To reduce the full rigour of the application of the rule a number of exceptions have evolved.

Exceptions to the hearsay rule in criminal cases

Hearsay evidence may be admissible at common law or through express statutory authority. Common law exceptions include statements in public documents, such as birth and death certificates, works of reference such as medical texts, and, though of limited contemporary relevance, dying declarations.

Sections 23 and 24 of the Criminal Justice Act 1988 represent one of the more important of the express statutory exceptions. Section 23 deals with first hand documentary hearsay, and section 24 with hearsay contained in documents created in the course of business or a profession.

Another statutory exception is the Police and Criminal Evidence Act 1984, s69 (1) which governs the conditions for admissibility of documents produced by computers where information is supplied to the computer by a human agent. Printouts from computers performing calculations or acting without human input are considered as forms of real evidence.

A strict insistence that all witnesses be present in court to give oral evidence would cause a great deal of inconvenience. Both s102 of the Magistrates Court Act 1980, and s9 of the Criminal Justice Act 1967 allow hearsay in the form of witness statements obtained by the police in the course of their investigations to be admitted *when both parties to litigation consent.*

It is unlikely that Article 6 of the European Convention would disallow such statutory exceptions, but may well disallow the common law ones.

Evading the hearsay rule

The courts have accepted that there are categories of highly relevant and probative evidence which should be admissible, in spite of the hearsay rules. Thus sketches made by officers on the directions of witnesses, and photofits are seen by the judiciary as forms of evidence to which the strict rules of hearsay do not apply[25].

---

24. Civil Evidence Act 1968 and 1972.

25. *R v Cook* [1987] QB 417, CA.

CONFESSIONS

A confession is any statement, made to any person, which may be in words or actions[26] and which is wholly or partly adverse to the person who made it[27]. There are a number of basic tensions in the issue over admissibility of confessional evidence. Unrestricted admissibility of confessional evidence would undoubtedly aid the efficient disposal of cases, but at the expense of the need to protect individual detainees from unwarranted and oppressive conduct at the hands of the police.

Confessional evidence was admissible at common law, as an exception to the rule against hearsay, on the basis that a person is unlikely to bear false witness against him or herself. This principle, however, provides scant succour to the psychologically vulnerable.

It is a fundamental principle of most civilised jurisdictions that any confession should be made freely, and with full knowledge of legal rights. It is on this principle that the statutory regulations[28] are predicated, particularly with reference to the exclusion of confessional evidence under ss76, 78 and 82 of the Police and Criminal Evidence Act 1984, and the care of detainees under the attached Codes of Practice.

Section 76 of PACE recognises the legitimate expectations of detainees to access to their legal rights, whilst also seeking to limit police malpractice. It has parallels in other jurisdictions such as the USA, where confessional evidence will be excluded if the accused has not been informed of his constitutional right to remain silent[29]. Under this section, if it is represented to the court that the confession was made or obtained under circumstances of oppression[30] or a consequence of anything 'said or done' liable to render the confession unreliable[31], the court will exclude this evidence *as a matter of law* unless the prosecution can show beyond reasonable doubt that it was not so obtained.

---

26. Such as nodding one's head or as in *R v Li Shu-Ling* [1989] AC 270, by the accused re-enacting the crime before police officers and video recorder.

27. Police and Criminal Evidence Act 1984, s82(1).

28. Criminal Law Revision Committee, 11th Report, the Royal Commission on Criminal Procedure 1978, followed by the Police and Criminal Evidence Act 1984.

29. *Miranda v Arizona* 384 US 436, 1966.

30. PACE s76 (2)(a). Oppression is a difficult concept, defined under the Act to include torture, violence or degrading behaviour (as it also appears in Art 3 of the European Convention on Human Rights). The courts will also consider subjective matters relating to the detainee since the effect of detention will undoubtedly differ between first time offenders and professional criminals.

31. PACE s76 (2)(b).

What is at issue is reliability, and as such the truth of the particular confession is not important. The judge must place himself in the accused's position at the time of the alleged confession. He must form an opinion, based on all the evidence, on the effects of what was 'said or done' on the mind of the accused and whether this would be likely to render any confession made by the accused unreliable.

The wording in s76 (2) (b) has been interpreted as requiring the application of some sort of external stimulus in the form of police impropriety, and not anything internal to the accused. As such, the courts have been reluctant to exclude confessions, later retracted, made by individuals who claim they confessed while suffering from drug withdrawal, as these are apparent inherent factors[32]. Furthermore, the confessions of substance misusers, made in order to get out of police detention and motivated by withdrawal symptoms, will not necessarily be regarded by the courts as unreliable[33].

Section 77(1) deals with the mentally handicapped, and states that special care is needed when convicting on their confessions. Confessional evidence may in exceptional circumstances be excluded even when there is no suspicion of police impropriety, as where the accused's mental state or physical condition is disordered.

Even if the prosecution is able to discharge the burden of proof for admissibility under s76, the judge still has a *discretion* under the distinct but overlapping provisions of s78 and s82(3) of PACE to exclude such evidence. This is likely if the judge is of the opinion that the prejudicial effect of the prosecution evidence far outweighs its probative value, and that by allowing it in it would have an adverse effect on the proceedings. This may be the case where there has been a substantive breach of the Codes of Practice under PACE. Both sections 78 and 82 have an application beyond confessions and can be invoked to exclude any relevant evidence.

The issue of confessional evidence has become increasingly important in forensic medicine. An increased awareness of the psychology of confessions has resulted in requests by the police for FMEs to assess detainees' fitness to be interviewed. Any true confession made at interview may be later regretted and retracted, with the accused arguing that he was labouring under a physical or mental handicap at the time of the admissions.

---

32. *R v Goldenberg* (1988) 88 Cr App R 285 (CA). These confessions may be excluded under the discretionary powers of ss78 and 82 PACE. The confession may also be excluded if the detainee has been *given* medication which may affect his mind at interview such as in *R v Sat-Bhambra* [1988] Crim LR 453, where the detainee was given Valium by an FME, prior to interview, to calm his nerves

33. *R v Crampton* (1990) 92 CR App R 369.

Conversely, false confessions made by innocent individuals labouring under psychological or psychiatric disability have led to more than one celebrated miscarriage of justice[34]. This issue is particularly acute in England and Wales where a person may be convicted on the evidence of his own confession alone, and in the absence of any other incriminating evidence[35]. In consequence, the medical assessment is most likely to be challenged in court where the confession is the only evidence against the accused. In Scotland and the USA, in contrast, independent corroborative evidence is always required in order to warrant a conviction.

OPINION AND EXPERT EVIDENCE

Witnesses in court should confine themselves to giving evidence which their senses have perceived directly (that is of fact), and not what they believe or think (that is opinion). To allow otherwise would be to usurp the role of the court by inviting it to accept that opinion rather than forming its own. While perfectly satisfactory in simple cases where the court is able to arrive at conclusions drawn from its own experiences, it is unlikely that the court is versed in the complexities of modern medicine and science[36]. Under these circumstances the court will admit the opinion evidence of those with the requisite expertise[37]. An expert must be suitably qualified in his or her particular field of science, or branch of medicine, and the jury should be directed not simply to accept the evidence because it is from an expert source.

Expert opinions may be based on personal experience of the facts in the case such as where the expert has examined the accused or a victim. Where there is no such contact, the expert may base his opinion on assumptive facts[38]. Experts are entitled to draw on their own experience, experiments, and any published[39] or

---

34. See Gisli Gudjonsson, *The Psychology of Interrogations, Confessions and Testimony*, John Wiley 1992 generally on the problems with false confessions and in particular the Broadwater Farm Riots in London in 1985 at 305, and *R v Ward* [1993] 96 Cr. App R 1 CA.

35. *R v Mallinson* [1977] *Criminal Law Review*, 161-162.

36. This is illustrated with regard to expert psychiatric evidence which the court will admit on issues concerning mental illness, but not for matters concerning how a particular individual would be likely to react under certain circumstances, given his personality.

37. *R v Turner* [1975] 60 Cr App R 80 CA.

38. The rule against hearsay operates to exclude a medical practitioner from giving evidence of past symptoms that have been described to him, as truth of their existence *(R v Bradshaw* [1985] 82 Cr App R 79).

39. *H v Schering Chemicals Ltd* [1983] 1 All ER 849, provided it is from a reputable source.

unpublished[40] data relevant to the case but of which they have no personal experience. These may, however, only be stated within the context of the expert's opinion, and therefore cannot be advanced by a non-expert as part of his defence.

SIMILAR FACT EVIDENCE

An accused stands before an English court of law with an unblemished character. During the trial the prosecution may not present evidence of the accused's bad character, previous convictions, or propensity to commit the sort of crime for which he stands charged. This is because it is feared that the jury would place undue emphasis on such facts which they may regard as conclusive evidence of his guilt. Such prejudicial evidence, it is argued, is irrelevant because there are many other individuals who share the accused's criminal propensities.

There may, however, be circumstances surrounding the accused's prior misdeeds that appear so like those in the case for which he stands accused, that to exclude them may result in an unjust acquittal. The judge will only allow such evidence to go before the jury if he is of the opinion that it has a 'positive probative' force, or a high degree of cogency[41], so as to assist the jury in appraising the accused's current circumstances in the light of past events. This degree of cogency would be supplied when there is a similarity between the offence charged and other crimes committed by the accused that is somehow 'striking', unique or forms a 'signature', so that common sense would render the similarity inexplicable on the basis of coincidence.

CORROBORATION

A person may be convicted in England and Wales on the evidence of just one witness. The potential dangers of this approach have been recognised and a corpus of law has developed which, under certain circumstances requires independent testimony (or corroboration) connecting the accused to the crime, in order to convict. An example of evidence that is capable of amounting to corroboration is the accused's failure to provide an intimate sample[42].

In some areas, corroborative evidence is sought as a matter of law, such as cases of speeding (Road Traffic Regulation Act 1984, s89). Previously, in cases involving sexual offences, it was mandatory for the judge to warn the jury about the dangers of convicting on the basis of uncorroborated evidence (a corroboration warning).

---

40. *R v Abadom* [1983] 1 All ER 364.

41. *R v Scarrot* [1977] 65 Cr App R 125.

42. Police and Criminal Evidence Act 1984, s62 (10)(b).

This requirement was swept away by s32 (1) of the CJPO 1994 whether the complainants be adults or children.

PROFESSIONAL PRIVILEGE AND DISCLOSURE

Some evidence is not admissible in court because it is privileged. Information concerning matters of national security fall into this category (Public Interest Immunity) and its exclusion from court is based on policy considerations. Professional privilege is the right to withhold certain types of information which pass between persons, one of whom is acting in a professional capacity. Legal professional privilege covers communications between client and lawyer for the purposes of giving or receiving legal advice, and communications between lawyer and/or client and third parties where the dominant purpose of which is for use in pending or contemplated litigation[43]. The rights and obligations of medical practitioners are discussed in the next chapter.

Reference

Woolf LJ 1995. Access to Justice: Interim Report to the Lord Chancellor on the Civil Justice System in England and Wales.

---

43. This common law principle is now codified under s10 of the Police and Criminal Evidence Act 1984; See *R v Central Criminal Court, ex Parte Francis & Francis* [1988] 3 WLR 989, HL.

PART II: SCOTTISH LEGAL SYSTEM

WDS McLay

HISTORY

The Treaty of Union of 1707 provided for the retention of a separate system of law in Scotland, particularly where this concerned private rights. The extent to which the Roman element in Scots law has persisted since, despite the loss of legislative understanding, is a tribute to the strength of a system based on principle rather than on precedent, which inspires Anglo-Saxon common law. Not only is Roman law influence still felt, it remains entirely competent to appeal to the ancient institutional writers' statements of valid law when apparent gaps are identified during a case. When a civil litigant appeals to the House of Lords (no such appeal is competent in criminal cases) the case is heard on the basis of Scots law. Since 1876 there has been always at least one Law Lord from the Scottish Bench.

Corroboration has long been a supremely important principle but, in civil cases, facts can now be proved by evidence from a single source. Hearsay evidence is competent, though not desirable (Civil Evidence (Scotland) Act 1988). In the criminal sphere, with a few statutory exceptions, an accused may not be convicted on the testimony of a single witness, nor by evidence from a single source, but corroboration is not required if the accused can be shown to have 'special knowledge' of a crime, that is to say, cannot have known material details unless he himself committed the crime. Another well known peculiarity of criminal evidence is that of mutual corroboration, now usually referred to as the *Moorov* (1930 JC 68) doctrine. Here a series of crimes, which could not be proved individually, may mutually corroborate one another, as in a series of individual sexual assaults against separate women – in other words, a course of conduct. The case of *HMA v Khaliq* (1984 SLT 137) where the accused was convicted of selling glue sniffing kits to children, often in exchange for stolen goods, is an example of the flexibility of the system. It was argued by the defence that such a crime was unknown to the law of Scotland. The court ruled that the act was a species of real injury and said that the law would always respond to new manifestations of criminality.

CRIMINAL JURISDICTION

Justices of the Peace, sitting in the District Court, deal with very minor common law and statutory offences, where they are advised on the law by a legal assessor. In Glasgow, many of the District Court cases are heard by stipendiary magistrates, whose powers in summary cases are the same as a sheriff sitting alone. Sheriffs, most of whom are advocates, are professional judges who hear both civil and criminal cases. Criminal cases are heard in the Sheriff Court either summarily or by a jury of fifteen (solemn procedure) when the accused (known as the 'panel') is charged on indictment. Minor exceptions apart, prosecution is a public duty under the control of the Lord Advocate, and the accused has very little choice of forum, nor does he pay costs if convicted. Some statutory authorities, for example the factory inspectorate, may institute prosecutions, but these are rare.

The Carol X case (*X v Sweeney* 1982 JC 70) is a rare instance of private prosecution. The Crown declined to proceed with a case where several youths were accused of rape on the basis of advice that the complainer's suicidal tendency might be exacerbated by the strain of a trial. She was later able to show that she had recovered, and was successful in an application to the High Court for a Bill of Criminal Letters, permitting her to mount a private prosecution leading to conviction. The Lord Advocate had disqualified himself from prosecuting, having acted publicly on the previous advice, but afforded Miss X the whole facilities of the Crown Office once the court had allowed her Bill. It is thought that, without such aid, bringing a private prosecution would be all but impossible. Legal aid is not available for such proceedings.

Trials for particularly serious crimes, including the 'pleas of the Crown' - such as murder, rape, treason - must be heard on indictment in the High Court. The High Court sits in Edinburgh, but the judges regularly go on circuit to other cities and towns as necessary. All serious cases in the locality, and certainly those where the penalty is likely to be greater than may be imposed by a sheriff (three years on indictment, although he may remit a convicted accused to the High Court for sentence if he considers his own powers insufficient) are included in a calendar to be tried before an appropriate sitting of the High Court. The jury's verdict is by simple majority. A *not proven* verdict has the effect of acquitting the accused; from time to time campaigns are mounted against the continuation of this verdict on the ground that it establishes neither guilt nor innocence, but the concept has found favour with the present Lord Chief Justice of England on the basis that no-one is ever tried on no evidence - the only question for the Court is therefore whether the case is proved or not. Strict time limits safeguard an imprisoned accused: committal to prison must be followed by the service of an indictment within 80 days, and the trial must begin no later than 110 days (40 days in the case of summary trials). From time to time procedural mistakes are made, and the accused must be liberated. The Crown may show cause why the period should be extended, but the Court will look critically at any such application.

Solicitors who have passed further examinations to satisfy the Court now have rights of audience in the Supreme Courts, where they are known as solicitor-advocates. They are recognisable in court by the lack of a wig. Sheriffs and High Court judges are addressed as 'My Lord' or 'My Lady' and magistrates as 'Your Honour'.

Appeal from any criminal court of first instance is to the High Court of Justiciary, in its capacity as Court of Criminal Appeal. Appeals are always heard in Edinburgh, the bench being composed of three judges, which may be increased to five or seven in particularly important or contentious cases. The right of appeal has existed only since 1926, partly due to the influence of Sir Arthur Conan Doyle, who took a great interest in the case of *Oscar Slater* (1928 JC 94) who was convicted of murder, but later exonerated by the new court. The House of Lords has no jurisdiction.

PROCURATOR FISCAL

(see also chapter 14)

The fiscal is a qualified lawyer and a member of the civil service. Each has a large measure of independence within his own sheriff court district. His office is situated within or near the sheriff court. The number of deputes, who perform much of the routine business, will depend upon the volume of work. The duties of fiscals include the assessment of evidence brought to him, usually by the police. He scrutinises reports and statements; he may instruct officers on further lines of enquiry; he ensures that expert opinion beyond the resources of the police force is obtained; he may interview (precognosce) witnesses, or have them seen on his behalf by clerks. Such a witness's statement to a fiscal is not given upon oath; inconsistencies between what he has said during precognition and what he subsequently says in court may not be referred to. Police statements may be put to officers if they say something different in evidence (a 'prior inconsistent statement'). During his preparations, the fiscal has power to bring witnesses thought to be prevaricating before a sheriff, when answers must be given under oath or affirmation.

He deals directly with *summary cases* by serving a *complaint* on the accused who may plead guilty or stand trial, usually at a later date. About two weeks before the trial, the accused appears at an *intermediate diet* to confirm his plea and to check on how well prepared is the defence. At this stage, a plea bargain may be struck between the accused's agent and the fiscal. The prosecution is led by one of the depute fiscals.

The procurator fiscal has a major role when complaints are made against police officers, so emphasising the separation of police and prosecution (see also page 38). His other weighty function concerns sudden death, whether or not in suspicious circumstances, considered in chapter 14.

THE CROWN OFFICE

Statements, reports and the written views of the fiscal form the *precognition* on which decisions about prosecution are made. In certain, mainly serious, cases the precognition is sent to the Crown Office in Edinburgh for consideration by one of the advocate deputes who, if the case merits trial in the High Court, has the responsibility of leading for the Crown. Some types of case are invariably considered personally by the Lord Advocate or the Solicitor General (both of whom are government ministers) and either may lead in particularly difficult cases, or where considerations of the public interest are especially important. When proceedings are to be taken on indictment, this document is served in the name of the Lord Advocate (the case is called 'HMA v So-and-so') and narrates the circumstances giving rise to the charge. It is unnecessary to name the crime alleged, although in suitable cases, the narration will include the phrase, 'and did murder him'. During a trial in the High Court, the fiscal acts as solicitor to Crown Counsel.

Cases may be sent back to the fiscal for further enquiry, the papers may be marked 'no proceedings' or the fiscal may be instructed himself to prosecute (on indictment if the matter is serious enough, or by way of summary complaint before a sheriff sitting alone). The fiscal has authority in more minor cases not to take proceedings; this power has allowed the development of diversionary schemes where, as a matter of public policy, it has been decided that measures other than prosecution could be more effective. By the end of 1996, for certain statutory offences, the fiscal will have extended powers to offer payment of a 'fiscal fine' to an accused instead of going to the expense of pre-trial procedure.

SOLEMN CASES

More serious matters are set out in a *petition* to the sheriff who grants a warrant for the detention of the accused, for his *judicial examination*, the summoning of witnesses and so forth. The judicial examination before a sheriff gives the accused an opportunity to make a declaration about the allegations; the prosecutor examines the accused with a view to eliciting denial, admission, explanation or justification and questions him about any alleged confession. The accused need not answer, but his silence may be commented on at his trial, unless he is silent on the advice of his solicitor (agent). The solicitor, too, may question the accused. Following this examination, the accused must be granted bail, unless accused of treason or murder, or there are objections from the Crown.

His next appearance in court is at a *pleading diet*, unless he is applying for bail after incarceration. If the accused is committed to prison at the judicial examination, the indictment narrating the alleged events together with a list of witnesses and productions (that is to say documents and material evidence such as weapons or stained garments) must be served with 80 days, to allow him or his solicitor adequate time to prepare his defence. Failure to serve the indictment timeously gives the accused the right to liberty forthwith. This requirement puts immense pressure on the police, forensic scientists and the fiscal, as does that other limitation on time - six hours - during which an arrested person may be statutorily detained by the police (s14 Criminal Procedure (Scotland) Act 1995, replacing s2 of the Criminal Justice (Scotland) Act 1980) before a charge is brought or the prisoner released. In preparing a defence, the solicitor is entitled to precognosce all the prosecution witnesses. This right is a main argument against the wholesale disclosure of unused evidence which has so exercised the English courts.

At a solemn trial the Crown, the prosecutor, in the person of an advocate depute (in the High Court) or the procurator fiscal (in the sheriff court) leads evidence first, calling witnesses in turn, with no preliminary statement. Witnesses are cited in advance, and will generally receive at least 48 hours notice. Medical and other expert witnesses should take care to ascertain exactly when to attend (the courts being generally aware of the other calls on the witnesses' time) and try to come to a suitable arrangement. Having said that, it is necessary to point out the over-riding nature of the duty to answer a citation timeously and to advise witnesses to keep closely in touch with the fiscal's office from which he received the citation.

When a witness seeking to be excused because of illness consults a doctor, the certificate must be issued 'on soul and conscience' or it is ineffective; even then, the certifying doctor may be called without notice to give oral evidence, or the fiscal may seek another opinion: it is essential, therefore, to give the matter deep thought before certifying. The same consideration applies when an accused attempts to postpone or evade appearance on medical grounds.

The oath is administered to a witness by the judge, both standing, and the witness remains standing in the witness box throughout his evidence in chief, cross- and re-examination. In most cases a doctor will have given documentary evidence in the form of a certificate or a report. He speaks to these, not solely from memory, and may (with the permission of the court) refer to notes made at the time of any examination. The judge may intervene to clarify points; it is not his function to ask questions on matters not raised by prosecution or defence. It endangers the evidence for the party calling the doctor if the doctor does not follow his Court oath and begins to answer questions he has not been asked. The witness should therefore not readily volunteer views. If he believes that the thrust of his evidence has been distorted by the manner in which questions have been put to him he should say so to the judge, who may offer a further opportunity to give evidence.

No doctor should usurp the Court's function by deciding for himself which information the Court should hear. Occasionally, either prosecution or defence will seek the Court's leave to have an expert witness sit in Court to assess the evidence of lay witnesses to the facts. He is not permitted to remain while an adversarial expert is testifying unless the parties' counsel agree to the contrary.

CRIMINAL PROCEDURE

The Criminal Procedure (Scotland) Act 1995 (CPSA 95) has very recently introduced major changes to the ways in which crimes are investigated and evidence gathered in Scotland. These changes are radical: doctors must be aware that their rights and duties in ordinary practice or acting under the auspices of the police have altered significantly. Any words or sounds heard, writings made before, during and or, after a medical examination (including, for instance, jottings made in a diary or at home, letters to general practitioners or hospitals) may now be used in evidence in any criminal trial in ways never before envisaged. Moreover, types of examination of the body previously thought of as sacrosanct to doctors can now be conducted by police officers in conditions which they dictate.

In Part II of the CPSA 95, under Police Functions, s18 gives police officers of the rank of inspector or above new powers to take, using reasonable force, *internal* samples, by means of swabbing, of saliva or 'other material'. They can also cut hair (except pubic hair) toe- and fingernails, take samples from underneath such nails and swab the body externally for blood or 'other bodily fluid'. Section 19 gives the police in the course of investigation or within one month of conviction, general powers to take samples of the type mentioned in s18 for the purposes of comparison with other samples. Section 20 allows the comparison, and thereby paves the way for creation of a national DNA database (see chapter 13). All of this can be done without the presence or participation of a doctor. These powers are not subject to any direct permission or review, so a doctor could now find his or her objections or refusals to take such samples overridden by the police.

It follows that it is entirely possible for a police doctor to have been excluded from seeing a suspect at a crucial stage of investigation, but be asked to attend at a different stage. At that stage the suspect may be in an entirely different physical or mental state. This possibility, when taken together with the important new exceptions to the 'hearsay' and 'prior statement' rules introduced by ss259, 260 and 261 CPSA 95, means that doctors must take the utmost care both for themselves and the suspect in observing and reporting the state of the suspect and anything the doctor may hear. These new exceptions only apply when the maker of the statement is dead, outwith the United Kingdom, missing or cannot reasonably be brought to Court or the Court allows him not to give evidence, say under the rule against self-incrimination.

So long as there is evidence that a statement was made and is contained in 'any document' or its making is in the 'direct personal knowledge' of a witness giving evidence (such as a doctor) that 'document' can be admissible evidence. Thus, as well as any formal note or report, any jottings may be admissible. Doctors may now find the defence or prosecution or both seeking an Order of the Court to search a surgery or home or both for 'any document' held by the doctor which may be held admissible. Further, although the rule against double-hearsay is preserved, it is quite possible in a serious case that anyone living or working with the doctor who may have seen the 'document' could be called to give evidence about its contents, when it was made and so on. It is important to note that the 'document' would be admissible just as much as the testimony of its author. But the situation could easily arise where the author did not give evidence, leaving the 'document' to stand alone. That situation could readily have civil consequences for doctors if the 'document' is founded upon but the accused is eventually found to have been wrongly convicted.

The standard of proof for those seeking to persuade a Court that, without such a 'document' a miscarriage of justice may ensue, is the civil standard of the balance of probabilities. Judges are therefore likely to be slow to refuse such motions.

CIVIL JURISDICTION

At common law, sheriffs retain the power to try a very wide range of civil causes arising within their district. Divorce, for instance, can now be litigated in the sheriff court. Solicitors and advocates may appear before a sheriff, but only advocates and solicitor-advocates in the supreme court. There, actions are pursued before a *Lord Ordinary* in the *Outer House* of the *Court of Session*. Appeals by pursuer or defender, whether from a decision of a sheriff (usually) or a Court of Session judge (always) are to the *Inner House*, which has two Divisions, the First and Second. These, chaired respectively by the Lord President and the Lord Justice Clerk, are thought to have equal authority. Further appeal may, at times, lie to the House of Lords. Most of these judges, the Senators of the College of Justice, sit in both criminal and civil courts. As head of the Criminal Appeal Court, the Lord President sits *qua* Lord Justice General of Scotland.

CHILDREN'S HEARINGS

These, set up under the Social Work (Scotland) Act 1968, replaced former juvenile courts, which no longer exist. Serious criminal cases involving youngsters are still heard by a sheriff or even the High Court, particularly when there is an adult co-accused. Children attend hearings with their parents. Although the facts alleged may constitute an offence, hearings form part of the civil law structure, and the child is not an accused. He or his parents may dispute the facts, where-upon the hearing is adjourned until the sheriff has heard evidence led by the Reporter (see chapter 7 on social work procedures in Scotland) and reached a conclusion, not on guilt or innocence, but on the truth or otherwise of the facts.

The main interest of hearings to police surgeons is in relation to child abuse, when doctors may appear to give evidence at such a 'proof' before a sheriff (see also chapter 7).

PART III: THE POLICE IN THE UNITED KINGDOM

C Strachan

THE DUTIES AND STRUCTURE OF THE POLICE SERVICE

In England and Wales the principal duties of the police were listed in the Report of the Royal Commission in 1962 (Cmnd 1728) as:-

- to maintain law and order and to protect persons and property;
- to prevent crime:
- to detect criminals and to play a part in the early stages of the judicial process, acting under judicial restraint;
- to decide whether or not to prosecute persons suspected of criminal offences;
- to conduct prosecutions for less serious offences;
- to control road traffic;
- to carry out certain duties on behalf of government departments; and
- by long tradition, to befriend any one who needs their help, and to cope with major and minor emergencies.

The style in which these duties should be undertaken is in the Statement of Common Purpose and Values published by the Association of Chief Police Officers (ACPO) in 1992: 'The purpose of the police service is to uphold the law fairly and firmly; to prevent crime; to pursue and bring to justice those who break the law; to keep the Queen's Peace; to protect, help and reassure the community; and to be seen to do all this with integrity, common sense and sound judgement. We must be compassionate, courteous and patient, acting without fear or favour or prejudice to the rights of others. We need to be professional, calm and restrained in the face of violence and apply only that force which is necessary to accomplish our lawful duty. We must strive to reduce the fears of the public and, so far as we can, to reflect their priorities in the action we take. We must respond to well-founded criticism with a willingness to change.'

The accomplishment of these duties is achieved within a tripartite arrangement. The Home Secretary has a wide range of powers to make regulations affecting pay, conditions, etc., of all police officers; to control the maximum spending on police forces, including the provision of a grant of 51% of each force's budget; and to provide or arrange for central police services such as training, scientific support and Her Majesty's Inspectorate of Constabulary. Since the passing of the Police and Magistrates' Courts Act 1994 (PMCA 1994) powers also exist to set policing objectives and performance targets for forces. Despite all this, the Home Secretary has no operational control of police and no accountability for police conduct.

Police authorities for all forces in England and Wales, apart from the Metropolitan Police and the City of London Police, are a composite body of nine local councillors, three local justices of the peace and, since the PMCA 1994, five 'independent' members selected by an arcane process between the first named members of the authority and the Home Secretary. The police authority sets objectives for its force and determines its budget, and it is its duty 'to secure the maintenance of an efficient and effective police force for its area'. It still has, however, no operational control of the police and no accountability for police conduct, save in respect of the selection, appointment and conduct of Assistant Chief Constables and Chief Constables, often on fixed term agreements.

For the Metropolitan Police, the Home Secretary is, uniquely, also the police authority. For the City of London Police, it is the Common Council of the City.

The Chief Constable of each force is solely responsible for the operational direction and control of his or her force. This reflects the position of every police officer as a constable holding office under the Crown (not an employee) and possessing original legal powers and duties.

There are 43 forces in England and Wales (including London), each of which has its own budget resources, management structure and support staff. Each force has total geographic responsibility for policing services within its area, unlike the systems of European countries or America, with Federal, state and local forces. Forces in England and Wales may now also accept gifts, sponsorship and special service agreements for the deployment of police officers.

In Scotland, the policing duties and structure reflect the long-standing differences in the legal system and administration of criminal law. The duties in the Royal Commission Report, above, are true of Scotland; but a more specific set of duties is laid out in the Police (Scotland) Act, 1967, whereby it is the duty of a police constable:-

– to guard, watch and patrol so as

i   to prevent crime;

ii to preserve order; and

    iii   to protect life and property;

  – to investigate and detect crime; and

  – to enforce traffic legislation.

All Scottish forces have policy statements which describe their intended quality of service, in support of these statutory duties.

The Secretary of State for Scotland has the same wide range of administrative and supportive powers as the Home Secretary (above), but he or she does not set policing objectives or performance indicators for Scottish forces.

Police authorities in Scotland comprise only local councillors for the authority or authorities within each force. They determine the budget of the force and have duties under the Police (Scotland) Act, 1967, to pay constables, and to provide and maintain such vehicles and other equipment, land and buildings as may be required for the purposes of a police force. They have no operational control of the police and no accountability for police conduct, save in respect of the selection, appointment and conduct of Assistant Chief Constables and Chief Constables, often on fixed term agreements.

Each Chief Constable of a Scottish force is in the same operational position as in England and Wales (above).

There are eight police forces in Scotland, each separately administered and with total geographic responsibility for policing services within its area. The arrangements for gifts, etc., set out for England and Wales do not apply in law in Scotland.

In Northern Ireland the framework of policing is contained within the Police Act (Northern Ireland) 1970. The powers of the Secretary of State for Northern Ireland are similar to those of his or her counterparts in England and Scotland. Additionally, he or she appoints the Police Authority for Northern Ireland, consisting of a chair, vice-chair and not less than 14, nor more than 20, members who must be representative of the whole community.

The authority in its turn is responsible for the provision and maintenance of the force, including ensuring that the Chief Constable is free from political pressure.

The Chief Constable of the Royal Ulster Constabulary (RUC) occupies the role of operational direction and control in a similar manner to English, Welsh and Scottish chief constables. There is one notable difference in the structure of the force, resulting from Northern Ireland's historical, political problems: in addition to 8,500 regular police officers, the RUC has 4,500 full-time or part-time reservists to augment its capacity. While peace lasts in Northern Ireland, this number may be expected to decrease.

THE INVESTIGATION OF CRIME, AND PROSECUTIONS

Since the Crown Prosecution Service (CPS) was established in England and Wales in 1986, the responsibility for detecting and arresting or summoning suspects has been clearly separated from the decision to take criminal proceedings against them. The CPS conducts all proceedings initiated by police in England and Wales, with the exception of cases prosecuted by the Serious Fraud Office, and other prosecutors who deal with revenue and trading offences and the like. All investigations are controlled by the provisions of the Police and Criminal Evidence Act, 1984 (PACE).

Scotland's legal system differs from the English in its law, judicial procedure and court structure. It has a system of public prosecutors (procurators fiscal) headed by the Lord Advocate, independent of the police; the police have no say in the decision to prosecute. All reports of crime and offences, from police or other agencies, are sent to the local procurator fiscal and will be prosecuted in a district court, sheriff court or the High Court. Highly significant changes, described in the earlier part of this chapter, have recently been introduced by the coming into force of the Criminal Procedure (Scotland) Act, 1995.

In Northern Ireland the system is closer to that of England and Wales, but minor, summary offences may still be prosecuted by the police. More serious cases are reported to the Director of Public Prosecutions for Northern Ireland.

OTHER OPERATIONAL MATTERS

There are many ways in which police forces co-operate to deal with crime and other operational matters which cross their boundaries. These include the National Criminal Intelligence Service (NCIS) to combat international, organised and specialist crime.

Arrangements to cope with major public order events or unforeseen major incidents are often co-ordinated through the Association of Chief Police Officers for England, Wales and Northern Ireland (ACPO) and its Scottish counterpart (ACPOS). Perhaps their most significant co-operation was in 1984 and 1985, to integrate large scale police deployments against striking coal miners and their 'flying pickets'.

It is also part of every local force's daily duty, however, 'to befriend any one who needs their help', and the majority of calls to the police turn out not to be crime but to be other problems. These include traffic accidents, sudden deaths and mental health problems, in many of which doctors may become involved. In the case of mental health, it will generally be an officer of Inspector rank who will handle the problem, particularly if a medical opinion is required. In the rare event of medical assistance being needed at a major incident or emergency, procedures exist to designate police officers responsible for casualties, rendezvous points, body identification and so on; and a doctor whose services may be called upon will need to identify such officers and work in accordance with the overall co-ordination they can bring to the scene (see chapter 16, page 302).

POLICE PERSONNEL

Recruitment to all British police forces firmly incorporates equal opportunities. Age limits have been raised well above the traditional 30 years of age in many forces and height limits have been reduced or abolished. Candidates accepted become probationary constables for their first two years of service, including considerable training. Most officers are now also trained to use an expandable baton for self-defence and the new rigid handcuffs. This training is linked with an understanding of personal space and body language, intended to make officers' approaches to violent situations more systematic and professional.

Promotion to Sergeant and Inspector, the principal supervisory ranks in a shift or geographical police working team, is by passing examinations and selection. Promotion to Chief Inspector and Superintendent ranks is by selection, and these officers have managerial roles in divisions or force specialist branches. The rank of Chief Superintendent, traditionally the head of a division, has been abolished by the PMCA 1994; but the Higher Rate Superintendent posts created in its place may still carry the old title by permission of the chief constable. Many officers who do not choose promotion as a development path will specialise instead, in criminal investigation, community involvement, traffic, dogs, mounted or other branches. Nearly all forces now have specialist officers to deal with crimes against women and children (although unit names vary widely) and a doctor will meet them when treating victims.

Civilian staff replace police officers in many posts which do not require police training and powers, and a doctor may also encounter such specialists as scenes of crime officers, laboratory staff, photographers, and (in England and Wales) coroner's officers.

COMPLAINTS AGAINST POLICE OFFICERS

Elsewhere in this work reference is made to doctors' ethical responsibilities towards prisoners, including injuries associated with the improper use of force. Such cases may lead to complaints or internal disciplinary action against police officers and a brief outline of that system may be informative.

In England and Wales, complaints and discipline matters must be proved against officers beyond reasonable doubt, as in criminal cases, even for a non-criminal allegation. Criminal allegations (for example, assault on a prisoner) are reported to the Crown Prosecution Service and non-criminal allegations (for example incivility) are reported to the Police Complaints Authority (PCA), an independent body who may also be called in for cases of unusual importance (for example an alleged gunman shot by police). Discipline reports are the responsibility of the deputy chief officer of each force.

In Scotland, complaints and discipline cases alleging criminality are all reported to a Regional Procurator Fiscal and must, as usual, be proved beyond reasonable doubt. Non-criminal complaints and discipline are handled on the balance of probabilities (the civil law burden of proof) and, although there is no PCA in Scotland, another new provision in the PMCA 1994 allows Her Majesty's Chief Inspector of Constabulary to direct a re-investigation of a complaint matter with a further report. With that exception, discipline reports are the responsibility of the deputy chief officer of each force.

In Northern Ireland there is an Independent Commission for Police Complaints, with ten members of the public providing an independent element broadly similar to the PCA. They review all cases, however, and can refer those implying criminality onward to the Director of Public Prosecutions for Northern Ireland.

OTHER FORCES

Apart from the principal forces of Britain described above, there are a number of others, distinguished by function or geography. They include the Ministry of Defence (at or near military bases), British Transport Police (for all Britain's rail network, including the London Underground system), and police for parks, ports or tunnels.

3

THE PRACTITIONER'S OBLIGATIONS

M Wilks, M Knight

INTRODUCTION

A police surgeon is called upon to undertake examinations in a wide variety of situations. Most people examined will be alive, and will therefore have certain rights, such as a right of confidentiality, and capabilities, which will include the capacity to give consent. It is the responsibility of the examining doctor to consider, in the individual case, where the boundaries lie between the (often conflicting) rights of the person examined, the processes of investigation, and the interests of justice.

This chapter aims to define the responsibilities of the police surgeon in an ethical context. Later chapters cover the practical aspects of clinical forensic medicine, and its many attendant complications and conflicts. In dealing with the individual case, many of the ethical considerations outlined here will be modified. Some may even be discarded. It is essential, however, for the clinician to be aware of broad principles, so that he can decide how closely he wishes to adhere to them. He will need to bear in mind that to depart from them without good reason may invite the interest of the General Medical Council, and of the civil or criminal courts. The ultimate test of any action is whether the doctor feels able to justify it to his peers.

Ethical principles define an accepted code of behaviour within a particular group, the group in this case being the medical profession. Ethical standards are not the same as moral standards, which represent principles accepted more widely within society. While ethical and moral behaviour will usually be within the law, there is no guarantee of compatibility between legal, moral, and ethical behaviour.

It must also be stressed that doctors will bring their personal moral opinions, formed through education, cultural background and religious beliefs, to bear on individual ethical issues. For police surgeons, it can be very easy, when dealing with detainees, for moral judgments about assumed guilt to interfere with impartiality. It is precisely because of this that absolute ethical principles are so important, as they provide a bench-mark for doctors in both the clinical work of examining prisoners, victims or injured officers, and in acting as an impartial expert in relationships with the police, the legal profession and the courts.

An essential feature of the police surgeon's role is that of 'dual responsibility'. This is not unique to forensic medicine. A doctor serving in the armed forces has a responsibility both to the individual soldier and for the safety and efficiency of a wider group, such as a regiment. The company medical adviser has a responsibility to a sick employee, but has to pay regard to the interests of the employer. In all cases of dual responsibility there is a conflict between the absolute confidentiality normally enjoyed by the patient and the wider interests of an institution.

In clinical forensic medicine this conflict is expressed in two distinct ways:

1. The majority of examinations undertaken will have a dual content – therapeutic and forensic. In most cases the doctor will have a responsibility of care which may involve the provision of actual treatment, or a decision to refer for further care. In addition, many, if not most, examinations involve the interpretation of clinical signs in an evidential context. Even the most minor of injuries may be the subject of detailed cross-examination in court, often considerably in the future. The doctor will be expected, using notes made at the time, to give an opinion on their appearance, age, and likely causation.

2. The doctor has a duty of confidentiality to the person examined. This is an essential feature of the doctor/patient relationship. However, the doctor also has an obligation to provide such details to the police as are necessary and appropriate for the investigation of crime, and, in the case of a person detained, for their safe care while in detention. This aspect of the dual relationship raises fundamental issues of confidentiality and consent.

Bearing in mind that, as doctors, we are subject to our own disciplinary codes, *the relationship between the forensic medical examiner and the person examined will be one of doctor and patient*. Although this may have little parallel with a consultation, say, between a patient and a general practitioner, it is essential that we start by considering that the contact between the forensic clinician and examinees, whether they be prisoners, victims or police officers, is a modification of that ideal consultation. With that starting point we can then highlight the differences, and from this see how the relationship is modified.

Traditionally, the ethics of the doctor/patient relationship are framed by four main principles. These are:

Autonomy
Non-maleficence
Beneficence
Justice

The first is autonomy. Autonomy is the capacity of people to choose freely and to control as far as possible what happens to them. Respecting this autonomy involves acknowledging the integrity of a person's choice, made according to the person's own values, conscience, and religious convictions. In recognising autonomy, the doctor implicitly agrees to two essential elements in patient care – the patient's ability to give or withhold consent, and the doctor's duty of confidentiality.

In clinical forensic practice, a prisoner's autonomy is clearly restricted by his loss of liberty. It may also be impaired by illness, intoxication and drugs, all of which restrict the capacity to make free choice. The loss of liberty also makes prisoners fearful and vulnerable, and often more acquiescent. It is part of the doctor's responsibility to recognise this, and take on a more interventionist – or paternalistic – role. The prisoner who is so drunk that he cannot appreciate the severity of a laceration, or the drug misuser whose request for medication should be denied because his recent drug history cannot be validated, are examples where free choice can be properly overridden. But it is essential not to confuse the loss of liberty with the loss of autonomy. A refusal to be examined or to be treated, if made in an informed way, must be respected. To take action in opposition to a refusal may lay a doctor open to a charge of assault.

There are, however, situations in which consent can be overridden, most notably in the case of intimate searches. These are dealt with in detail later.

The second principle is non-maleficence, which reminds us that, while the price of doing good may be to do harm, there should be both a minimisation of harm, and an outcome in which there is a balance in favour of good. In practical terms it is a principle that obliges the doctor to respect a patient's dignity and privacy.

The third principle, beneficence, is a wider concept than simply doing good. We are doctors because we seek to care. As civilised humans, we adopt the assumption that our society is essentially compassionate, and that those with more will try to help those with less. In the context of forensic medicine, those with less include people with less information, and, crucially, with less liberty.

The final principle is justice. We all have a moral obligation to act fairly in respecting rights, to obey laws, and to act in accordance with general moral principles. As forensic physicians, each of us will bring our own moral perspective of justice to bear on any particular case. We cannot help it, nor should we be concerned about it. What matters is how it affects our actions. To bring personal moral judgments to bear on our management of individual cases undermines our capacity to be impartial, and is unethical. The police surgeon is called upon to provide a wide range of duties. These responsibilities should, and normally will, be clearly set out in the contract held with the police authority.

These have traditionally been grouped in accordance with their specialist (forensic) content, a higher fee being paid for those duties requiring more skill. A lower fee is paid for those examinations that have more therapeutic content, such as an examination for fitness to detain. These distinctions are less clear in practice, for almost all examinations have both therapeutic and forensic content, and what usually distinguishes the higher from the lower rate examinations is the time they take. In recent years, police surgeons have felt that an examination to determine fitness for interview, as an example, may have important implications for the integrity of statements given at interview, and its importance should be accorded more recognition.

In the course of his duties, and apart from his clinical and forensic responsibilities, the clinician will have a professional relationship with a wide variety of people and disciplines. These include solicitors, barristers, social workers, lay visitors, court officers, and criminal justice units. The degree of confidentiality of information held by the doctor will always influence the extent of disclosure to these different groups.

THE LEGAL FRAMEWORK

Let us now consider those laws and legal processes that are relevant to forensic practice. The most important legislation in England, Wales and Northern Ireland is the Police and Criminal Evidence Act 1984 (PACE). Under this Act, the Home Secretary issued Revised Codes of Practice in 1995, regulating police practice in a number of areas. Code C relates to the detention, treatment and questioning of persons by police officers. In this context 'treatment' refers to overall care, and embraces more than the medical aspects of detention. This Code determines, and tightly regulates, the work of the custody officer in the care of detained people. Scrupulous attention is required if prisoners' rights are not to be disregarded or overridden, and a knowledge of this Code is an essential requirement for a good working relationship to be established between the custody officer and the forensic clinician.

As examples, para 8.10, referring to the detention of people who are drunk, requires that they are visited, and roused, every half hour. Paras 9.2 to 9.9 deal specifically with medical treatment. Familiarity with these paragraphs will enable the doctor to give advice to the custody officer which is either consistent with, or complimentary to, his normal responsibilities.

Code D defines police procedures in relation to the identification of persons. In particular it contains references to the mentally impaired, appropriate adults, and the taking of samples, both intimate and non-intimate.

Other legislation bearing on the work of the forensic clinician include the following:

Data Protection Act 1984

Access to Health Records Act 1990

Access to Medical Reports Act 1988

The Misuse of Drugs (Notification and Supply to Addicts) Regulations 1973

The Public Health (Control of Disease) Act 1984

The Public Health (Infectious Disease) Regulations 1988

National Health Service (Venereal Disease) Regulations 1974

The National Health Service Trusts (Venereal Disease) Directions 1991

The detention of an individual against consent raises questions of personal liberty and human rights. The Declaration of Geneva (1948) is an international statement of the duties and responsibilities of doctors. There are moves to redraft this in time for the meeting of the World Medical Association's meeting in 1998 – the 50th anniversary of the Declaration. It could then be more widely adopted as a bench mark for doctors, and might replace the Hippocratic Oath as a basic set of principles. Acceptance of the fundamental ethical principles of autonomy and justice require doctors to be alert to potential or actual abuse of prisoners, and to ensure that appropriate representations are made (BMA 1992).

CONSENT

A general principle of English law is that a patient always has the right to withhold consent to medical treatment, even where such a refusal may involve declining life-saving treatment. In his judgement in *Re T* [1992] 4 All ER 649 Lord Donaldson, the Master of the Rolls, stated that "Doctors faced with a refusal of consent have to give very careful and detailed consideration to the patient's capacity to decide at the time when the decision was made. What matters is that the doctors should consider at that time he had a capacity which was commensurate with the gravity of the decision he purported to make. The more serious the decision, the greater the capacity required. If the patient has the requisite capacity they are bound by his decision. If not, they are free to treat him in what they believe to be his best interests."

This illustrates two essential questions facing the doctor:

Is the consent for therapeutic or for forensic examination?

Is the consent valid?

Examinations of prisoners, victims and officers will, in almost every case, have both therapeutic and forensic content. The proportion of one compared to the other may be small, but it will nearly always be there. One of the most important reasons for keeping accurate and comprehensive notes is that information, derived from what at the time was a therapeutic examination, may have to be reinterpreted – often months later – in the form of a statement or in evidence at court.

In respect of prisoners, Section 9 of Code C of PACE lists the circumstances in which the custody officer is obliged to seek medical assistance whether or not he is asked to do so by the detainee. He will do so when the detainee appears to be suffering from a physical or mental illness (para 9.2(a)), is injured (9.2(b)), does not show signs of sensibility or awareness (9.2(c)), fails to respond normally to questions or conversation - other than through drunkenness alone (9.2(d)), or otherwise appears to need medical attention (9.2(e)).

In these circumstances there may be limited consent, or none at all, for the examination, and the doctor has to proceed on the basis of *implied* consent, that is, on the assumption that a person suffering from an illness would wish to have that illness treated, particularly if there was a risk to life. The doctor can proceed as far as is therapeutically necessary, and, during the course of the procedure, will gather information that may be of forensic value, and useful to the investigation of crime. The doctor, by virtue of his position as a clinician advising the police, is free to give an opinion on the forensic content of his examination, but is not free to take samples or material without consent.

The custody officer is obliged under para 9.3 of Code C to seek medical advice if the detainee appears to be suffering from an infectious disease, or, under 9.6, if a detained person has in his possession, or claims to need, medication relating to a heart condition, diabetes, epilepsy, or a condition of comparable seriousness. In these circumstances, the doctor will obtain consent for an examination to assess the prisoner's fitness for detention, and there is unlikely to be any forensic content. When a person in custody requests the presence of a doctor, and therefore has some expectation of examination and treatment, there will be an assumption of implied consent. Such a right of request exists under para 9.4 of Code C, and includes the right to be examined by a medical practitioner at the prisoner's own expense. There are those, such as Robertson (1992), who feel that "normal doctor/patient rules clearly do not apply in this situation". However, most doctors will try to apply the normal rules that govern the doctor/patient relationship to the best of their ability in what is an abnormal clinical situation.

More detailed issues of consent apply where the doctor is called to examine a detainee in order to assist and advise the police on the collection of evidence with respect to an alleged crime. Such evidence will be obtained by an examination to assess the presence – or absence – of injuries, and to interpret the significance of the findings. It may also involve the taking of samples, the analysis of which may confirm or refute an allegation, for example, under the Sexual Offences Act 1956. In these circumstances the doctor is obliged to be specific about his role, and to emphasise that his responsibilities to the police include the interpretation of relevant clinical findings in an evidential context, but that his responsibilities to the prisoner/patient include keeping confidential those matters that are not, in the doctor's opinion, immediately relevant to the case. The term 'immediately' is important, as it reminds us that in later statements or evidence in court, the doctor may not be free to judge the relevance, or 'materiality', of his findings. This is dealt with later in the section on disclosure.

Since the consequences of acting without consent may be damaging to the doctor, both in terms of the law, and in the eyes of the GMC, many forensic clinicians prefer to obtain consent from prisoners in writing. Consent forms need to make clear that the subject understands the nature and purpose of any examination or investigation undertaken. An example, designed by Dr S Robinson, is shown below. It is arguable whether consent in writing offers

---

CONSENT FORM

Name .... Address ....

....

D.O.B.. ....

I consent to a medical examination, including the taking of samples, if appropriate on myself

or/my ....

in connection with/allegations of..

as explained to me by Dr. Robinson

I also consent to the consultation/examination:-
        a) being recorded in writing/audio/video
        b) involving the use of photographs which may be used in teaching
        c) findings being disclosed to the police/social services/other

I also understand that anything I tell the doctor may have to be produced and declared if so ordered by a court.

Signed... Date..

WITNESS
Signed... Date..

(name/address/relationship of witness)

....

I confirm that I have explained the purposes of the "examination"

Signed .... Date ....

---

a greater protection to the doctor than that given verbally. There is therefore no requirement that consent should be written, but the fact that consent has been given orally should always be recorded in the doctor's private notes.

Consent must be given in writing in the custody record (Code D 5.1(2)) in the case of intimate samples, and can be overridden in the case of intimate searches by police officers.

INTIMATE SAMPLES

Sections 62 and 65 of the Police and Criminal Evidence Act 1984 defined intimate and non-intimate samples. However, PACE was amended by section 58 of the Criminal Justice Act 1994, which redefined samples[1] as follows:

> An intimate sample means a dental impression or a sample of blood, semen or any other tissue fluid, urine or pubic hair or a swab taken from a person's body orifice other than the mouth. A non-intimate sample means a sample of hair (other than pubic hair) which includes hair plucked from the root, a sample taken from under a nail, a swab taken from any part of a person's body including the mouth but not any other body orifice, saliva or a footprint or similar impression of any part of a person's body other than a part of his hand.

In redesignating mouth swabs as 'non-intimate', the Criminal Justice and Public Order Act has followed the example set in Northern Ireland, where the status of saliva and mouth swabs was moved from the intimate to the non-intimate category by Schedule 14 to the Criminal Justice Act 1988.

Sections 62 and 63 of PACE respectively describe the circumstances in which these samples can be taken. The sample should be taken only if an officer of the rank of superintendent or above authorises the taking of such samples, which he may only do if he has reasonable grounds (a) for suspecting the involvement of the person from whom the sample is to be taken in a serious arrestable offence, and (b) for believing that the sample will tend to confirm or disprove his involvement.

Section 62 demands that intimate samples can be taken only (S 62 (1)(b)) '.... if the appropriate consent is given'. With respect to non-intimate samples, s 63(1) indicates: 'Except as provided by this section, a non-intimate sample may not be taken from a person without the appropriate consent'. Section 63(3) goes on to indicate the circumstances in which a non-intimate sample may be taken without the appropriate consent in that the person from whom the sample is to be taken must be held in police detention or held in custody by the police on the

1. See Code D §5.11.

authority of a court and the authority has been obtained from an officer of at least the rank of superintendent.

A further difference between intimate and non-intimate samples concerns the person who will take the samples. Section 62(9) states that: 'An intimate sample, other than a sample of urine or saliva, may only be taken from a person by a medical practitioner'. Thus all non-intimate samples, and urine and saliva, can be taken by police officers or civilian scene-of-crime officers.

By redefining mouth swabs as non-intimate, the need for the attendance of medical personnel, and for consent to the taking of samples, has been avoided, thereby opening the way to the use of DNA in the identification of a perpetrator of a crime, and to the establishment of DNA databases.

It should also be noted, in accordance with a general policy shift on the right to silence, that para 5.2 of Code D of PACE states that: 'Before a person is asked to provide an intimate sample he must be warned that if he refuses without good cause, his refusal may harm his case if it comes to trial'. While it is not part of the doctor's obligation to interpret the law, he will be aware that the operation of this clause will increase the vulnerability of the prisoner, and therefore emphasises the need for an unambiguous statement of the doctor's role. In contentious cases the doctor may wish to supplement the prisoner's written consent in the custody record with his own consent form.

The doctor will also need to be aware that para 5.6 of Code D states that '...reasonable force may be used if necessary to take non-intimate samples.'

It seems probable that most detained persons would prefer a doctor to take non-intimate samples with consent, rather than for a police officer to do so without consent. However, good practice dictates that a doctor taking a sample does so with full, informed, and valid consent.

Intimate body searches

Section 55 of PACE 1984 allows for intimate body searches to be carried out under certain circumstances. These powers present the medical practitioner with a considerable ethical dilemma.

The Act distinguishes between two groups of material for which a search can be authorised. Referring to prisoners, Section 55(a) deals with '..anything which (1) he could use to cause physical injury to himself or others; and (2) he might so use while he is in police detention or in the custody of the court...' This section is designed to cover items such as weapons, sharp implements and other similar dangerous material.

Section 55(b) deals specifically with drugs, and states '...that such a person (1) may have a Class A drug concealed upon him; and (2) was in possession of it with the appropriate criminal intent before arrest,...'

The difference between these sub-sections determines the difference in the location, and type of search, and who is authorised to undertake it. A search for a weapon may be carried out at a police station, hospital, registered medical practitioner's surgery, or some other place used for medical purposes (s8). An intimate search for drugs may not be carried out at a police station, and therefore must be performed on 'medical premises' (s9). It is recommended that all searches be carried out by a 'suitably qualified person', defined under the Act as a 'registered medical practitioner or a registered nurse'. However, in extremis, a search under s55(1)(a), for example for a weapon, can be carried out by a police officer providing that that police officer is of the same sex as the examinee.

Class A drugs, as defined under the Misuse of Drugs Act 1971, include a wide range of substances, including the opiates, but excluding cannabis.

The 'appropriate criminal intent' is defined under s55 (17) of PACE as '....an intent to commit an offence under (a) section 5(3) of the Misuse of Drugs Act 1971 (possession of controlled drug with intent to supply to another) or (b) s68(2) of the Customs and Excise Management Act 1979 (exportation etc., with intent to evade a prohibition or restriction)...' An intimate search for drugs can therefore only be authorised if a senior police officer has evidence to suggest that the detainee is a purveyor of drugs, not merely a user.

A medical practitioner seeking to conduct an intimate search, properly authorised under section 55, would, in the first instance, seek the consent of the detainee. The dilemma for the doctor arises if such consent is refused.

Zander (1990) correctly points out that a doctor or nurse cannot be compelled to carry out searches of body orifices where there is no consent. However, he goes on to say, "...consent to such a search by the suspect is not essential and force could therefore be used to carry out the search - presumably even if it is being carried out by a medical practitioner or nurse." This view was supported by a Home Office draft circular (1988) which held that 'In s55 of PACE there is no mention of consent or the absence of consent in respect of constables or qualified persons. Under this section, therefore, a qualified person is empowered to act without the consent of the person concerned. It was not the intention that the power of a superintendent to authorise a medical examination should be frustrated because the suspect could not be restrained'. There is therefore an expectation that medical personnel will be asked to carry out searches of body orifices without consent, despite both the ethical difficulties this would cause, and the potential harm and technical difficulties inherent in such a procedure.

The Home Office Circular continues (para 37): 'Provided suitably qualified persons conducting intimate searches do not use unreasonable force, or cause injury through negligence, they will, in the Secretary of State's view, be protected from complaints arising from searches. On normal principles if a procedure is provided by Act of Parliament for carrying out that which would normally be unlawful, then those acting under the procedure will have a defence to any proceedings, civil or criminal, brought against them.'

It appears that doctors conducting such searches without consent, despite the 'assurances' given by the Home Office, would be inviting proceedings under all three elements of the so-called 'triple jeopardy', criminal proceedings for assault, civil proceedings for the tort of battery, and disciplinary proceedings before the General Medical Council. To date, these matters have not been tested before any of these Courts or Tribunals.

The British Medical Association (1986) jointly with the Royal College of Nursing provided guidelines for doctors and nurses with regard to intimate searches: 'In the surroundings of the police station where a refusal to perform an intimate search may imply guilt, it is very unlikely that the health professional will be able to obtain freely the consent of the suspect to perform an intimate search. However, except on very rare occasions, an intimate search should not be performed without the subject's acquiescence having first been obtained.' In relation specifically to searches under s55(1)(a), the guidelines insist that: 'We are not convinced that there are sufficient grounds for an intimate search if a non-acquiescing subject is believed to have concealed upon him an object or substance which will not harm others but only himself', echoing the definition of the 'appropriate criminal intent' under s55 (17)(a) of the Act.

Havard (1989) gave similar guidance: 'Doctors should not take such (intimate) samples unless the person consents, and they are not required to do so under the Act. Refusal to consent may provide corroboration of evidence subsequently given in court and adverse inferences can be drawn from refusal when there is no good cause for it'.

In the same year the BMA resolved that '... no medical practitioner should take part in an intimate body search of a subject without that subject's consent'.

In personal correspondence, the GMC (1988) has indicated that although 'the Council cannot undertake to offer advice on the interpretation of the law....the Council's Committee on Standards of Professional Conduct and on Medical Ethics has endorsed guidelines issued by the British Medical Association and the Royal College of Nursing in connection with the implementation of the Police and Criminal Evidence Act'. The GMC thus gave a clear indication of the view it would take should a doctor appear before it accused of misconduct in relation to an intimate search.

The Medical Protection Society (1990) in promising to support and assist members challenged after an intimate search, added: 'Provided that the medical practitioner does not use unreasonable force or cause injury through negligence, we believe that the police surgeon would be able to defend himself successfully against any complaint laid with the GMC'.

The doctor's defence would be based on the presumption that the examination was carried out because the police officer had formed the view that the drugs were being secreted with the appropriate criminal intent to supply another with a controlled drug; a forced search would then be justifiable in the public interest. The doctor could claim an analogy with disclosure in the public interest, as referred to by the GMC[2]: 'Disclosures may be necesssary in the public interest where a failure to disclose information may expose the patient, or others, to a risk of death or serious harm....'

It seems likely that, with the problems presented to society by the increase in illegal supply of drugs and drug misuse, this issue will be tested before long in the courts, or by the GMC.

CAPACITY

In assessing a detainee's fitness for detention and/or interview, the doctor will make judgments about that person's ability both to give consent, and to understand and answer questions put to him at formal interview. This raises the issue of capacity, which has been extensively covered in a document issued jointly by the BMA and the Law Society (1995). In addition, the Law Society (1994) has issued a wide-ranging consultation document on consent and the criminal law. What matters to the clinician in advising the police is whether or not a person detained has the capacity to give consent, and to understand the procedures applied to him. If the doctor is content that a detainee is fully aware, and therefore fully capable, then the interview may proceed, and consent for investigation and examinations, whether performed by the police or by the doctor, will be valid. It must be remembered that any suggestion that a person detained did not understand what was happening to him might have serious consequences later on if the matter proceeds to trial. The doctor may wish to set a time limit on the extent of the fitness for interview, or may give directions regarding reassessment.

Appropriate adults

However, a person may not be competent to give consent for a number of reasons. These include age, and either physical or mental illness. The Codes of Practice of PACE recognise a range of circumstances in which an appropriate adult should be present during the cautioning, searching or interviewing of

---

2. General Medical Council 1995 Confidentiality at §18.

vulnerable suspects, in particular juveniles and persons who are mentally disordered. Prior to PACE, such persons could be interviewed only if their parents, guardian, or other independent person were present. Following research done for the 1981 Royal Commission on Criminal Procedure, and on the recommendation of the Commission, Codes C and D set out a requirement for an appropriate adult to be called and to attend the police station in cases of arrest of juveniles and persons who are mentally disordered.

These arrangements were reviewed by the Home Office (1995). The Royal Commission on Criminal Justice, reporting in 1993, expressed concern that this arrangement was often inadequate, that certain categories of vulnerable persons were not receiving appropriate representation, and that many appropriate adults were unclear as to their proper role.

The review concluded that there should be improvements in the following areas:
- appropriate adults should be independent of the police;
- they should be in a position to advise and explain to a vulnerable person their rights while in custody;
- they should be in a position to assist the person in the exercise of those rights;
- they should help to ensure that a vulnerable suspect is treated properly while detained.

Under the PACE Codes of Practice, persons aged 17 are not treated as juveniles, and are therefore not entitled to the assistance of an appropriate adult. The review has suggested an amendment to PACE to alter this position.

Unfortunately, the review group states (p.10) '... the decision to call an appropriate adult ... is one for the custody officer, not for the forensic medical examiner, who may not have expertise in mental health issues'. The Home Office has been advised that a custody officer is not trained in the assessment of mental illness, and that, because the forensic examiner is so trained, he will be familiar with the working of the Mental Health Act. A note of caution should be introduced when dealing with juveniles. It is clear that persons under 16 are competent to give consent for medical treatment. However, it should not be assumed that this consent extends to the provision of forensic samples. In these cases an appropriate adult should be present to oversee consent.

CONFIDENTIALITY

The principle of medical confidentiality extends back to the Hippocratic Oath, but was restated in guidance from the GMC[3]: 'Patients have a right to expect that

---

3. GMC 1995 *op.cit.* §1.

you will not disclose any personal information which you learn during the course of your professional duties, unless they give permission ...'

An action for breach of confidentiality has always been possible under civil law. In the controversial case of *AG v Guardian Newspapers Ltd* (2) [1988] 3 All ER 545 (the so-called Spycatcher case) the general principle was stated by Lord Gough: 'I start with the broad general principle ... that a duty of confidence arises when confidential information comes to the knowledge of a person (the confident) in circumstances where he has notice or is held to have agreed, that the information is confidential, with the effect that it would be just in all the circumstances that he should be precluded from disclosing the information to others'.

While the view of the GMC, and the likely view of the civil courts, would be a severe censure of a doctor who knowingly disclosed confidential information about a patient to a third party, it must be stressed that, in the matter of medical records, there is no absolute privilege. However, the very clear circumstances, currently being reviewed and debated by Parliament, under which clinical material can be disclosed, make it essential that police surgeons start from the basis of absolute confidentiality, and develop a view, in the individual case, on the extent of legitimate disclosure, whether informally to a custody sergeant or investigating officer, or formally in a custody entry, statement or report.

A major bearing on the extent of confidentiality that can be accorded to a prisoner is the dual role of the forensic examiner, referred to earlier. By virtue of being required by the police to attend in both a therapeutic and forensic capacity, the doctor necessarily is expected to make a report to the police. In relation to a detainee's fitness to be detained, the information given must be relevant to that person's likely period of detention, the sole purpose of the information being to safeguard that person's well-being while in custody. In relation to an examination for evidential purposes, the doctor's duty is to provide to the police that information that he feels is material to the investigation. At this early stage he should not impart information that does not seem relevant. The relevance of information held may change, and may need to be disclosed, but this occurs at a later stage, and is governed by legally enforceable procedures on disclosure.

Confidentiality in the custodial situation

A major conflict for the doctor examining a detainee is in balancing confidentiality with personal safety. It is by no means uncommon for doctors to be threatened or assaulted by prisoners. Sensible guidance on this issue is set out in the joint British Medical Association/Association of Police Surgeons booklet (1994) on the health care of detainees. The advice can be summarised as follows:

• It is good practice for a prisoner to be accompanied by an escort, usually a police officer;

- the escort should remain within calling distance, but out of earshot;
- a doctor should never examine a person (including police officers) of the opposite sex without a chaperone present.

The doctor will be required, or expected, to make records of his examination. In many instances a note will be made in the custody record giving a brief summary of the advice given regarding a person's detention. Such a note may, in relation to victims of assault, injured police officers, and injuries sustained by detainees, briefly outline the injuries, to assist investigating officers. In London, forensic medical examiners enter such details in a 'Book 83', whose circulation as an administrative record makes confidentiality impossible. The BMA/APS booklet gives clear advice on how this record should be completed.

In addition to a station-based record, the doctor will keep private notes. These include written notes, recordings, drawings, and photographs. A doctor should be entirely free to keep those records he thinks appropriate, including photographs, but, in the case of the latter, he may wish to advise investigating officers of his intentions. In addition, the consent of the subject is essential. It must be remembered that, in the case of serious crime, police photographs will normally be available.

When making private notes it is essential that the record be complete. Although these notes do not have absolute privilege, it is bad practice, and unhelpful both to the investigation and to the case in court, for potentially relevant information to be omitted. The doctor may well feel that certain matters are irrelevant to the case, but in the absence of an overview of the entire investigation and evidence, such a judgement may well be flawed.

Paragraph 1 of *Confidentiality*[3] states clearly the view on security of records taken by the General Medical Council: doctors who are responsible for confidential information must "make sure that the information is effectively protected against improper disclosure when it is disposed of, stored, transmitted or received".

It is difficult to comply with this apparently straightforward principle in the abnormal clinical situation between a doctor and a detainee to which the Police and Criminal Evidence Act applies. Para 9(c) of Code C requires that 'If a medical practitioner does not record his findings in the custody record, the record must show where they are recorded'. There is therefore an expectation within the Codes that confidentiality will be breached to the extent that clinical findings will be available on the custody record, and therefore available to all who see that record. These might include lay visitors, the Crown Prosecution Service, court staff, and the person detained.

Paragraph 2.5 of Code C states: 'The person who has been detained, the appropriate adult, or legal representative who gives reasonable notice of a request to inspect the original custody record after the person has left police detention should be allowed to do so'. In practice, such persons are often supplied with a copy. There therefore exists a wide variety of people who may have legitimate access to a record containing clinical material. When making entries, doctors should be aware of the possible circulation of the record used.

Paragraph 9.4 of Code C makes reference to the right of a detainee to be examined by a practitioner of his own choice. Bevan and Lidstone (1991) state: 'The custody record can conveniently be used if the person is under arrest. A police surgeon will naturally enter his findings on the custody record, but a general practitioner need not do so because of the confidentiality with the patient.' There is therefore an assumption that a duty of confidentiality lies with the detainee's own general practitioner, but no such duty lies with the police surgeon. As mentioned earlier, other legislation governs the confidentiality of, and access to, records (Panting 1992).

Data Protection Act 1984

This ensures that information relating to an individual is obtained fairly, kept up to date, and stored securely. The individual whose data are stored has rights of access enabling him or her to check the accuracy of the information. No information referring to those in custody, whether held by the police or the doctor, should be held on computer without appropriate registration under the Data Protection Act 1984. The only exception to this rule is where information is held for word processing purposes only.

Access to Medical Reports Act 1988

This came into force on January 1st 1989. Under the Act, a patient has a right of access to any medical report prepared for insurance or employment purposes by a doctor who is or has been responsible for the patient's care provided that allowing the patient to see the report will not endanger his or her physical or mental welfare or disclose information about another person who is not a health professional.

Since the Act applies only to reports prepared for employment or insurance purposes, the contents of a statement to the police regarding a detainee are not subject to the Act. If, however, a police officer were to be examined, for example following an injury on duty, such a report would be for employment purposes and the Act would apply if the doctor was or had been responsible for the police officer's medical care. If the Act did not apply, the findings would still be subject to the normal rules of confidentiality, but the patient or police officer would not have the right to see the report before it was sent to the employer.

Access to Health Records Act 1990

This came into force on November 1st 1991. Its main purpose is to enable patients to have access to their own medical records made after November 1st 1991, the patients already having access to computerised records under the Data Protection Act 1984. Hand-written notes, which are by definition clinical records, made at the time of an examination at the police station, are subject to the provisions of this Act. Consequently, either prisoners or police officers who are the subject of those records will have a prima facie right of access. There are, however, exceptions. Under both the Access to Medical Reports Act, and the Access to Health Records Act, the doctor need not disclose if he considers that to do so would be likely to cause serious harm to the physical or mental health of the patient, or of any other individual.

In addition, in the case of persons under 16, access should only be granted to a child if the child is capable of understanding the implications of the application for disclosure. If the child lacks the necessary capacity to consent, the record holder should only disclose the information to a third party (such as a parent) if he or she believed it to be in the child's best interest. While such a legal framework may seem to the humble clinician to represent a dangerous minefield, a straightforward observance of the basic principles of consent and confidentiality will ensure that the doctor complies with the GMC's guideline[4]: 'You may release confidential information in strict accordance with the patient's consent, or the consent of a person properly authorised to act on the patient's behalf'.

With appropriate consent in place, the forensic clinician is free to share information with the police, from whence it will be disseminated to other agencies such as the Crown Prosecution Service, and prosecuting and defending counsel. This principle also applies to the victims of crime.

However, we here must enter a note of caution. In the earlier section on consent, the doctor was invited to consider, when obtaining consent, how extensive that consent is, and, therefore, how free the doctor is to disclose the information obtained. It must be remembered that the consent of a detained person, or of a victim of assault, may not be fully 'informed'. This is particularly true when we consider the victim of a serious sexual assault, who will be tired, frightened and confused, and who may be under the influence of alcohol or other substances. Such a person is incapable, at the time, of making decisions regarding the dissemination of highly confidential information. In such a case, 'best practice' dictates that a further approach is made at a later date to obtain detailed and informed consent to disclosure. These issues underline the whole problem of disclosure, the law relating to which is, at the time of writing, in a state of change.

---

4. GMC 1995 op.cit §2.

DISCLOSURE

Several recent high-profile cases, including *R v Saunders* (unreported) 29 September 1989 (the 'Guinness' case), *R v Ward* [1993] 1 WLR 619; 2 All ER 577 CA, and *R v Keane* [1994] 1 WLR 746 have highlighted the issue of 'unused' or 'undisclosed' material. A firm onus is placed upon the prosecution to identify evidential material which, though not forming part of the prosecution case, should nevertheless be disclosed to the defence.

Such material will include the hand-written record, and private notes, made by a doctor following an examination. It may also include other confidential information, such as reports from probation officers, social services, and health carers.

The issue of disclosure was refined in *R v Keane* by Lord Taylor of Gosforth CJ (page 752): 'The prosecution must identify the documents and information which are material ... Having identified what is material, the prosecution should disclose it unless they wish to maintain that public interest immunity or other sensitivity justifies withholding some or all of it. ... If in an exceptional case the prosecution are in doubt about the materiality of some documents or information, the court may be asked to rule on that issue.' The court then has the responsibility of conducting a balancing act in deciding between the rights of the defendant for a fair trial, and the obligations of the keeper (here, the examining doctor) of the material to maintain confidentiality.

Firm guidance has been issued by the Crown Prosecution Service (1995) to Branch Crown Prosecutors that police surgeons' hand-written notes should be regarded as 'unused material', and should be passed to the defence, provided that the materiality test, as stated in *R v Keane*, is met. Consequently, police surgeons are now often approached by both police and Crown Prosecutors to disclose their hand-written notes, either immediately following an examination, or shortly afterwards. These notes may contain highly sensitive information, which the source may wish to keep confidential at all costs. Examples of such material include a previous history of sexual abuse in a victim of rape or a history of infidelity of which the partner of the victim was unaware.

There is a clear conflict between the need for the doctor to respect confidentiality, and the requirement to disclose. If a doctor accedes to a general request from the police to disclose, he faces severe penalties from the GMC. The GMC's stance remains unchanged, and is set out in the new booklets issued in 1995[2]. At para 18, it states: 'Disclosure may be necessary in the public interest where a failure to disclose information may expose the patient, or others, to risk of death or serious harm. In such circumstances you should disclose information promptly to an appropriate person or authority'. While stating in paragraph 19, that '... disclosure is necessary for the prevention or detection of a crime', the GMC is quite clear, in paragraph 21, that: 'In the absence of a court order, a request for disclosure by a third party, for example, a solicitor, police officer, or officer of a court, is not sufficient justification for disclosure without a patient's consent'.

The doctor's position in relation to the GMC is therefore unequivocal. In the absence of consent, he should not disclose unless directed to do so by a court. If he does disclose without consent, he faces the possibility of disciplinary procedures for serious professional misconduct.

In an attempt to resolve this dilemma, and following the publication of a Government consultation paper (Home Office 1995) on disclosure, the BMA set up a working group, which included representatives from the Association of Police Surgeons, the GMC, the Law Society, the Crown Prosecution Service, the police, and the medical defence bodies. As a result of this discussion, the BMA and the APS have jointly issued guidelines (1996). This emphasises that the duty of confidentiality owed by police surgeons is the same as that owed by any other doctor. It rehearses the GMC's position, and warns doctors that the Crown Prosecution Service, in taking the view that police surgeons form part of the prosecution team, expect full disclosure of material. Doctors are encouraged to be explicit about their role, particularly when obtaining consent from detainees, and from victims of sexual offences, and, if the Crown Prosecution Service requests further information, the specific consent of the patient should be obtained. Finally, it acknowledges that in the event of a court order, disclosure must be made.

However, these guidelines are likely, as their name suggests, to be temporary. In November 1995, the Government introduced the Criminal Procedures and Investigations Bill. The role of police surgeons in relation to new disclosure procedures envisaged in the Bill is far from clear, although, in response to questions in the House of Lords, the doctor's confidential relationship with his patient, and his independent status in relation to the police, appears to be secure. In addition, it seems likely that procedures involving the testing of the materiality of evidence, including a pre-trial hearing for this purpose, may be proposed. Advice to doctors on the implication of the new Bill will be issued by the BMA once it becomes law.

References

Bevan V Lidstone K. 1990 *The Investigation of Crime: A Guide to Police Powers*. para 7.110, p.405 Butterworth, London.

British Medical Association 1986. Guidelines for Doctors and Nurses who have been asked to help in connection with the implementation of Section 55 of the Police and Criminal Evidence Act 1984 (intimate searches). BMA, London.

British Medical Association 1992 *Medicine Betrayed* page 187. BMA, London

British Medical Association/Association of Police Surgeons 1994 *Health Care of Detainees*. BMA, London.

British Medical Association/Association of Police Surgeons 1996 *Interim Guidelines on Confidentiality for Police Surgeons*. BMA, London.

British Medical Association/Law Society 1995 *The Assessment of Mental Capacity*. BMA, London.

Crown Prosecution Service 1995 Casework Standards Division Advice No 2. CPS.

General Medical Council 1988 Personal correspondence.

Havard JDJ 1989 The Responsibility of the Doctor. *British Medical Journal*, **299**: 503-508.

Home Office Circular 1988. Police and Criminal Evidence Act 1984; parts I, X, XI and related matters, para 36.

Home Office 1995 Disclosure: A Consultation Document. Cm 2864. Presented to Parliament May 1995. HO, London.

Home Office 1995 Appropriate Adults Review Group.

Law Society 1994. *Consent and the Criminal Law*. Consultation Document 139. Law Society, London.

Medical Protection Society 1990 Personal correspondence.

Panting G (The Medical Protection Society). 1992 Personal correspondence.

Robertson G 1992 Evidence to the Royal Commission on Criminal Justice, *Role of Police Surgeons – Research Study No 6* HMSO, London.

Zander M 1990 *The Police and Criminal Evidence Act 1984*, p149. Sweet and Maxwell, London.

4

CLINICAL EXAMINATIONS IN THE POLICE CONTEXT

R Bunting

When assessing injury and complaint, the forensic medical examiner is often faced with the probability of multiple cause. By reading this chapter, or this book, the doctor will not be transformed into an expert examiner, but should become aware of some of the possibilities and pitfalls. Familiarity with the criteria to apply to these cases comes essentially with experience, experience which can only be obtained by practising the art thoughtfully and assiduously, with frequent referrals to texts and discussion with colleagues.

Your observations and conclusions must be converted to a readable, accurate and cogent report. The final act is to present your evidence in court, a topic discussed in the next chapter.

GENERAL CONSIDERATIONS

Examinations fall into two broad categories:

  i To ensure the safety and well-being of the detainee.

  ii To help the police in the investigations of an alleged crime, when the examinee may be a suspect or a victim.

Although these two often overlap, specific informed consent must be obtained for each category. A detainee may agree to be examined for one purpose, but not the other. Information obtained during an examination in the first category may also have important evidential connotations.

You may ask the detainee if he knows why he is in custody, and why he is being examined in order to assess his understanding of the situation, but you must not discuss the alleged crime, except insofar as that is part of a clinical examination.

You may ask for an explanation of injuries or marks, but if the explanation appears to implicate him in the crime, you must remind him that he is still under caution.

The importance of the doctor's ethical and legal approach to examinees is covered in chapter 3, and the care of detainees in chapter 6.

FACILITIES FOR EXAMINATION

Examination facilities should match those available in the National Health Service, but experience shows this not always to be so. Every effort should be made to bring shortcomings to the notice of police authorities.

The surgeon should have the exclusive use of a room set aside solely for examinations. It should be of adequate size, comfortably heated and well ventilated. The desk must provide storage for writing materials and all the appropriate forms, but be separate from a working surface for the processing of samples. It is preferable to have colour corrected lighting of high quality. An adjustable, mobile light should allow detailed examination of the person, whether standing, seated or lying on the couch. A secure telephone must be available. Comfortable chairs for the doctor, examinee and any accompanying person improve the atmosphere.

In the interest of confidentiality, police officers are excluded, unless there is a risk of violence. However, an officer ought to be within calling range. A chaperone is essential when a detainee of the opposite sex is examined. An exhibits officer may be needed to assist with any labelling at the sampling stage. In Scotland, there is a requirement to have an officer present to corroborate the taking of samples.

Adequate sound-proofing will prevent conversations from carrying to anyone outside the examination room. In laying out the room, take care that the doctor cannot be trapped by a potentially violent detainee. An accessible panic button provides some comfort to the doctor.

Hand washing and toilet facilities should be available en suite. The room must have a refrigerator and deep freeze dedicated to the storage of samples.

Not all detainees or victims require medication, but some preparation must be made for the supply of analgesics, dressings or specific treatment if required. Forces vary in their readiness to supply medicines. It is preferable for the doctor to carry his own emergency supplies or to have a means of having medication dispensed on private prescription without any great delay. NHS prescriptions may not be issued. When giving drugs from the bag, the doctor becomes the dispenser and must record the origin, batch number, and use by date.

Instruments kept at stations will depend on the preferences of the doctor and the type of examinations or treatment likely to be carried out. Disposable equipment is to be preferred, but satisfactory arrangements for sterilisation of other instruments are essential.

Any equipment kept in examination rooms must be securely stored. The basic items listed below are considered essential, although local practice may necessitate some variation; for example, suturing material and instruments are only needed if the police station is remote from an Accident and Emergency Department.

Examination kits (general and special)

Sterile syringes and needles (forensic science laboratories may specify the pattern)

Needles and needle holders

Sterile dressing packs, 5 x 5 cm and 10 x 10 cm

Assorted adhesive wound dressings

Micropore tape

Elastic bandages

Triangular bandages and safety pins

Clinical thermometer

Hibitane individual sachets (or similar)

Plastic receiving dish and gallipot

Plastic or dumb-bell sutures

Proctoscopes and vaginal specula

Dressing scissors

Forceps

KY Jelly

Disposable gloves

Brooke airway

Separate containers for sharps and contaminated materials

DOCTOR/PATIENT RELATIONSHIP

The nature of the environment (usually a police station or police examination suite) and the antecedents (a crime is alleged) render the doctor/patient relationship abnormal. It is not difficult to be aware of this when faced by many offenders, but it is quite easy to forget when dealing with a victim or plausible stories of mistakes or mitigating circumstances from a detainee.

The surgeon must always be aware that the examinee is a fellow human being: be open minded on all issues, but maintain a high index of suspicion. As much as possible of the information gleaned by interview or examination must be tested. The surgeon must always ask himself, "Do the physical findings fit the explanation offered; is the story plausible?"

Alternative solutions should be considered and tested by questions or detailed examination to see if this or that hypothesis fits the facts. Try putting yourself in the place of the suspect or victim and imagine how you would account for any findings which might suggest mitigating circumstances. Remember, people do lie and malicious complaints are made in the attempt to shift blame in preparation for any future enquiry or court hearing.

Stressed suspects or victims may catastrophize events. In order to get a clear picture of what happened, you must always move on from the general to the specific whenever possible. Clinical interviews and examinations cannot, and must not, be rushed.

Call-out response

Most doctors contracted to police authorities are working on a part-time basis. They have other demanding jobs, usually in general practice. However, the job of police surgeon/forensic medical examiner carries its own special responsibilities.

The police are constrained by the Police and Criminal Evidence Act (PACE) and by their own manpower problems. Delays in examinations lead increasingly to complaints from detainees or their legal representatives which can obscure the criminal issues when the cases come to court. Most importantly, physical evidence may be lost.

On receiving a call, make every effort to contact the initiator of the call at the earliest opportunity to establish details of what is required and the degree of urgency. Negotiation and diplomacy go a long way to smoothing over difficulties, and allowing the investigations to proceed in a more relaxed fashion.

BEGINNING THE INVESTIGATION

Having fixed the time and place for the examination, get there on time. Liaise with the relevant officer. This will usually be the custody officer in a station who, in turn, may contact others having an interest in the case (Criminal Investigation Department, Social Services). When attending a scene away from a police station, contact the senior investigating officer present or the senior scenes of crime officer.

Whether at the station or elsewhere, find out why you have been called and what is required of you. You need not be bound by the police requests; it may be necessary to discuss the issues using your own knowledge and experience. Simply taking a blood sample because that is all you were asked to do when a little thought and discussion would have indicated a thorough clinical search, can lead to embarrassment in court. The police surgeon may, at his own discretion and with appropriate consent, carry out a full examination in any type of case if he feels it is required.

When body samples are to be obtained, the necessary consent from senior officers provides for the safety and well-being of the detainee. The relevant police officer will state that he has "reasonable grounds to believe that the samples will tend to confirm or disprove the person's involvement in the offence and therefore give my authority for the taking of such samples". The detainee's consent must be informed and (preferably) in writing. The detainee may refuse to provide samples, but will be warned, "if you refuse without good cause, your refusal may harm your case if it comes to trial."[1]

You must always think ahead in every case when considering the scope of your interview and examination. Ask yourself, or an investigating officer, where this case may lead and then act appropriately.

Clinical records

Clinical notes must be contemporaneous. Ideally they should be written as the history and examination proceeds. The detainee can see that a record is being kept.

Conversations which may turn out to be contentious ought to be recorded verbatim. It is not unknown for defence counsel to ask you in the witness box exactly how his client replied to specific questions. Generalisations or a precis of the history and of examination may lead to difficulties in court. Your report and opinion have to be firmly based on recorded information. The shorthand, "...Examination (or part of examination) - NAD" may not be adequate. You may know the extent of your examination, but the court does not know if it is not recorded. It is becoming more common for either side to request a view of the original notes and a Judge may order this.

If notes are kept in a bound, hard-backed book, the danger of being accused of additions or wholesale changes in the interval from examination to court is minimised. A 19 x 25 cm plain, artist book is easily carried and allows diagrams to be interspersed in the narrative. Separate printed body sketches are available. These should be used to indicate the patterns of injuries, each injury being numbered. The numbers should be those recording the description of the injury

---

1. For a full discussion of this topic, see chapters 2 and 3.

in the contemporaneous notes, and the same numbers will be used when writing a report for the courts. These diagrams must not be relied upon as the sole source of information.

Some forces use printed booklets into which the information is recorded. These may be good aides memoires for the inexperienced, but the doctor using such a book must have control of the completed booklet. Questions of confidentiality may arise if this is passed on to the Crown Prosecution Service or the police. Do you have a copy or other contemporaneous notes? (See also chapters 2 and 3.)

Clinical history

Only now are you ready to continue with the clinical history and examination. The extent of this history and examination will depend upon the circumstances of the case. The detainee in a cell asking for some form of sedation may not require the detailed attention which must be given to a victim or perpetrator of a serious crime. The scope of the examination must be assessed by the doctor.

The name, address and date of birth of the detainee and information about the circumstances of the arrest and any other information regarding the detainee may be obtained from the custody officer. Prior knowledge of this helps in assessing the orientation and lucidity of the detainee when interviewed. Ask the custody officer specifically whether or not an interview is pending.

Depending upon the circumstances of the examination, you may ask the detainee what is wanted or expected of this examination or if there is any complaint. Complaints may refer to illness, injury or the conditions of detention.

The medical history includes past illness or injury, current medication, substance abuse and alcohol consumption prior to arrest. The detainee may be asked to describe how he came to this examination and if he understands why he is there. Explanations about causation of injuries, marks or general condition should be accepted and recorded without further discussion. The level of awareness, mobility and co-ordination are noted during the interview and subsequent examination. Where a detainee is asked to copy a short text in assessing level of intoxication, it may be necessary to ask about educational attainments.

Further investigation and the help of an approved social worker and Section 12 approved doctor may be required if a mental health problem appears probable (see chapter 10). The need for the attendance of an appropriate adult at any subsequent interview must be considered (chapter 6).

A more detailed examination or even referral to hospital may be necessary if questioning leads to the suspicion of an occult injury or intercurrent medical condition.

Clothing

Detectives or scenes of crime officers may have arrived on the scene before the doctor and confiscated clothing to preserve trace evidence. Ask to see the retained clothing if you feel this is relevant to your assessment.

If the person is dressed in clothes worn during an incident, establish with the investigating officers what clothing may need to be retained for forensic examination. It is important to know the routine adopted by your force. In any event, enquire about and record clothing worn. This may influence your interpretations of bodily marks or injury. If trace evidence is being sought, undressing is done on the sheet of paper provided in the examination kit. The order in which garments are removed should be recorded so that any transfer of evidence may be assessed by the forensic scientists.

Preliminaries and general examination

Having recorded the history, explain to the client exactly what you are going to do. The order in which the examination is performed will depend upon the circumstances. Do not home in on specific areas of damage or complaint. Start off with simple and probably familiar procedures, such as pulse, blood pressure and auscultation of the chest, for this can make the more detailed examinations easier to accomplish. Notes about general hygiene, nutrition, height, weight, muscularity or mobility may have relevance to your assessment.

Significant information can be obtained when doing this general review. For example, while attention is being given to some other part of the body, supposedly injured areas may perhaps be seen to move fluently and cause no distress. This is particularly relevant when examining for a complaint against the police. The undressing process necessary during the general examination gives adequate access for viewing, assessing areas of injury and assessing co-ordination. When performing these examinations, thought should always be given to the comfort and modesty of the individual.

The general and specific parts of the examination will inevitably overlap. It is most important to remember that any complaint calls for a full viewing of the body. The localised injury may be genuine, but, as in all medico-legal matters, there may be a hidden agenda. Finding additional injuries where there is no complaint may put an entirely different interpretation on the case.

If you do not consider that an area of the body needs to be examined, or the client will not allow an examination, this must be specifically referred to in the notes.

SPECIFIC FORENSIC EXAMINATION
Fitness to detain and to interview

Among the commonest examinations performed in a police station are assessments of fitness to be detained and to be interviewed. These topics are included in chapter 6, but physical injury is dealt with below. A particularly difficult task is to examine detainees and others who have made complaints against the police; some preliminary remarks will be made about these.

Examinations in cases of complaint

Complaints are often made by a detainee that undue violence was employed during an arrest or that treatment after arrest was not given. There may be allegations of violence by other parties in a criminal act. When examining a distressed victim, you must not disregard your critical faculties. The examining doctor may become the subject of complaint, but not be aware of this until giving evidence in the witness box.

The examination procedures remain the same. Fully informed consent must be obtained, preferably in writing. The client must be aware that a report will go to the police, the Police Complaints Authority or to the Crown Prosecution Service. Copies for the client's solicitor will normally be available through these sources.

A brief chronology of events leading to the complaint must be obtained as related by the client. Following a violent arrest, an attack or a public order situation, it may be difficult for the client to remember details, but every effort must be made to get specific facts relating to the complaint. Lack of details in the client's story may be due to the confusion of the situation, but may also be due to deliberate obfuscation.

The examination must be in a good light, using ancillary lighting for difficult areas. The whole body surface should be minutely inspected. If an area is left out, the notes should contain a reference to this. Any failure of the client to co-operate should be noted.

If there is total non-compliance by the detainee, the doctor should observe behaviour, signs of any distress and fluency of movement and record these observations. It can be useful at times to observe discreetly movements to and from the detention room.

The newcomer to forensic medicine must be aware that it is often the smallest abrasions or petechiae that are important. A central examination suite may be graced with an efficient illuminated magnifier, but all police surgeons should carry at least a loupe or other lens to examine surface markings. This may yield clues as to the causative agent or the direction of force.

Description of injuries must be accurate and the correct terminology used in the notes, but these terms will have to be interpreted for lay persons when the statement is written. The different categories of injury are fully described in chapter 8. Positioning of lesions must be unequivocal, so use body diagrams or sketches. It is poor practice to depend on notes written on body diagrams as the sole source of information. Marks or injuries should be numbered and related to the written notes.

Having examined individual marks or injuries, step back and observe any marks as groups or patterns. The ultimate significance of such patterning may only become apparent when you are considering your notes and diagnosis away from the tension of the scene. You cannot then go back and check, you must have adequate and accurate notes in front of you.

Decide if photography is required. In many cases, the police may have called the scene of crime photographer, but make it clear which views or significant marks you wish to be photographed. In any event, a well documented, carefully observed description of any injury or group of injuries is worth many photographs. It is worth recounting this in court when appropriate. Counsel can be very imaginative when drawing conclusions from photographic exhibits.

If marks appear difficult, don't hesitate to ask for another opinion either on the actual injury or on photographs. This is of particular importance with presumptive bite marks. Bite marks are not always crescentic with broken lines indicating dentition. It will depend upon the area being bitten. Can the tissue be accommodated in the mouth? Teeth can be used as a weapon without actually biting. These marks can be difficult to interpret – don't forget the forensic odontologist.

Fingernail marks are not always crescentic with the concavity facing towards the perpetrator. They can, under certain circumstances, be straight abrasions or even reversed concavity, depending upon the mobility of the receiving tissues. If you have limited experience with injuries, don't make assumptions. Discuss the marks with colleagues who have experience before committing yourself to a written report.

The whole process cannot be rushed. Look, record and look again. You only have this one opportunity to get it right.

Police arrest techniques

It is well worth discussing the methods current in your force with the training sergeant or physical training instructors. They are only too willing to demonstrate the various movements, allowing you to see and perhaps experience the stresses that can be imposed upon the body. This will give useful insight into interpreting injuries. The techniques usually rely upon inflicting pain to control violent behaviour. This will occasionally stress joint capsules and related structures which must be recorded. In some subjects such techniques may exacerbate problems from old injuries or age related degenerative changes. Obtaining a complete medical history becomes important.

Examination kits

Having looked and recorded, decide if samples need to be taken. Police forces in the UK generally have a series of prepared examination kits. These usually contain body diagrams, instruction sheets, all sampling materials, envelopes, bottles, needles, syringes and swabs. When only limited sampling is required (perhaps blood for DNA or drugs, mouth swabs or hair samples) individual small examination kits are made up to save cannibalising the more comprehensive and therefore more expensive kits. In any event, the procedural requirements and the necessary consents before samples are taken must be complied with.

Ultraviolet light is often advocated to search for body surface stains. Under ideal conditions of adequate blackout and a suitably powerful light, this should show biological (semen, saliva) staining. In practice, adequate blackout is difficult to obtain and the weak fluorescence of biological staining is often ousted by the vigorous background radiation of fibres, detergents and other debris. Do not rely upon it. Swab where the victim indicates, where dried surface particles are seen on careful examination and swab elective sites (nipple, breasts, thigh, vulva, hands) as a routine if the case suggests it.

Moistened swabs may be used to collect stains or surface debris. Inadequate sampling is common. Make use of the whole surface of the swab by rolling it around. Use two swabs if there is enough material (labelled as one specimen). Larger debris (hair, fibres, vegetation) can be picked off with forceps, packaged and labelled.

The head and neck

Palpate the scalp. Tenderness, swellings, depressions and even unsuspected bleeding can be found by this means. Congealed blood can be missed in dark hair. Inspect the surface of the scalp. Flicking the hair through the fingers, as in flicking the pages of a book, can give a good idea of colour changes in the scalp. Look for bald patches and broken hairs. If an area is dirty or bloody, clean it. Remember to take swabs if it seems necessary before cleaning, then inspect the site.

Look at the ears. Inside - think of barotrauma from closed blows to the ears. Outside - crushing the pinna on the mastoid process may cause obvious deep bruising, but occasionally only very faint, scattered intradermal bruising.

Is the face symmetrical? Is there any swelling, redness or surface marking? Check conjunctivae (including the lower sac) for subconjunctival or petechial haemorrhages. Check for asymmetric eye movements, pupillary abnormalities and nystagmus. Is there any evidence of nose bleeds (you have to look in the nasal cavity!)? Is the airway patent?

Examine the lips for asymmetry due to swelling, for abrasions, bruising or lacerations. Look inside the lips and on the buccal surface of the cheeks for evidence of crushing against the teeth. Check the jaw and teeth for pain, loose or damaged teeth or irregularity of dentition.

Facial injuries tend to be by blows from fists or hands. The bruising occurs at the point of contact and is usually more marked when skin is crushed against subcutaneous bone. Occasionally the skin is lacerated over bony prominences (orbital ridges, malar bone, nose, over teeth and jaw), the subcutaneous bruise then spreading by pressure and gravitational flow. In a fresh complaint, the time interval between injury and examination must be recorded.

Flat hand blows generally do not crush tissue, but force out blood from capillaries where the fingers land and cause intradermal disruption of capillaries at the edges of the lesion. This produces the tramlining effect of intradermal bruising between the fingermarks; often centrifugal force produces the greatest impact pressures at the extremity of the hand or where the fingers wrap around a curvature of the face. This effect is often seen in flexible rod, electric flex or rope injuries to the skin.

Check the neck for tenderness and swelling by palpation and for any marks, especially ovoid subcutaneous bruises caused by fingertip pressure. Do the discrete marks show a pattern of hand gripping? A single mark on one side with several vertical in-line marks on the other side of the neck may indicate which hand was used.

Neck holds or locks by police or assailants may imprint overlapping red marks or intradermal bruising in a "linen fold" pattern of marks. The imprinting arises from folds of cloth covering the neck or the arm of the assailant which in turn may imprint their surface pattern of folds and weave. Finally, check for cervical movements. Soft tissue damage may be caused by acceleration/deceleration injury in road traffic accidents, but also by blows to the head, by falls, or by violent avoidance of blows.

The limbs

Check for shoulder, elbow, forearm and hand ranges of movement. Capsular and ligament stresses to joints from forced rotation or hyperextension are not uncommon.

Bruising may be of any type, but look for grip marks especially on the medial aspect of the upper arm which bruises easily. Again, the disposition of bruises around the arm may indicate how the arm was held.

Bony injury must be excluded. This is of particular importance in the hand which may have been used as a weapon. Always check and record the dominant hand.

Handcuff injuries are perhaps the most common cause of complaint. Injuries can occur if they are overtightened, but this should not happen with the new quick-cuffs if double locked. Injuries include circular red marks, usually more prominent over the ulnar and radial borders or styloid processes. There may be superficial abrasions; occasionally the abrasions are deep enough to draw blood. Bruising, if it occurs, is usually subcutaneous due to the crushing action of metal on subcutaneous bone. Chip fractures around the styloid processes have occurred. It is possible to fracture a bone by self-inflicted, voluntary muscular action and this may occur in violent prisoners, especially when drugged or drunk.

In the lower limbs, pain, tenderness, loss of function (mainly weight bearing) and sensory changes should be recorded. The legs are often the target for kicks.

The trunk

Bruising, abrasions, lacerations and other injuries can occur anywhere. The whole body, with due thought to comfort and modesty, must be carefully examined in a good light. Each individual mark must have its position described in relationship to fixed body parts. It must be measured, its direction or disposition recorded and the nature of the injury accurately described.

The same principles apply as described in head and upper limbs. Crush marks will be accentuated over bony landmarks. Bruising will move with gravity and muscular activity. Surface markings may carry the signature of the causative agent.

Over the trunk be especially careful of penetrating wounds. Differentiate laceration from incision and especially stiletto wounds. Consider what may be happening below the integument due to penetration of the weapon or to transmitted forces. Don't forget to undertake a normal clinical examination for swelling, tenderness, rigidity or guarding. Always look at groups of marks to see if a pattern emerges. Do marks sweep around body contours as in flexible rod or flex injuries? Has the body rolled or been dragged? Look at surface markings with a lens to see if a direction of force can be ascertained. Do the marks form a coherent pattern as in seat belt marks? Does the imprinting or patterning suggest a particular type of weapon?

The genitalia

As part of a general examination for injury, inquiry must be made about genital symptoms. In a general examination of assault, the possibility of a concomitant sexual element must be considered and it may be necessary to inquire about, for example, male rape as part of a violent assault. If this area of examination is not pursued, record the omission and reason in your notes.

How was the injury caused?

The marks seen will depend upon:

1. *The nature of the inflicting weapon*

   The relatively soft flat of the hand, a clenched fist, metal objects, road surfaces, brick, concrete: the list is long and each may leave its own signature on the body.

2. *The relative mass and the velocity*

   A 70 kg body free falling or propelled to hit a static object, a flailing fist or a baseball bat used double handed will each transmit different amounts of energy causing a great variety of wounds and marks.

3. *The covering of the body or surface of the object*

   The covering, its type and thickness will modify the transference of energy and therefore the mark left. It may also cause the transfer of material from weapon to body or vice versa, and imprint its signature or that of the covering material.

4. *Obliquity of contact*

   This modifies the degree of trauma and also its signature.

5. *Area of body affected*

   Muscular areas and other soft tissue may "give" under impact and mark much less easily. Subcutaneous bone may trap interposed soft tissues and leave more obvious damage. Transmitted energy may damage deep tissues or remote organs.

6. *Personal characteristics*

   Age, body mass, sex, general health, degree of mobility and athleticism may all modify the effects of trauma.

Having described the marks and considered the dynamics of the possible causation, you must now consider how this fits the explanations offered. If no explanation is offered, you will still need to come up with a plausible hypothesis which fits the known facts. The permutations are enormous. If you haven't thought of the variations and formed an opinion, the other side certainly will. Putting yourself into the scenario and playing the "what if?" game on how you would explain signs and symptoms if you were the detainee can give you useful insight into a case and suggest lines of questioning or further examination.

Flexibility and a readiness to concede to reasonable alternatives will be most helpful to the courts, either at the report stage or during a court appearance.

However, the doctor needs to have enough conviction to stick to reasonable alternatives. To quote Lord Denning, "An explanation may be possible, but not in the least probable."

It is often helpful to inspect an alleged weapon or to view the site of an incident after the examination. The head injury allegedly caused by a constable appears less plausible when blood and hair are found on the windscreen frame of a stolen car, as do allegations of a kicking supposedly delivered by three or four officers in the back of a police van, when examination reveals fixed rows of narrow seats in the van.

SUMMARY

Every effort must be made to get the descriptions correct. Examinations should be performed in a good light. An illuminated magnifier is an asset, or at least a good quality hand lens of x10 or x15, together with an auriscope, an ophthalmo-scope and a focusable pen torch. A measuring device (ruler, tape or callipers) and body charts are helpful. Photography is desirable. If it is not provided by a profes-sional scene of crime photographer, some thought should be given to a suitable camera and lighting arrangement (ring flash is preferable) and arrangements for confidential processing. The author has found no advantage in examining for bruises with ultraviolet light: the eye is insensitive to this frequency. However, the migration of melanocytes may be captured on panchromatic film and show sites of old bruises. The necessary techniques are within the province of the specialist.

Justice is not served when the doctor describes an injury inaccurately, allowing its attribution to become doubtful. There are rarely second chances in forensic med-icine: you must get it right first time.

When assessing wounds of any kind, the doctor may consider self-infliction. These may occur in para-suicide, in mental illness or with a deliberate intention to mislead. Some idea of motivation may emerge during the interview or medical examination. The appearance of such injuries may be obvious, but occasionally problems of interpretation may arise when they are extensive and life-threatening and allegedly done by another person. This type of self-inflicted injury usually occurs in accessible areas of the body, but areas of difficult access must not be dismissed. The injuries are often concentrated on the side opposite to the dominant hand. The observed angulation of the wound may favour self-harm rather than an outside attacker. Injuries to eyes, ears, mouth and nose are often avoided. Marks tend to appear deliberate, superficial, of equal depth throughout, multiple and parallel. The victim may not show serious injuries such as lacerations or extensive bruising, but one must not under-estimate a determined deceiver. The apparent victim may be playing for high stakes such as a cover for injuring or killing some other person and he may prevail on another to injure him deliberately. Self-harm in police cells with a view to involving the arresting or custody officers is not unknown. A careful examination of the victim and the site of the supposed incident, a thorough search for "weapons" by the police and careful consideration of all aspects of the case, are required.

Inferences from the circumstances and the past medical history, accompanied by self-inflicted wounds, usually allow one to diagnose para-suicide. Old linear scars and amateur tattoos may indicate previous self harm. Mentally disturbed persons may inflict severe and bizarre injuries on themselves.

At the other extreme, the examiner should be aware of injuries which could be "defence injuries". Any conflict where injuries may occur is a dynamic situation; the victim may raise hands and arms to protect the face or roll into a ball to protect vital areas. Weapons may be grasped. A little thought will indicate the type and areas of injury.

Often the appearance of the victim leads to an intuitive diagnosis, but this should not be an excuse for a lack of careful examination and documentation of the injuries. The medical report, if required, must be firmly based on the written contemporaneous notes.

In conclusion, this chapter offers ideas for the general clinical assessment of detainees and victims. The doctor will rarely arrive at a textbook diagnosis in clinical forensic medicine. Often the person who knows the truth about a particular encounter will be unwilling to share that knowledge and may be intent on misleading the examiner.

For this reason the interview, the examination and the recording of information need to be as detailed and as exhaustive as possible.

Further reading

Police and Criminal Evidence Act 1984 Codes of Practice (1995) HMSO.

Health Care of Detainees in Police Stations 1994 BMA Medical Ethics Committee and Association of Police Surgeons. (A new edition is in preparation.) BMA, London.

Knight B 1991 *Forensic Pathology.* Edward Arnold, London.

Mason JK 1993 *The Pathology of Trauma.* Chapman and Hall Medical, London.

Gresham GA 1978, *A Colour Atlas of Forensic Pathology* (Wolfe Medical Atlas 12) Wolfe Medical Publications, London.

5

THE DOCTOR IN COURT

M Clarke

Almost all doctors attend court as a witness at some time. Forensic clinicians are likely to have to attend court more frequently than any other members of the medical profession. The forensic clinician has a vital role to play in the judicial system of the United Kingdom, and he or she should not undertake any aspect of clinical forensic medicine unless prepared to go to court and accept from time to time the personal inconveniences that this may cause.

The importance of the doctor's evidence cannot be overstated. The doctor is regarded by lawyers and others as a trained observer and capable of giving an impartial opinion. This may have enormous significance in matters as varied as the interpretation of injuries sustained by a drunk at the time of arrest, to the assessment of the condition of a child suspected of having been sexually abused.

On the whole, the courts endeavour to list cases and call doctors so as to cause as little inconvenience to the doctors as possible. However, the demands of the court take precedence over all other commitments, and a doctor may be required to return from holiday to give evidence essential in a case. To minimise inconvenience, it is advisable to keep those concerned with listing cases, both at local police level (Administration of Justice Department) and at the Court Listing Office, updated on problems of availability.

A doctor may be called to give evidence as a witness of fact. For instance, the doctor may have seen a road accident occurring and can describe what happened. The doctor's evidence will not depend on his professional expertise, and will be limited to recounting what he or she saw of the accident. The doctor may have been involved as a casualty officer in the treatment of a person injured in the same road traffic accident. The casualty officer will be called to give evidence as a professional witness regarding the injuries sustained by the accident victim. Similarly, a forensic clinician may be called as a professional witness, to give evidence of the results of examinations carried out at the request of the police or other authority. An expert witness is a person who, because of depth of experience, is asked to give an opinion on the observations of others; in the case of the accident, the expert witness will not have observed the accident, but may have seen the photographs, and will usually not have examined the patient, but will have had access to all relevant documentation including photographs and X-rays if appropriate.

A forensic physician becomes competent through adequate training and through work experience. The more work undertaken, the greater the accumulation of experience. The more forensic work undertaken, the more frequent the cases which require the doctor's attendance at court. A busy forensic clinician is at risk of working much of the night and spending most of the following day in court.

STATEMENTS

However, it is not always necessary for the doctor to attend court in person to give evidence. If a case proceeds to trial, the forensic clinician will be asked to provide a statement (often referred to as a Section 9 Statement). A statement is a report which, in England and Wales, includes the statutory declaration shown in fig. 1. Unless instructed otherwise, reports for the police should be submitted in statement form. Police forces have headed statement papers with continuation sheets, plain for typewritten statements, lined for handwritten. Handwritten

---

STATEMENT OF WITNESS

(Criminal Justice Act 1967, s.9)

(Magistrates Court Act 1980 - s. 102)

(Magistrates Court Rules 1981 - r 70)

Statement of ....

Age of Witness (if over 21 enter "over 21") ....

Occupation of Witness ....

This statement (consisting of .... pages each signed by me) is true to the best of my knowledge and belief and I make it knowing that, if tendered in evidence, I shall be liable to prosecution if I have wilfully stated in it anything which I know to be false or do not believe to be true.

Dated the .... day of .... 19 ....

Signature ....

Figure 1 – Front page of statement paper

Continuation of Statement of:	Page No ....

Figure 2 – Continuation sheet of statement paper

statements should be submitted only in an emergency - lawyers delight in questioning the clarity of a doctor's handwriting! It is not necessary to use the police paper for statements, provided the statutory declaration is included and the format is followed. In addition to the signature acknowledging the serious consequences of making a knowingly false statement, the bottom of the first sheet of the statement and each subsequent sheet are also signed, with the signature on the last sheet being placed immediately below the last paragraph.

The use of a word processor ensures that the statement will be read through to check for errors and sense before being printed, and corrections can easily be made after the first draft. A copy of any statement made to the police or other interested parties must always be kept. The statement is usually the only information the lawyers have about what the doctor might say, and the order in which the medical observations are to be presented.

Statements are not for other medical practitioners. Statements will be read by lay people – the police, the Crown Prosecution Service and the lawyers. If the doctor's statement is agreed by both the prosecution and the defence, the statement may also be read to the jury. For this reason it is essential to use everyday language which will be clearly understood; if no appropriate expression exists for a medical word or term, the nearest English word or phrase should be used with the medical term also included but put in brackets, for example "black eye (periorbital haematoma)". Sometimes doctors have to attend court and give evidence just to explain in plain English what their statement means. Clear, concise and comprehensive statements reduce the necessity to attend court.

A statement may be requested weeks or months after an examination. A busy doctor will see many cases and cannot be expected to remember the details of one of a number of similar cases. The doctor must rely on the contemporaneous clinical notes made at the time of or immediately after the examination. It follows that if the record of examination findings is full and comprehensive (including negative observations if appropriate) the doctor will be able to complete a statement which will include all possible relevant information (see chapter 4).

Setting out the statement in paragraphs gives it a professional appearance, making it easier for the reader of the statement to find his or her way about, and easier to refer back to a particular point. Interpretation is impeded by allowing the history taken prior to the examination to run into the clinical details.

The first paragraph should contain the doctor's qualifications and appointments, with relevant experience of special interest to the case. Next should come an explanation as to how the doctor became involved in the case, for example, as a forensic physician called by the police to examine a person in custody, or as a duty casualty officer.

The name, age and date of birth of the person examined now follow, with the name printed in capitals; whenever the examinee's name appears in the statement it should be in capitals. The address of the person examined should not be included. As a security measure, current practice is not to include the addresses of witnesses, including medical witnesses, in statements. The times the examination commenced and ended must be included, as must the place of examination; if in a police station or a hospital, the exact room should be specified. The purpose of the examination should then be indicated, as should the name of the person who gave consent to the examination, the taking of samples or photographs, and the making of a report. The names of those present during the examination must also be included. The role of other medical personnel present during the examination should be explained.

The next paragraph should include details of the complaint which led to the examination, with a note as to who gave the history (complainant, relative, police officer). As far as the court is concerned, this is hearsay, but clearly any opinion expressed by the doctor will take into consideration the history as given to the doctor. It may be that the doctor will have to revise his or her opinion in the light of further information, perhaps only becoming available during the trial. When giving evidence, the doctor may have to detail the complaint as recounted at the time of the examination. It is a matter for the court whether this evidence is given by the doctor. It is proper to summarise the history of the complaint in the statement, provided that the full contemporaneous notes taken prior to commencing the examination are available at the trial.

Reference should be made to past medical history, even if only to record that it did not appear relevant to the case. For example, the court should know of a long-standing handicap or chronic illness, for this could render the person less able to defend himself against assault. During the discussion prior to commencing the examination, the doctor will have explored current medication, use of illicit drugs and alcohol intake, and will report in the statement any relevant information.

Then follow the details of the examination. The use of numbered paragraphs for describing the findings is strongly commended. If many injuries are recorded on body sketches, the injuries should be numbered there, with the corresponding numbers inserted in the text; photocopies of the body sketches should accompany the statement. In describing injuries, the site of the injury should precede the description of the nature of the injury followed by the measurements (see chapters 4 and 8).

Negative findings should always be recorded in the contemporaneous notes, and frequently be included in the statement. In particular, after injuries have been listed, a note indicating that the remaining body surfaces were examined and showed no injuries should be added. The presence or absence of tenderness or discomfort can also be of significance.

At a suitable place in the statement, usually towards the end, any specimens taken should be listed, together with their reference numbers. The time at which the specimens are handed to another person, and that person's name, must also be recorded.

Finally, at the end of the statement comes the opinion, given a heading of its own. The opinion includes an indication of the age of injuries, the conclusions to be drawn from injuries, marks or stains, and whether the findings are "consistent" or "compatible" with the complaint. Absolute dogmatism at this point can be disastrous; at the time of the examination, the doctor learns only part of the story of the incident. He may not hear of other explanations until in the witness box, and may then have to concede that the new explanations of the clinical findings are as likely or even more probable. A specimen statement is shown in fig. 3.

ATTENDANCE AT COURT

In a civil case, decisions are made on "the balance of probability", a less strict standard of proof than that required in criminal cases. The standard of proof in criminal cases is such that the prosecution must satisfy the jury, upon the whole of the evidence called by all parties, of the accused's guilt, "beyond reasonable doubt". In England and Wales, the jury is often instructed that they "must be satisfied so that they are sure of the guilt of the accused."[1]

Any person charged with a criminal offence is entitled to legal advice and representation; it is the duty of the custody officer to ask the detained person whether he requires to consult a solicitor as soon as detention begins. The police may not question a detained person who wishes to speak to a solicitor until he has done so (except, for instance, if there are reasonable grounds to believe that delay will involve an immediate risk of harm to persons or serious loss of, or damage to, property)[2].

The duty of the defence lawyers is to test the prosecution case by examining the evidence presented by the prosecution witnesses. There is "no property in a witness"; although the prosecution may be calling a witness, the prosecution does not own that witness or what he will say. A doctor due to appear as a prosecution witness may very occasionally be called to a conference with the solicitor and

---

1. Archbold 1995 *Criminal pleading evidence and practice* Re-issue volume 1: 4-389, 4-394. Sweet and Maxwell.

2. Police and Criminal Evidence Act 1984. Revised (1995) Codes of Practice, Code C §6 et seq.

STATEMENT OF WITNESS
(Criminal Justice Act 1967, s.9)
(Magistrates Court Act 1980 - s. 102)
(Magistrates Court Rules 1981 - r 70)

Statement of...................................... Desmond Beckett ....

Age of Witness (if over 21 enter "over 21") .... Over 21 ....

Occupation of Witness ..... Divisional Police Surgeon ....

This statement (consisting of ...... 3 ...... pages each signed by me) is true to the best of my knowledge and belief and I make it knowing that, if tendered in evidence, I shall be liable to prosecution if I have wilfully stated in it anything which I know to be false or do not believe to be true.

Dated the .... 2nd .... day of .. .. January .... 19 96.........

Signature .... D. Beckett ....

I am a Divisional Police Surgeon and General Practitioner. I hold the qualifications Bachelor of Medicine, Bachelor of Surgery, Member of the Royal College of Surgeons, Licentiate of the Royal College of Physicians, the Diploma in Child Health, and the Diploma in Medical Jurisprudence. I have been a police surgeon for more than twenty-five years. I practise from the address given on the reverse of this sheet.

On 1st January 1996, at the request of WPC 4478 Brown of the County Police Force, I attended Main Street Police Station, Anytown. There I saw and examined BARBARA SMITH, age 14, date of birth 18th April 1981. The examination was made in the police station medical room between 2.15 a.m. and 3.0 a.m.

Present throughout the examination were Mrs. Julia Smith, BARBARA SMITH's mother, and WPC Brown. Consent to the examination, the taking of certain samples and the making of a report to the police was given by Mrs Smith. BARBARA SMITH also consented to the procedures.

BARBARA SMITH told me that on her way home from a party after midnight on 1st January 1996, about an hour before the examination, she had been struck on the head by a man, and had fallen to the ground. She said that she had a pain on the left side of the head and about the right knee. She said she was feeling very upset and shaken.

D. Beckett

Figure 3 – Specimen statement

Continuation of Statement: Desmond Beckett   **Page No.. 2 ...**

There appeared to be no significant features in her past medical history. She is not on regular medication, and does not take illicit drugs. She said that she had had a few glasses of wine during the evening, but could not remember how many.

On examination I noted the following:-

1.   BARBARA SMITH was fully conscious and co-operative throughout the examination. She appeared upset, and had a brief weep whilst giving the history of the alleged assault.

2.   I noted that there was blood on the left side of the head and neck, and on the left side of the blouse and cardigan she was wearing. There were smears of dirt on the right side of the skirt, the outer aspect of the right shoe and the right sock.

3.   5 cm above the top of the left ear, there was a 3 cm deep laceration which gaped. The injury ran downwards and backwards. This injury had bled. There was an area of swelling and tenderness surrounding the injury.

4.   There was some superficial abrading of the palm of the right hand, which was dirt stained.

5.   On the outer aspect of the right knee, there was an abrasion 3 cm x 6 cm, running vertically. There was some dirt staining about the injury, which had bled slightly. This injury appeared tender.

6.   Examination of the remaining body surfaces revealed no other evidence of recent injury.

7.   I noted that BARBARA SMITH's breath smelled of alcohol. The whites of the eyes were injected. The pupils were of normal size, and reacted briskly to light. There was no nystagmus; nystagmus is an abnormal rapid movement of the eyes, present in certain illnesses, and in intoxication with certain drugs including alcohol. The pulse rate was within normal limits at 90 beats per minute. BARBARA SMITH's behaviour and co-ordination throughout the examination were normal.

I took the following specimens during the examination and handed them to Det. Con. 2211 Jones at 3.15 a.m.

DB1   Venous blood (EDTA vial) (Freeze)

DB2   Venous blood (EDTA vial) (Refrigerate)

DB3   Venous Blood (RTA vial) (Refrigerate)

DB4   Scalp hair from region of injury

DB5   Random samples of scalp hair

D. Beckett

Figure 3 – continued

Continuation of Statement: Desmond Beckett   **Page No.. 3 ...**

OPINION

The injuries noted above were consistent with having been caused within a few hours of the examination. The injury to the left side of the head was consistent with having been caused by a blow from a blunt instrument. The injury to the right knee was consistent with having been caused by ground contact.

The injuries were consistent with having been caused in the manner described to me by BARBARA SMITH

Although BARBARA SMITH had taken alcoholic drink, there was no clinical evidence of significant impairment due to drink at the time of the examination. The reddening of the whites of the eyes could have been caused by crying.

At the end of the examination I made arrangements for BARBARA SMITH to be seen at the Hospital Casualty Department.

(DB1 is for DNA profiling, DB2 for grouping, DB3 for blood alcohol)

D. Beckett

Figure 3 – continued

barrister representing an accused person prior to the trial, and the evidence to be adduced discussed. Any doubts about the propriety of attending such a conference can be resolved by discussion with a senior colleague or with a representative of the doctor's defence organisation. The doctor is entitled to a fee for attending the conference.

Forensic clinicians with a moderate to heavy workload will soon find that they are required to attend the Crown Court with some regularity. Other courts which may require a doctor's presence are the Coroner's Court, the Magistrates Courts and the County (civil) Courts. Attendance at the civil courts will usually be in connection with an action for compensation, or, increasingly, in relation to child care.

Doctors at court will soon find that much of their time in court is spent in non-productive waiting. Many of the decisions regarding a case are not taken until the morning of a trial. The doctor's evidence may be agreed between the prosecution and the defence after a wait, without the doctor ever seeing the inside of the courtroom. The doctor's evidence will then be read to the jury, as is permitted if it has been submitted in "Section 9" format.

There are several ways of keeping to a minimum the time spent at the courts. The most important is to ensure the highest standard of statement making; a first class, impartial report, dealing with all reasonable alternative explanations for injuries or other findings, will usually (but not always) be agreed without the doctor ever having to attend the court hearing. A first class statement depends inevitably on a high standard of examination and documentation at the time.

Increasingly, requests are made (usually by the defence) for copies of the doctor's original notes. This is a perfectly proper exercise. The defence lawyers are entitled to test the quality of the medical evidence; there is no privilege in a doctor's examination notes. If the doctor feels that there are matters which do not assist the case and should not be brought into the public arena, the doctor may express a wish to reveal the notes only to another named doctor acting for the defence (General Medical Council 1995). A steadfast refusal to produce the notes made during an examination will usually result in the doctor being called to court to explain the circumstances. It is worth remembering when making notes during an examination that the original notes may be subjected to relentless scrutiny, and discrepancies of time and clinical details between the notes and the eventual statement exploited. It is generally agreed, at least among lawyers, that doctors are incapable of writing clearly, and no opportunity is lost in court if difficulties are encountered in interpreting a doctor's squiggles, a great source of innocent, if embarrassing, legal merriment.

The doctor may be instructed to attend court before the trial begins. This gives the opportunity for the doctor to speak to the prosecuting counsel and through him to the defending counsel; arrangements can then be made for the doctor to be called at an agreed time during the trial. Medical evidence is usually taken towards the end of the prosecution case, or whenever it fits logically in the proceedings. With agreement of the defence and the judge, the medical evidence may be taken immediately after the complainant's evidence. Counsel who know that the doctor is immediately available by telephone or radio can plan accordingly.

If attendance at court is going to cause difficulties in the doctor's medical practice, contact should be made with the appropriate police Administration of Justice Department or with the Crown Prosecution Service. If warned to attend court by telephone, a note should be made of the contact telephone number in case of difficulties. Usually the courts make every effort to accommodate the doctor. It behoves the doctor to be philosophical about delays at court; the doctor who always emphasises his importance and the irreplaceable value of his or her time lost hanging around court will impress no one, will find he spends even more time waiting, and will get a witness summons to attend court on the day of planned departure on holiday.

Witness summonses are issued by the Crown Courts or the magistrates courts, and are signed either by an officer of the court (for Crown Courts) or by the clerk to the justices or by a justice of the peace (for magistrates court). The request for the summons may originate from the court itself, the Crown Prosecution Service or from a solicitor acting in the case. The summons gives the name of the defendant, and requires the presence of the named witness at the court, giving the date of the hearing and the time to attend court and adds "on subsequent days until the court releases you". Failure to attend court as a witness without just cause may be treated as a contempt of court, the penalties for which include fines and imprisonment. In recent years a few doctors have been obliged to pay substantial penalties for contempt of court.

Attendance at court should always be at or before the time instructed. An excuse for a late arrival due to some unforeseen event will be more readily accepted if a reputation for promptness has been established. Dress should be appropriate for the occasion, the doctor being the representative of a learned profession attending to give evidence in a forum where decisions of the utmost gravity are made. Men should be dressed in a dark suit and suitable tie; women should be dressed equally soberly and with restraint in the use of make-up. Giving evidence can be a strain even for those who are frequently in the witness box; no resort to alcohol should be made – the smell may drift across the courtroom as far as the judge. Many find that they are better able to give evidence if they are keyed up.

All original notes must be taken into court, together with any relevant photographs, X-ray or laboratory reports, and copies of any statements or reports already submitted. A doctor who has neglected to bring the correct documents with him may find himself sent away to retrieve them in the middle of a trial, to be further discomfited on return to court by legal wit in an endeavour to diminish the value of the medical evidence, if that is appropriate for the defence case. The records should be read through, preferably the night before giving evidence, and again before going into court. If difficulties are anticipated, for instance in interpreting a finding, the textbooks should be referred to (and if necessary taken into court) and the matter discussed with more experienced colleagues.

If the doctor has not attended a particular court before, it is advisable to familiarise oneself with the layout of the court, and establish the relative positions of the witness box to the judge, to the jury, to the dock and to the area used by the lawyers. Whilst modern courts have a similar layout, older courts can have some interesting variations. The witness box in Lancaster Crown Court is raised substantially above the court floor, rather like an elevated pulpit in church! (In that same court, a branding iron is fixed to the prisoner's dock, used to impress the letter M on the malefactor. It is not currently in use.)

Witnesses of fact and professional witnesses are not allowed in court until it is their turn to give evidence. During the period prior to adducing evidence, the prosecution lawyer outlines the facts of the case to the magistrates or to the jury, and then the complainant and other witnesses who might be required before the medical evidence are called.

On entering the witness box, the witness is sworn. This is a particularly solemn moment – the penalties for perjury are severe. The witness can indicate to a court usher before approaching the witness box the nature of the oath he or she wishes to take – whether it be on the New or the Old Testament, on the Koran or other holy book, or whether the witness wishes to affirm. The oath will be administered by an usher or other court official, or in Scotland, by the judge.

One of the lawyers sitting in the body of the court (usually a solicitor in a magistrates court or a barrister in the Crown Court) will rise to begin the questioning of a witness. In the Crown Court it is the custom for the defence barristers to sit closest to the jury, with their instructing solicitors behind. The representative of the Crown Prosecution Service sits behind the prosecuting barrister. (For Scottish procedure, see chapter 2.)

The magistrates or the jury usually have no idea who a witness is or what his or her involvement is in a case apart from what has been said in the prosecution opening of a case. The doctor will therefore be asked to identify him- or herself, and to list qualifications. This is the point where nervousness can play its greatest part. It is wise to have asked the usher beforehand to ensure that there is a glass of water available on the witness box from the beginning of the evidence. The doctor may also be asked to give an address; for security purposes it is advisable to give the practice or hospital address. The doctor should then ask the judge or the chairman of the magistrates if reference can be made to original notes made at the time of the examination; permission is rarely withheld.

After the preliminaries, the doctor gives his evidence in chief. The doctor should speak slowly and clearly, addressing the back row of the jury (or the magistrate) in a voice loud enough for all those in court to hear, and using everyday language. It is tempting to reply to the questioner, but answers should be directed to those who are to decide the guilt or innocence of the accused, the jury or the magistrates. The judge and lawyers, but usually not the magistrates, will have copies of the doctor's statement, and it will be convenient for the doctor to follow the same order of evidence as given in the statement. Notes are made of evidence given during the proceedings by the lawyers and the judge or magistrate. Evidence may be tape recorded or recorded by a stenographer. It is advisable to watch the judge's pen so that the judge is able to record all the medical evidence without asking the witness to pause.

In evidence in chief, leading questions are not usually permitted. However, prosecution and defence may have agreed much of the medical evidence, and the witness is then led through the agreed evidence. Whilst giving evidence in chief, points may occur to the doctor which may clarify an observation. Such additional points may be made, with caution.

After evidence in chief, the lawyer representing the defendant rises to cross-examine the witness. Contrary to the procedure during evidence in chief, the defending lawyer is able to ask leading questions. (A leading question is one formed in such a way as to suggest the answer – "Did James Brown attack the deceased?" rather than, "Who attacked the deceased?") The defence is seeking to establish that reasonable doubt exists in the evidence presented, and may properly employ a number of tactics to diminish the value of the doctor's evidence in the eyes of the jury. Obtuseness, affected indignation, belittlement ("That's only your opinion, doctor") or sarcasm may all be used. Should counsel step outside the proper bounds, the judge will intervene. Questioning is designed to elicit more information, or to put a slant more helpful to the defence on the evidence. The doctor must not be upset by the questioning, or take the defence attack personally; he should continue his evidence as concisely and briefly as possible, repeating answers if need be, and not volunteering information unless requested. Attempts to score off the barrister should be avoided; the barrister will always win that type of exchange.

The doctor should not be drawn into areas outwith his experience or expertise, as this will soon be shown up, and cast doubt on the value of the other medical evidence. The witness can always ask for a question to be repeated, which gives time to consider a reply. "I don't know" is an answer which indicates honesty, not ignorance. Admit omissions; an examination of a drunken driver may not require the use of all the tests ever described. Sufficient tests must have been done to ensure the accuracy of the diagnosis, and the driver's safety in custody. This can be explained to the court, for the cross examining barrister must give the witness the full opportunity to reply.

The defence will put points to the medical witness which must be conceded – there are few observations in medicine which are capable of only one explanation. By adding if appropriate, that alternative explanations were considered, and, on balance, the witness prefers the conclusions already expressed, the witness gives a good impression of fairness.

Finally, there may be questions asked in re-examination by the prosecuting barrister, usually related to points opened up by the defence. The judge or the presiding magistrate may then ask questions. Judges dressed in black with a sash are addressed as "Your Honour". Judges dressed in red and judges at the London Central Criminal Court (Old Bailey) are addressed as "My Lord" or "My Lady". Magistrates are addressed as "Sir" or "Ma'am" or "Your Honour".

On the conclusion of giving evidence, the doctor before leaving the box should ensure that he has been released from Court. The judge will usually indicate that this is so, but there will be occasions when the doctor is required to stay and listen to subsequent evidence, to advise the prosecution on the evidence given by defence medical experts, and possibly to be recalled to give further evidence.

DEFENCE EXPERTS

The defence are entitled to seek expert medical advice to assist in preparing their case. Increasing use is being made of defence medical experts, particularly in the more serious trials. They are drawn from the ranks of senior and experienced doctors who with the passage of time have gathered expertise in the particular problems in a case. Thus a professional witness who has examined a rape case or a driver accused of having been under the influence of drugs may find that a senior forensic clinician is advising the defence. The defence expert has the advantage of seeing all the relevant documents and considering them at leisure; he has the disadvantage of not having seen the patient at the crucial time of the examination.

If the defence do not call "their" expert to give evidence, but rely on the expert's report, for instance, in formulating questions in cross-examination, the expert's report does not have to be disclosed. However, if it is intended to call the defence medical expert to give evidence, the expert's report must be disclosed to the prosecution before the trial starts. The prosecution medical witness is entitled to, and should, see this report before giving evidence, preferably several days before the trial commences; it is always worthwhile asking, prior to going into court, if the defence are calling their expert. If they are, the doctor should insist on seeing the defence expert's report, and insist on having the time to study the document. The sight of an eminent colleague sitting behind a defence barrister listening avidly to all a medical witness says, and occasionally scribbling a note to pass to counsel, can be disconcerting.

The defence expert may be required to sit in court from the beginning of the trial, usually behind but close to the defence barrister. Complainants and other witnesses frequently give evidence from the witness box which differs from what is in their statements. If the defence expert is sitting in court, the prosecution may require "their" doctor also to sit in court until the end of the medical evidence. The defence expert will usually give evidence at the end, but sometimes at the beginning, of the defence case. However, in a change of procedure within the last few years, the defence expert may be called to give evidence immediately after the prosecution medical evidence. This has the advantage that the jury can consider the medical evidence in one piece.

Confidence in the quality of the examination and honesty in the witness box will be sufficient to get through what may seem to be (and occasionally is) an ordeal. Many doctors express indignation after a trying session in the witness box – they forget that it is not they who are on trial, but the man or woman in the dock. The doctor is not judge and jury, merely the impartial presenter of part of the case, called usually by the prosecution, but in effect giving evidence on behalf of the court rather than for one particular side. The impartiality must be continued outside the court, and personal views on what was or what should have been the outcome of a case kept to oneself.

Increasingly, prosecution doctors and defence medical experts are requested to confer where there appears to be a divergence of opinion to see if the divergence can be narrowed, or to isolate the points of difference. This may result in an agreed statement being read out to the court, thus saving trial time, doctors' time and public money. However, the doctors should not discuss the case until instructed to do so by their "side". How a case is presented in court is a matter for the lawyer making the presentation. "Live" evidence with cross-examination, even when the content of the doctor's statement has been agreed, can make a bigger impact with a jury than the reading aloud of a medical statement by a non-medical person.

FEES

Payment for professional witnesses in England and Wales is claimed from the Crown Prosecution Service on a form used only for that purpose; the form may be sent with the initial instructions to attend court, or will be handed to the witness by the CPS clerk. If for some reason the form is not produced, write to the CPS, quoting the case number on the list displayed outside the court. Payment is determined in two hour bands, counting from the time of leaving home or practice and returning there. Alternatively, but not in addition, payment may be claimed for the cost of employing a locum, subject to proof of employment being supplied. Mileage rates are less than those paid by the police to police surgeons.

Fees for expert witnesses should be negotiated with solicitors before the doctor accepts instructions, and confirmed preferably in writing. Most cases are funded by the Legal Aid Fund, and the approval of the Legal Aid authorities has to be obtained by the solicitor before the instructions are confirmed. An estimate has to be given by the doctor what the fee for the study of documents and the preparation of a report is likely to be; this can be difficult if the papers are not to hand, and it is advisable to give an upper limit within which one can work. Guidance on fees is given in the Lord Chancellor's recommendations on fees for expert witnesses.[3] On completion of the report, the fee note is sent with the report to the solicitor, but will not usually be paid until the solicitor is paid at the conclusion of the case.

Expert witness's fees for attendance at court in legally aided cases, together with travelling and accommodation expenses, if incurred, are also in accord with the Lord Chancellor's recommendations. Claims are submitted on Form 5113A (Professional witnesses expenses sheet) obtainable from the Crown Court office, and returned on completion to the Cash Office of the appropriate Crown Court. If the expert has attended court, but not given evidence, and thus not come to the attention of the court clerk, it is advisable to request the instructing solicitor to enclose with the claim form a letter confirming the attendance at court.

---

3. Lord Chancellor's Department. Guide to Allowance under Part V of the Cost in Criminal Cases (General) Regulations 1986.

Fees for attendance at court are usually promptly paid to professional and expert witnesses. However, many months may elapse before fees for the preparation of defence medical reports are paid. After six months, the expert should send reminders of outstanding accounts. Eventually, it may be necessary to invoke the Solicitors' Complaints Bureau of the Law Society[4], or even to sue through the small claims procedure of the County Court[5] before payment is received.

Further reading

Duties of a Doctor 1995 General Medical Council, London.

Gee DJ and Mason JK 1990 *The Courts and the Doctor.* Oxford University Press.

4. Victoria Court, 8 Dormer Place, Lemington Spa, CV32 5AE (tel: 01926 820082).

5. County Court Summons. Form N1.

6

CARE OF DETAINEES

S Robinson

INTRODUCTION

The forensic clinician treats patients in an unusual environment, that of detention. This automatically imposes a need for certain skills and knowledge in addition to those of basic medicine. Training in primary health care is an obvious requirement; competence is not restricted to general practitioners, for other fields of medicine may well provide the sound basis of practice needed.

The additional demands made on forensic clinicians include the problems of treating patients many of whom are reluctant to report their history faithfully. The doctor lacks previous knowledge of the patients and faces a dearth of information from other health care sources, partly because of the unsocial hours during which clinical problems often present. Patients in the closed community of detention interact and may be manipulative. The short time most prisoners spend in police custody restricts treatment plans and reduces the opportunity for clinical monitoring.

The 'fitness to be detained' examination is full of potential problems; time spent in explaining the independent role of the forensic medical examiner is time well spent. Emphasis should be put on the health and welfare of the patient, but the doctor must also be honest about the potential evidence gathering aspects that may arise. Honesty with the patient is never unrewarded, even if the patient then withholds consent for any disclosure to the charge officers or the court. Any delay in disclosure by the doctor will then be seen to be founded on sound ethical grounds. In the United Kingdom, the doctor/patient relationship is not based on absolute privilege; disclosure may be ordered by a court. In some circumstances the doctor feels a need to disclose confidential information immediately (see chapter 3).

Mandatory reading for all police surgeons is the booklet *Health Care of Detainees in Police Stations*[1] – compiled jointly by the British Medical Association (BMA) Ethics Committee and the Association of Police Surgeons. Various aspects of the booklet are addressed throughout this chapter. It should forever be borne in mind by the forensic practitioner that any examination may entail both therapeutic care and forensic intent. This chapter deals almost exclusively with therapeutic care, but evolution into an evidence gathering exercise requires any consent to be re-assessed.

CLINICAL NOTES

Poor note keeping is the downfall of many a practitioner. The crucial importance of good records in clinical forensic medicine has been emphasised in previous chapters. In dealing with detainees, the dimensions of liberty and justice are added to the doctor's ordinary concern for the preservation of health, the reduction in morbidity and the prevention of mortality. From among the many cases seen, the physician cannot present any one with candour, honesty and accuracy without relying on clear and accurate clinical records.

Contemporaneous notes are still most often handwritten, but the physician who uses dictated records must remember that the tape forms the contemporaneous note. Reference by a witness to any other document may be restricted by the court. For computerised records, registration under the Data Protection Act 1984 is required in the UK. That Act empowers the Data Protection Registrar to remove those particulars of any individual whose data retention constitutes a contravention of any of the data protection principles.

SOME GENERAL CONSIDERATIONS

In looking at the general aspects of detention in custody, this chapter refers to a small number of specific conditions which have particular relevance to the forensic practitioner; it cannot replace textbooks of internal medicine. Much of the chapter is reproduced from *Principle of Forensic Medicine* (Robinson 1996) with the permission of Greater Manchester Police.

On arrival at a custody area the clinician should discuss with the custodian all the circumstances of the arrest and proposed detention which may have any bearing on the health and welfare needs of the patient. The need for this becomes obvious throughout the remainder of the chapter.

---

1. A new edition is in preparation.

Necessary immediate assessment, care and treatment of, for example, the unconscious patient aside, all detainees should be examined in a properly appointed medical room (see chapter 4). They should be given the attention of the doctor in private whenever possible, but this stance must be modified in the circumstances considered below.

Juveniles in custody should have a parent or other appropriate adult present. It is unlikely that the treatment needs of a juvenile in police custody would fall outside the understanding of the patient, therefore the child may give valid consent. Rarely, a child under the age of 12 years may be in custody and it is considered that under that age the child will not have reached sufficient maturity (Brazier 1992).

When a detained person of the opposite sex is being examined, a chaperone of the same sex as the patient should be used. It is courteous to introduce the chaperone to the patient, and to seek approval for his or her presence. If the patient refuses to have the chaperone present the doctor must carefully consider the position before commencing any examination. It is sometimes possible to have the chaperone within sight but out of immediate earshot, and this can be acceptable to the patient who has doubts about the advisability of a non-medical person being present, particularly if that person is a police officer.

The request of a patient to have a solicitor present at the examination should present no problem to the skilled forensic clinician. However, no undue delay which may affect appropriate care or the financial burden to the authority responsible for remunerating the physician should be contemplated.

The safety of the physician must be considered, and with this in mind the custody officer's opinion must always be taken into account and the presence of a police officer accepted if deemed appropriate.

Joint interviews with an approved social worker, in the case of a patient suspected of mental disorder, or with another physician are, of course, entirely acceptable. On this point, chapter 10 should be read as well as the references to mental health later in this chapter.

TREATMENT PLANS

Whatever decision is made about the health care needs of a specific patient, the clinician has a duty to disseminate the information to enable that care to be provided. In addition to discussing the medical advice with the patient (a prime requisite) communication with other physicians who are likely to be involved with the patient, and with the custody staff, is vital. Specific consent should be sought at the outset.

Notes or letters to other police surgeons, hospital doctors or general practitioners will be needed in all cases where continuation of treatment, or further clinical investigation, are required. Such missives should be sealed in an envelope, ideally addressed to the appropriate doctor, and a copy kept by the referring doctor in the contemporaneous notes.

The situation regarding custody staff is somewhat different. A police officer cannot be expected to care for a patient in custody without the appropriate advice. Clinical detail need not be divulged, but medication schedules, diet, frequency of cell visiting (including the observations required) and clinical review periods should all be indicated in writing for the custody staff. The doctor should be satisfied about arrangements for the custody of medicines and their administration. Consideration has to be given to the health and safety of the custody staff and other detainees. Someone with open pulmonary tuberculosis is not an ideal patient to keep in a potentially crowded custody suite. However, the practice of declaring specific patients to be infectious disease risks on the basis of presumed or previously declared hepatitis B or HIV status, for example, has been shown to be fallacious (Payne-James et al 1994).

Common sense has to prevail in deciding that a prisoner with a defined condition is fit to be kept in cells. Were you in general practice would you be happy to keep this patient at home or does he need hospital admission? Police officers are not trained nurses, can only perform basic tasks of care and should not be expected to make the more sophisticated observations.

In dealing with patients suffering from the conditions specified below it is safer, if in doubt, to refer to hospital. A death in police cells is taken very seriously and investigated thoroughly. The enquiry may reveal that a patient received treatment at a level less than reasonable. Criminal prosecution could follow (Brahams 1992).

Any detainee needing medication should be prescribed a sufficient quantity for his stay in custody. The prescription should be a private one, paid for by the police (Home Office 1950). If the detention is to last longer than 7 days (which occurs when prisoners are remanded to police custody by a court, or are contained because of the lack of prison accommodation), it is sensible for the medication to be reviewed at the end of this period and a further prescription issued if necessary. The patient's condition may indicate earlier review or this may be requested by the custody officer; the important factor is clinical need.

SPECIFIC CONDITIONS
Heart disease

Most patients seen with heart disease are well controlled on regular medication and present no problems. They are likely to have a chronic condition such as angina, cardiac failure or a stable arrhythmia such as atrial fibrillation. Regular medication may be continued or prescribed in the normal way, and the custody record annotated with drug dosage and times of administration. Simple advice can be given to custody staff such as, "Please ring me if the patient gets worse," as indicated by chest pain, breathlessness or sweating.

The most difficult complaint to assess is chest pain. It is obviously important to decide whether it is cardiac or has some less life-threatening cause. In chest pain of cardiac type, the problem is to differentiate angina from infarction. The police surgeon must record a detailed history of the type of pain, the clinical examination of the heart, blood pressure and pulse rate, with any evidence of cardiac failure. The basic values apply as in general practice: refer to hospital if in any doubt, sending a letter with the patient.

Where medication is needed, it should be prescribed in the doses and at the times that the detainee would normally take it outside custody. If the detainee is on symptom led medication such as a nitrate, he should be allowed to keep that in his cell unless there is a specific reason not to do so. Doubt as to the identity of the medication, or regular abuse of any medication are examples of the need to restrict access to drugs.

Epilepsy

Most epileptics seen in police custody are well controlled and know their own disease well. However, many prisoners do not take their medication as prescribed and some have a high incidence of fits. As with cardiac disease, hospital referral is safer when the doctor would not feel confident in managing that patient at home.

The history should elucidate:
- The type of epilepsy and the type or frequency of fits.
- When the prisoner last had a fit.
- The medication taken, in detail.
- When the last dose was taken.
- What doses are necessary for that day and subsequent days in custody.

One self limiting fit in custody is probably acceptable if no precipitating factor is found during clnical assessment. A detainee who has had a fit should not be released until any post–ictal state has resolved. A prisoner having more than one fit needs hospital review. If the fit is the first ever, this needs hospital investigation as one would in general practice. Police officers are capable of immediate first aid and should be instructed to put the patient in the recovery position and inform the doctor.

It is worthwhile recording clearly the type of epilepsy if this can be determined. Epilepsy is a group of syndromes, constituting 'a chronic brain disorder of various aetiologies characterised by recurrent seizures due to excessive discharge of cerebral neurones' (World Health Organization 1973). As the police surgeon often has little history from the patient and none available from previous doctors, the seizure type classification attempted should be a simplified one (Porter 1984) acknowledging the difficulty of differentiating, in particular, generalized seizures. The importance of attempting to make a diagnosis may extend beyond immediate treatment. Automatisms do occur, particularly in some complex partial seizures, and recognising such a diagnosis could save much police time where, for example, the alleged offence is shoplifting. Of course the presence of epilepsy does not exclude criminal activity.

Treatment of epilepsy in custody is difficult, for the patient's account of his medication schedule may be totally unreliable; some epileptics in custody exhibit chaotic treatment compliance; some have a personality disorder and may have substance abuse problems as well. The claim that the patient is on oral temazepam or diazepam as an anti-epileptic should be treated with disbelief. It may be that an oral benzodiazepine in the form of clobazam is used as an adjunct in epilepsy with an associated anxiety state, when the treatment will probably need to be continued. Clonazepam is the only benzodiazepine used as a long term anti-convulsant; it may be used in all forms of seizure (British National Formulary 1995) but particularly in absence attacks and myoclonus (Isselbacher et al 1994).

To miss a single dose of anti-convulsant medication while in custody overnight should make little difference, yet it could be extremely risky to miss medication if the epilepsy is brittle. Many anti-convulsants have a long half life, but both carbamazepine and valproate have a short half life of about 12 hours. These drugs are best given in divided doses and, to avoid side effects, can be administered up to four times a day. To prescribe doses of these drugs thus is unlikely to cause any side effects. Phenytoin is the only problem drug from the aspect of toxicity, if the patient claims to be on a what would usually be considered a high dose which is continued or even increased.

A further complication is the habit of some patients to bolt all and every drug in their possession when the police officer knocks on their door prior to arrest. With all anti-convulsants, if the patient is in custody for an extended period of time, serum levels should be obtained. The custody record must be clearly written and annotated with the name of tablets and the time when doses are to be administered.

Diazepam remains the drug of choice for status epilepticus and can be administered intravenously or rectally. It is useful to carry rectal diazepam for use in a prisoner who is fitting in the cells. Any patient in custody who has needed parenteral anti-convulsant therapy for status epilepticus, even if conscious post-ictally, should be referred to hospital.

Diabetes

The only likely problem in non-insulin dependent diabetics is hypoglycaemia, if tablets are taken and food not provided, but this should not occur with proper care. The history taken should include any complications, the name and dosage of tablets and the time at which the tablets are due. Recommendations for feeding should be conveyed to the custody officer.

It is easy to measure blood sugar with any of the commercial testing sticks, or an electric meter. Ideally, every diabetic staying in custody should have blood sugar measured at least once, especially if he is to be interviewed. This may be waived if the patient is clinically well, non-insulin dependent, and only to be in custody for a short period, say less than four hours.

The insulin dependent diabetic is more difficult to control in custody. Any diabetic who is unstable, with hypo- or hyperglycaemia, needs hospital assessment and sometimes in-patient care. Once stabilised, the patient may be returned to police custody. There is a need to consider the particular circumstances of the arrest, such as recent pursuit or substance abuse: particularly in the case of an undernourished patient, hypoglycaemia may be induced. Hypoglycaemia may also be precipitated by alcohol. A prisoner may over- or under-dose on purpose to cause problems. It is preferable for the surgeon to supervise the patient in drawing up and administering insulin on the first occasion in custody to be sure that the patient is competent. Once again, clear instructions must be left to notify the doctor of changes in condition, for example pallor, sweating, confusion.

Asthma

Decisions on fitness for detention depend on medical assessment, following the basic principles of the British Thoracic Society (BTS) guidelines (Woodhead 1993):

- Control of Symptoms – Specific questions about frequency of symptoms, presence of wheezing, breathlessness, coughing or chest tightness, diurnal and activity variations.

- Current Medication – The type of medication, delivery systems, and dosage; the use of symptom led medication and the ability to use the relevant delivery systems should be recorded.

- Examination – As well as basic cardiorespiratory examination, it is helpful to test the peak expiratory flow rate (PFR) and compare the result with the predicted rate and the best level recorded by the patient, if known.

The medication schedule should be written out for the custody staff. If the asthma is well controlled, no change to the medication should be made. Occasionally the clinician will see a detainee whose asthmatic symptoms are controlled by medication that is not in line with BTS advice, when it may be appropriate to discuss the principles of treatment, and encourage the patient to seek a further consultation with his general medical practitioner if released, or the prison medical officer if remanded or detained. If the patient is remanded into police custody for more than a few days, the police surgeon may undertake such rationalisation of treatment.

If changes of medication are needed to establish control, it is recommended that the BTS stepwise approach, shown in the box below, is used. Any change in medication should be explained in detail to the detainee, reassurance being given and any fears addressed.

MANAGEMENT OF CHRONIC ASTHMA		
step 1	Occasional use of relief bronchodilators	Inhaled, short acting agonists prn [*] If needed ›1/day check technique, if ok ➡ **step 2**
step 2	Regular inhaled anti-inflammatory agents	Inhaled, short acting agonists prn [*] + beclomethasone or budenoside 100-400 µg bd [*] or try cromoglycate or nedocromil, but resort to steroids if no improvement is obtained with these
step 3	High dose inhaled steroids	Beclomethasone or budenoside 800-2000 µg daily via a large volume spacer or for those with difficulty with inhaled steroids, a long acting agonist or sustained release theophylline. Possibly try cromoglycate or nedocromil
step 4	High dose inhaled steroids and regular bronchodilators	Inhaled, short acting agonists prn [*] + beclomethasone or budenoside 800-2000 µg daily via a large volume spacer + a sequential therapeutic trial of one of:- inhaled long acting agonists sustained release theophylline inhaled ipatropium or oxitropium long acting agonist tablets high dose inhaled bronchodilators cromoglycate or nedocromil
step 5	Addition of regular oral steroids	Inhaled, short acting agonists prn [*] + beclomethasone or budenoside 800-2000 µg daily via a large volume spacer + one or more long acting bronchodilators + regular prednisolone tabs in a single daily dose
[*prn = as required; bd = twice daily]		

Rescue courses of oral steroids may be required for the treatment of chronic asthma, allowing the detainee to remain fit to be detained, in these circumstances:

• Symptoms and PFR get progressively worse by day

• PFR falls below 60% of best

• Sleep is regularly disturbed by asthma

• There is diminishing response to inhaled bronchodilators

In these circumstances, a single dose of between 30-60 mg of prednisolone must be given immediately and each morning until two days after control is re-established. A sufficient supply of oral steroids must, therefore, be prescribed. As well as giving the oral steroids, adjustment to maintenance medication should be made in line with the stepwise approach.

If the detainee is leaving custody an appropriate written summary should be made available for the patient to take when property is returned, or transmitted to the patient's general practitioner. It is often convenient to send such information by facsimile to the practice.

Acute asthma may be treatable in custody, but requires careful assessment. The BTS "steps" protocol (Woodhead 1993) gives detailed guidance, but the doctor must consider the best interests of the patient, the police and himself before deciding not to recommend referral to hospital.

HEAD INJURY AND ALTERED CONSCIOUSNESS

A detailed history must be taken about how the injury occurred and at what time:

• Was the patient knocked out and if so for how long?

• Can this be independently corroborated?

• Was there diplopia?

• Has he vomited since?

• Is the conscious level varying?

• Remember the lucid interval in extradural haemorrhages.

• Remember the time lapse with subdural haemorrhages; the elderly and the neglected (alcoholics and malnourished) are more likely to get subdural haemorrhage (Bannister 1985).

The examination will include a full central nervous system (CNS) examination including examination of the fundi. Areas of contusion and lacerations of the scalp may give an indication of the severity of the initial impact, but the lack of severe visible trauma does not exclude significant brain damage. Remember contra-coup injuries.

Major symptoms and signs for concern are:

- Pupil inequality
- Variable consciousness
- Localising neurological signs
- Diplopia

The head injury/intoxicated patient represents an assessment dilemma. Guidance from the Royal College of Surgeons (1986) sets out criteria for skull X-ray, hospital admission and consultation with a neurosurgical unit. These criteria, modified after McLaren *et al* (1993), are shown in table 1.

It is worth noting that post-traumatic amnesia with full recovery is not an indication for admission. Any patient sent home should be given written instructions about possible complications and appropriate action (see example in fig. 1 which was designed to assist custody officers, but conveys the essential information).

Alcohol intoxication, as well as predisposing to a risk of trauma (Rix & Rix 1983) can also potentiate the symptoms of brain damage by causing a change in vascular tone and thrombocyte function, with a consequent risk of haemorrhage (Brismar *et al* 1983). Brismar also drew attention to similar problems caused by abuse of intoxicants other than alcohol, as did McLaren (1993) who included abnormal

CRITERIA FOR SKULL X-RAY AFTER RECENT HEAD INJURY
1. Loss of consciousness or amnesia at any time.
2. Neurological symptoms or signs other than mild headache, dizziness or blurred vision.
3. Cerebrospinal fluid or blood from nose or ear.
4. Penetrating injury of scalp or periorbital bruising or swelling.
5. If any of the above cannot be reliably excluded.
6. The elderly.

CRITERIA FOR HOSPITAL ADMISSION AFTER RECENT HEAD INJURY
1. Confusion or any other depression of the level of consciousness at the time of examination.
2. Skull fracture.
3. Neurological signs of headache or vomiting.
4. Difficulties in assessing the patient e.g. the young, epilepsy.
5. Other medical conditions e.g. haemophilia.
6. The patient's social condition or lack of responsible adult/relative.
7. Alcohol or drug intoxication.

Table 1

HEAD INJURY INSTRUCTIONS FOR CUSTODY OFFICERS

If a detainee after a head injury:-

1. Becomes unconscious

2. Becomes increasingly sleepy

3. Complains of increasingly severe headache

4. Complains of blurred or double vision

5. Vomits

6. Has a fit

The medical officer must be contacted immediately. If immediate response from the physician is not obtained the detainee must be taken to the nearest Accident & Emergency Department at once.

Figure 1

behaviour and not just a history of alcohol consumption in his definition of the intoxication group.

What constitutes a head injury? Most drunks in custody seem to have some form of injury. The problem is to differentiate between a cranial injury and a minor scalp or facial injury. Bleeding from the nose may only be due to damage to the nose and not the cranium or its contents. To some degree common sense must be used, but only after a detailed clinical appraisal allowing the physician to show that any craniofacial injuries satisfy the conditions to exclude them from the guidelines summarised in table 1.

Concussion is a transient and immediate loss of consciousness, which may only last a few seconds, associated with a period of post-traumatic amnesia which may last considerably longer. It should be remembered that about 3% of patients who have had concussion will have an intracranial haemorrhage. The risk is increased in the presence of a skull fracture (Isselbacher et al 1994).

The assessment of other forms of altered consciousness is equally important. If the patient is unconscious the decision is easier, but assessment of the degree of altered consciousness in the patient who is not comatose is more difficult. In a series of 500 patients (none, of course, being in custody) only 149 who presented as stupor or coma of unknown aetiology were due to drug poisoning of one form or another (Plum & Posner 1982).

Restricted neurological signs such as amnesia may reduce the total content of consciousness but are not normally regarded as an altered state of consciousness. It is vital for the police surgeon to record accurately the level of consciousness. Labelling of the conscious level does not carry reliable agreed terminology for all levels, one of the problems being that altered consciousness does present as a continuum rather than stepped sequential conditions. Nevertheless, a forensic clinician often has to produce a meaningful assessment in court at a later date and must rely on notes which are themselves meaningful. Such a degree of assessment becomes even more important in the case of examination for fitness to be interviewed which is dealt with later. It is important, therefore, for the physician to use terms which are explicit or at least consistent, for example the following defined by Plum & Posner (1982):

Coma	eyes closed, unresponsive even to noxious stimuli
Stupor	capable of being roused by vigorous and repeated stimuli, lapse back into 'deep sleep' mode on ceasing stimulation
Obtundation	torpor, reduced alertness and interest in environment, slow response to stimuli, and increased sleep
Delirium	floridly abnormal with disorientation, irritability, fear, sensory misperception and sometimes visual hallucination – may get lucid intervals
Clouding of consciousness	reduced wakefulness or awareness, may have irritability alternating with drowsiness; attention reduced; misjudgement of sensory perceptions, reduced rate and quality of cognition
Clouding of consciousness with confusion	as above but more advanced state with at least minor disorientation to time and place, faulty memory, with prominent drowsiness

Proper instructions must be left for the custody staff. The medication, dose and frequency of dose, or preferably specific times the medication is to be given, should be written out for each patient. Even though the discussion above has highlighted the diagnostic dilemma faced by trained physicians, there is still an expectation of simple guidelines on the risk of late complications of head injury for lay people. The typical instructions given when a patient is discharged from casualty (fig.1) are all one can expect a police officer to carry out. Information on medication should be included whenever a patient is discharged with these care instructions. The ever valid advice for the clinician is: take no risks, for fatality and morbidity occur too often.

INTOXICATION AND DRUG ABUSE

Substance misuse is dealt with in chapter 9, but it must be remembered that acute or chronic abuse of a substance may mask other conditions which will require proper clinical assessment.

FITNESS TO BE INTERVIEWED

Paragraph 12.3 of Code C to the Police and Criminal Evidence Act (PACE Code C) states, "No person who is unfit through drink or drugs to the extent that he is unable to appreciate the significance of questions put to him and his answers may be questioned about an alleged offence in that condition except in accordance with Annex C. [See Note 12C]"[2] The note states, "The police surgeon can give advice about whether or not a person is fit to be interviewed in accordance with paragraph 12.3 above." There is no mention of the police surgeon being involved with regard to fitness for interview in any other condition, including mental health disorders.

There is mention of calling the police surgeon, and immediately so, if a person brought to the police station appears to be suffering from a mental illness or is incoherent except through drunkenness alone in C9.2 and Annex E of the PACE Codes but there is no mention of involvement with fitness for interview. As fitness to be interviewed is a relatively new area of clinical forensic work, parameters for such an assessment are not yet based on specific research; lacking set protocols, the forensic clinician in attendance must rely on clinical judgement.

The Victoria Police Forensic Medical Officers' Manual (1992) written and compiled by Drs David Wells, Edward Ogden, Simon Young and Faika Jappie, states, "You do not have to make a definitive diagnosis. You simply need to establish :-

1. Is (s)he mentally alert and orientated to answer questions?
2. Is (s)he physically well enough to answer questions?"

Experience suggests that rather more is required. No apology is made for reiterating the need for complete and comprehensive contemporaneous records.

GENERAL ASPECTS

Fitness for interview should be considered as a forensic examination, not a therapeutic one, requiring the appropriate consent. The forensic clinician must be prepared to assess patients for potential vulnerability during interview: false confessions have attracted much publicity. It must be remembered that not everyone interviewed is in detention. Not everyone interviewed is a suspect. A police surgeon may be asked to assess an individual who is a complainant or a non-participating witness to the alleged events.

---

2. Annex C is discussed on page 108.

In assessing someone's fitness for interview, consider

- the likely verbal rigour and its propensity for harm;
- the interviewee's capacity to recall and recount the 'facts';
- any undue suggestibility of the subject (it should be remembered that most people are suggestible to a certain extent).

As a point of principle, the detainee should always be asked for any objection or comment on the subject of interview. Many will wish to be interviewed as soon as possible, in order (or in hope) that they will then be released to go about their daily business.

Even though much of the text will refer to a "detainee" for the sake of simplicity, the information and opinion that follows applies equally to any interviewee, whether a suspect or not, except, of course, to any specific issues about custodial care.

CLINICAL ASSESSMENT OF INTERVIEWEE

Physical illness

Any detainee suffering from physical illness should be stable before interview takes place. It is difficult to be specific, but hypertension may serve as an example. Some hypertensive patients are stable at a theoretically hypertensive level. It behoves the clinician to establish, if possible, the 'normal' state for that patient, if a higher blood pressure reading than expected is obtained. This, of course, can be a difficult or even impossible task in the middle of the night, in which case the doctor's clinical judgement must be exercised. If a patient is on medication the treatment protocol should be ratified and written up on whatever is the accepted format for care instructions for detainees.

The detainee who is injured or suffering from a musculoskeletal disorder needs assessment, then any appropriate analgesia. The *British National Formulary* (BNF) describes both aspirin and paracetamol as particularly useful for musculoskeletal pain and pyrexia, the former to be used (if not contra-indicated in the individual) where anti-inflammatory properties are required. The BNF points out that any combined analgesic containing an opioid has no substantiated benefit over the simple drugs, if the dose is low, and carries all the side effects of the opioid if containing a higher dose. Visceral pain is, however, more responsive to opioid analgesics. Care must be taken not to give an opioid analgesic in a dose which may cause drowsiness during the interview, particularly in a patient unused to strong drugs. In police surgeon practice the above example infrequently presents. The specific case of drug misuse is dealt with below.

Examination

The examination should be preceded by the taking of a full medical history (including family, social, and past medical/surgical/obstetric). Details of medication should include any alcohol or illicit drugs used. For illicit drugs, it is of help to use the regional database forms as part of the medical record. These are available from the Regional Drug Database Centres (for a list of the addresses see Robinson 1996). The history should include habitual use of, as well as intake in the last 24 hours. It is worthwhile to remember that some readily available herbal preparations are taken for their euphoric effect.

Enquiry about nutritional state must include when and what food was last taken. During a full clinical examination, particular attention is paid to stigmata of drug abuse and/or withdrawal.

Anyone about to be interviewed or asked to sign anything will require access to spectacles (or contact lenses) if these are normally worn. For the same reason, inquiry should be made about any hearing deficit and habitual use of a hearing aid.

The CNS examination should include locomotor function, co-ordination, temporo-spatial orientation, cognitive function and short-term memory recall.

Clarke (1991) referred to Kipling's 'five men' (who, where, when, what and how) as sufficient to establish orientation in space and time. These are readily translated into Where are you? What day is it? What time is it? Why are you here? Who are you (what is your name, where do you live)? Who is that (identification of police officer, doctor, another prisoner)? The classic questions of naming the Prime Minister, and/or a recent news item, remembering a name and address given to the detainee a few minutes before, and taking serial 7's from 100 are all suitable tests of cognition.

The depth of the assessment is important. Gudjonsson (1995) develops the subject based on a case where he gave evidence as an expert. The accused had been declared fit for interview by a doctor and a consultant psychiatrist, and was attended by an approved social worker as the appropriate adult (see below). After expert evidence by Gudjonsson the interview statements were declared inadmissible by the judge. There was no question of improper behaviour by the police in interview technique, but it was apparent that the medical assessment had not been adequate to meet all the needs specified above.

Psychiatric problems

Any indication of depression, thought disorder, delusions or abnormal behaviour should be examined more deeply (see chapter 10). Depression, other than mild, may be accompanied by psycho-motor retardation, and poor memory. Anxiety and agitation often co-exist. A careful assessment must be made before declaring any apparently depressed patient fit for interview.

Anxiety itself can be induced in the innocent by interrogation (Gudjonsson 1992) and should not therefore be taken to preclude interview. The degree of anxiety, however, should be assessed and discussed with the patient. Such a discussion itself may resolve much of the anxiety without further interference. Many of the unpleasant symptoms of anxiety may be controlled by a small dose of a beta blockade preparation which should not affect cognitive function.

Patients with active severe disease such as mania, psychosis and schizophrenia-like disorders will not be fit for interview.

Alcohol

The mere label of alcoholism does not bar the patient from interview, but alcohol intoxication is another matter. It has been suggested by Clarke (1991) that the level set by the Road Traffic Acts of 80 mg of alcohol per 100 ml of blood should be a level above which a patient is unfit for interview, but this opinion appears to have no sound basis. The individual response to any level of blood alcohol concentration (BAC) varies, so to set an arbitrary limit of a BAC of 80 mg % in connection with fitness for interview cannot be supported. Survival with a BAC of about 1500 mg % (Williams P, personal communication) shows that massive tolerance may develop. Measurement of breath alcohol could be helpful, but such a reading would be only one facet of a comprehensive clinical evaluation. Routine use of such devices was considered to enhance the practice of forensic medicine, but not replace it (Rogers et al 1995).

It has recently been suggested by Robertson et al (1995) that the idea quoted above from Clarke "... has considerable merit... and if no medical or drug related complications are suspected, there is no reason why doctors need be involved in the procedure as the police are perfectly capable of using the instrument themselves." Though the caveat of medical and drug problems is mentioned by Robertson, the suggestion itself must rely on the police officer's opinion that there is no clinical abnormality. Such would not be a pathway of safety for the patient. Clarke does suggest the need for clinical re-assessment, even when the BAC has dropped to the acceptable limit. The decision on fitness for interview should be made on a clinical assessment.

Drug addiction

In relation to fitness for interview, the two important questions are:

1. Was the withdrawal complex severe enough to invalidate the recall of the witness or to result in distress sufficient to lead to false confessions?

2. Did administration of the dependency substance adversely affect the cognitive function of the interviewee?

Gudjonsson *et al* (1994) found that the consumption of alcohol or illicit drugs up to 24 hours prior to arrest did not appear to have significant effect above mental health, memory and suggestibility, previous criminality and literacy and IQ as factors affecting the interview. One reason why this should be so was that substance abuse shortly before arrest may have had relatively little effect on the subject's mental state (see also Sigurdsson & Gudjonsson 1994).

Gudjonsson's research involved up to one hour to assess each detainee. Police surgeons have neither the time nor the psychological skills to do such an assessment, but a comprehensive and detailed examination by the physician is appropriate.

If an opioid abuser is showing significant signs of withdrawal, including those signs which are difficult to mimic, such as gooseflesh, tachycardia, increased bowel sounds and pupillary dilatation, he is unlikely to be fit for interview without therapy. It may be that the detainee will be released after interview, and the physician has a responsibility to the patient to expedite the interview, rather than allow him to languish in custody for an unreasonable time, until his symptoms allow him to be interviewed. Such an end may be reached by the administration of a small dose of methadone, and physeptone tablets are easily carried in the medical bag for this purpose. However, the treatment decision is one that can only be made by the physician in attendance and other treatment options are available.[3]

Is there a window of opportunity for completing an interview? When the clinician declares a detainee fit for interview, that declaration is valid at the time of writing, and that must be made clear there and then. In the vast majority of cases the examination findings should hold fast for 3-4 hours, as long as a new event such as a fall in the cell or a change in symptoms does not intervene. If the interview is delayed for any reason beyond that time scale the interviewee must be re-assessed.

If the detainee is declared not fit for interview, and interview will be required at some stage, the police surgeon should indicate a time when the patient can be re-assessed clinically. A detainee, late at night, with a degree of intoxication and fatigue, may be better left to sleep overnight; the clinician may wish to indicate a time for interview to take place without re-assessment. It is safe to do this only with a known individual, lest other mental problems be masked by the transient symptoms and signs.

---

3. *Guidelines for the Clinical Management of Substance Misuse Detainees in Police Custody.* HMSO 1994. ISBN 0 11 321807 9.

RESPONSIBILITIES OF FORENSIC CLINICIAN

Appropriate adult

The appropriate adult was born fully grown but seemingly immature with PACE in 1984. The role appears to be increasing, probably as a consequence of heightened awareness of the need for appropriate adults, rather than a change in the dimensions of their responsibilities.

The appropriate adult is recommended for juveniles (PACE Codes C 1.7 (a)) and for a person who is mentally disordered or mentally handicapped (PACE Codes C 1.7 (b)). Sections 1.4 and 1.5 of the Codes, immediately preceding the above sections, indicate that if the custody officer is suspicious or is informed in good faith that either apply, then the detainee shall be treated as though the category did apply.

The responsibility to call an appropriate adult lies with the custody officer. The clinician should make it clear, however, to the custody officer whenever he or she believes an appropriate adult should be involved. It may be all too easy for a busy custody officer to assume that when a detainee has been passed fit for interview by a police surgeon, significant mental disorder does not exist, unless the doctor has so indicated.

The research by Nemitz & Bean (1994) appears to indicate that this reliance on the police surgeon is an active if informal reality. The clinician should certainly express an opinion one way or another, any doubt tending towards a recommendation for the involvement of the appropriate adult.

The responsibilities of an appropriate adult are laid down in the PACE Codes in C paragraph 11.16 where it is clearly stated that the appropriate adult is not just an observer but should also advise the person being questioned, observe whether or not the interview is being conducted properly and fairly, and facilitate communication with the person being interviewed. In the case of a juvenile the parent can act as the appropriate adult.

ANNEX C

Annex C of the PACE Codes C is designed to avoid delay in gaining necessary information which otherwise is "... likely (a) to lead to interference with or harm to evidence connected with an offence or interference with or physical harm to other people..." This annex allows vulnerable subjects to undergo urgent interviews, overriding the safeguards designed to protect them. The urgent interview must end as soon as the information which will avert the risk mentioned above is available.

The police surgeon should be aware of Annex C, as clinical assessment for fitness to be interviewed may be requested after the urgent interview has taken place.

References

Bannister R 1985 *Brain's Clinical Neurology* 6th Ed. Oxford Medical Publications, Oxford, p281.

Brahams D 1992 R v Salim and Saha. *Lancet* **340**:1462.

Brazier M 1992 *Medicine Patients and the Law*. Penguin, p341.

Brismar B, Engstràm A, Rydberg U 1983 Head Injury and Intoxication: A Diagnostic and Therapeutic Dilemma. *Acta Chir Scand* **149**:11-14.

British National Formulary 1995 30th Ed. British Medical Association and the Royal Pharmaceutical Society. BMA, London.

Clarke MDB 1991 Fit for Interview? *The Police Surgeon* **40**:18.

Commission on the Provision of Surgical Services, *Report of the Working Party on Head Injuries* 1986 Royal College of Surgeons of England, London.

Gastaut H 1995 for World Health Organization quoted in Scambler G 1989 *Epilepsy* London, Routledge.

Glaus RA 1975 Suggestibility in young drug dependent and normal populations. *British Journal of Addiction* **70**: 287-293.

Gudjonsson GH 1992 *The Psychology of Interrogations, Confessions and Testimony*. Wiley, Chichester: p25-27.

Gudjonsson GH 1995 Fitness for interview during police detention: a conceptual framework for the forensic assessment. *The Journal of Forensic Psychiatry* **6**: 185-197.

Gudjonsson GH, Clare I, Rutter S 1994 Psychological characteristics of suspects interviewed at police stations: a factor-analytic study. *Journal of Forensic Psychiatry* **3**: 517-525.

Home Office Circular 1950 HO17/50.

Isselbacher KJ *et al* 1994 *Harrison's Principles of Internal Medicine* 13th Ed. McGraw Hill, New York.

McLaren RE, Ghoorahoo HI, Kirby NG 1993 Skull X-Ray recommendations of the Royal College of Surgeons Working Party in practice. *Archives of Emergency Medicine* **10**: 138-144.

Nemitz T, Bean P 1994 The Use of the "Appropriate Adult" Scheme (A Preliminary Report). *Medicine Science and the Law* **2**: 161-166.

Payne-James JJ, Keys DW, Dean PJ 1994 Prevalence of HIV risk factors for individuals examined in clinical forensic medicine. *Journal of Clinical Forensic Medicine* **2**: 93-96.

Plum F, Posner JB 1982 *The Diagnosis of Stupor and Coma* 3rd Ed. F.A Davis, Philadelphia, p2.

Porter RJ 1984 *Epilepsy 100 Elementary Principles* Vol 12 Major Problems in Neurology Saunders, London: p14-41.

Rix KJB, Rix EL 1983 *Alcohol Problems, A Guide for Nurses and other Health Professionals*. Wright, Bristol: p65.

Robertson G, Gibb R, Pearson R 1995 Drunkenness among police detainees. *Addiction* **6**:793-803.

Robinson SP 1996 *Principles of Forensic Medicine* Greenwich Medical Media, London.

Rogers DJ, Stark MM, Howitt JB 1995 The Use of an Alcometer in Clinical Forensic Practice. Presentation at 44th Annual Conference of Association of Police Surgeons.

Sigurdsson J, Gudjonsson GH 1994 Alcohol and drug intoxication during police interrogation and the reasons why suspects confess to the police. *Addiction:* Nordic Journal of Psychiatry **94**: 915-917.

Woodhead M 1993 *Thorax* **48** Supplement S22 BMJ Publishing Group London.

7

CHILDREN

R Roberts

Child abuse is common and has been so throughout history. It has frequently gone unrecognised, but increasing awareness of its incidence has sometimes led to overdiagnosis, perhaps contributed to by a lack of understanding of forensic principles. It cannot be emphasised enough that a detailed understanding of the different types of injury and their causation, the natural history of healing and changes in appearance, as well as knowledge of precise definitions in law are essential. It is important to maintain objectivity with regard to the pattern and possible causation of injuries while caring for the child and its family with skill and compassion.

Children who are non-accidentally injured are commonly taken to hospital and may be admitted, when a full investigation of the child's background and past history, together with a full and careful physical, social and psychological assessment is made. In addition, the blood is screened for clotting defects and a full skeletal survey may be performed.

The forensic physician may be asked by police, social workers or paediatricians to examine a child where non-accidental injury is suspected. In these cases the injuries are often relatively minor, yet assessing their significance accurately, although vital for the further well-being of the child, can be much more difficult than evaluating gross injuries. It is a tragedy when the significance of a minor injury is not appreciated and the child is left at risk only to be maimed or killed later. It is no less true that the trauma and damage to the child and his family of a wrong diagnosis of abuse may be catastrophic.

NON-ACCIDENTAL INJURY [1]

The risk factors for non-accidental injury, including unwanted pregnancy, social isolation, scapegoating of a sometimes handicapped child, drug and alcohol

---

1. With only a few changes, this section has been reprinted from the first edition of *Clinical Forensic Medicine* with the permission of the author, Dr James Hilton.

abuse, are well known, as are the pointers which should raise suspicion, namely

a) Is the history consistent with the injury? A careful look must be taken into the mechanism of the injury and a commonsense judgement made on the credibility of the explanation given. In this respect, the development of the child must be considered – would it be capable of the actions or movements described?

b) Multiple injuries of differing ages: bruises of different colour are unlikely to have been caused at the same time from the same accident.

c) Discrepancies in varying and changing explanations: it is quite common for the story to be changed if the abuser thinks that the original one is doubted.

d) Delay in reporting, sometimes of hours and sometimes of days: a concerned parent is more likely to seek medical advice soon after any accident.

e) The parents may seek help from different outlets or become afraid and withdraw.

f) Denial and collusion: the denial is invariably strong and is supported by both partners; the abused child becomes part of the conspiracy and only rarely implicates the parents.

Diagnosis

The behaviour of the child may be significant: whether he shows fear of one parent or the other, or is unwilling to make eye contact (eye avoidance). He may cringe with a wary and hunted look, the so called look of frozen awareness. This is not always present, but is striking evidence of chronic abuse when seen. Excessive compliance during the examination is also a clue; an abused child may seek comfort and affection from comparative strangers.

A diagnosis of child abuse should not rest on evidence of injury alone, nor should unilateral decisions be made, particularly when it comes to decisions on returning a child home. The results of all strands of the investigation are best co-ordinated through the case conference.

Types of injury [2]

It is important to strip search the whole body in every case; marks may be hidden by long sleeves and high necked jumpers. It is also helpful to view the whole picture rather than concentrate on individual injuries: for example, bruising on more than one side or plane of the body is significant. Bruising is also important because frequently it precedes more serious injury. The examination should include the inside of the mouth and lips, behind the ears, the palms and soles and in between

2. Most illustrations in this section were drawn by Ms D Lytton from photographs.

fingers and toes. The object causing the injury – bruise or abrasion – may leave the pattern of its shape.

a) *Spot Bruises*. Caused by harsh finger tip pressure, 0.5-2.5 cm in size, there may be clusters corresponding to the fingers of the grasping hand. Look for the thumb-print on the opposite side of the arms (fig.1) or commonly, if the child is shaken, there will be finger bruises on the trunk in front and thumb marks on the back and vice versa.

b) *Slap Marks*. Found often on the face, where they may involve the ear (look behind, at the drum, and at the other ear) and on the trunk and buttocks. There may be clear lines of petechial haemorrhages (fig. 2).

c) *Knuckle Punches*. These show as rows of three or four roughly round bruises, a favoured site being on the back and particularly over the spine (fig. 3). Where the skin covers bone, a rounded swelling will also be present, for example on the side of the head or over the facial bones.

d) *Instruments*. Bruising from the use of belts, straps, canes, pieces of wood, hair brushes and electric flex (which wraps around limbs) will all leave recognizable marks (fig.4). These are frequently to be seen on the buttocks and thighs, and may involve the genital area. Look for grip marks on the arms where the child has been held roughly, and also for defence injuries on the hands and arms.

e) *Bite marks*. Human bite marks are distinctive, crescent shaped lines of discoloration. A bite made by a child has a narrow arch and is smaller than one made by an adult, which often involves teeth behind the canines (fig.5). Animal bites are characterised by puncturing and tearing of the tissues, unlike the human whose bite compresses, so causing the distinctive bruises (see also chapter 15).

f) *Pinch Marks*. These may form a butterfly-shaped bruise with one wing (caused by the thumb) larger than the other (fig. 6). If near the lip, the under-surface of the nose may be scraped by the finger nail, or the frenulum torn.

Some bruises are in themselves highly suggestive of abuse. These include black eye (fig. 7), bruised ears, bruising on the inner side of the thighs, bruised face in babies under 18 months of age and central spinal bruising. Other significant injuries to note include:

a) torn frenulum in babies commonly caused by roughly forcing a bottle into the mouth or bruised lips and displaced teeth with bleeding gums;

b) friction burns of prominent areas such as the chin and cheeks from dragging over carpets and furniture;

c) hair pulling leaving bald patches;

d) marks around the mouth and face indicative of gagging;

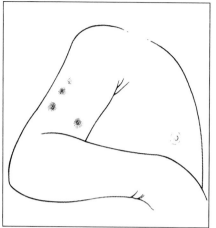

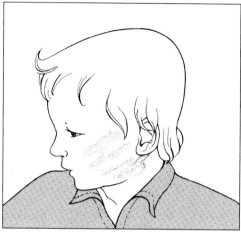

Figure 1 – Grip marks on right arm caused by squeezing with an adult right hand which has encircled the limb from its inner aspect

Figure 2 – Slap marks on the side of the face: an outline of individual fingers is often seen.

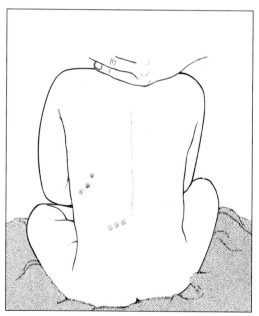

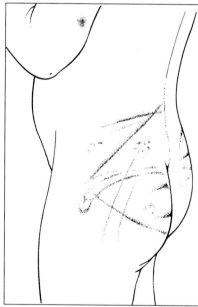

Figure 3 – Rows of bruises left by knuckles

Figure 4 – Typical site of weals and bruises caused by canes, belts and other instruments. The loop of a doubled, flexible instrument such as a dog lead may leave rounded impressions, as seen here on the upper thigh.

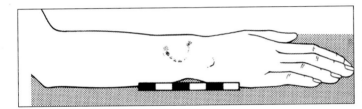

Figure 5 – Pattern of bruises caused by biting.

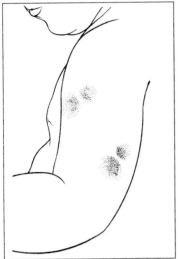

Figure 6 – Pinch marks (see text).

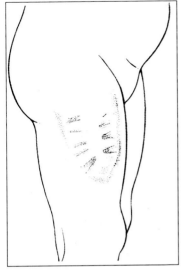

Figure 8 – Burns from an iron applied to the thigh.

Figure 7 – Black eye (a much more graphic description than 'periorbital haematoma').

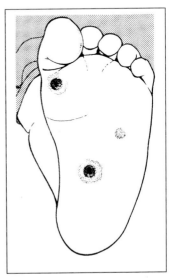

Figure 9 – Cigarette burns on the sole (see text).

e) encircling marks on the wrists and ankles where the child has been tied up, perhaps to a chair;

f) pinch or ligature marks round the penis and scrotum.

Burns and scalds

Approximately 10% of abuse involves burning, but it can be very difficult to show that some burns were inflicted deliberately. The heat source will leave an unmistakable pattern on the skin, for example the outline of a flat-iron (fig. 8). The degree of heat generation must be considered; the depth of the burn may indicate how long the contact must have been maintained to produce the marks. The burn may be in an accessible position, and the ability of the child to draw away from the heat source is another important factor. Other abuse injuries may be present.

Cigarette burns give a round, punched out lesion of the expected size when applied at right angles to the skin (fig.9). Such injuries are caused when a lighted cigarette is held deliberately against the skin for at least a few seconds, not when the child accidentally brushes against the cigarette, nor when the cigarette is dropped accidentally on the child. Cigar and match stick burns may also occur. They are often full thickness, and leave characteristic scars. Frequently found on the arms and legs, they may be seen in other situations such as the genital area or even between the toes. Dipping into hot water is seen especially on the hands when a 'tide' mark may be apparent, or a 'stocking' distribution from dipping the feet. Areas of scalding round the upper thighs with clear, unaffected areas on the buttocks arise when the child is forcibly sat in hot liquid (see fig. 10).

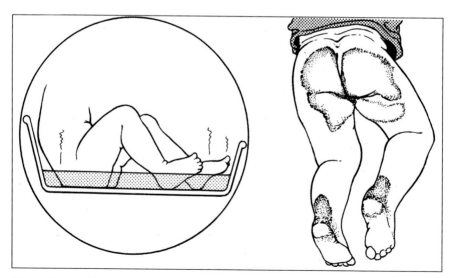

Figure 10 – Scalding

Bone and joint injuries

Injury to the skeleton may result from a severe fierce outburst or may indicate increased violence to the child. Not all fractures are apparent on clinical examination, and some small children can have quite serious bone injuries without showing much external sign. This is notably so in skull and rib fractures, and also in long bone fractures in small babies. A skeletal survey is essential in every case and may reveal old healing fractures in the seemingly straightforward case. Fracture of the ribs in infants rarely, if ever, occurs accidentally whereas, over the age of five years, abuse fractures are uncommon.

A closely detailed history of the incident should be taken, and the X-rays examined by a specialist. The mechanism of the fracture should be worked out in consultation with the radiologist or orthopaedic surgeon. The age of the fractures is estimated from the amount of callus already formed, although skull fractures pose difficulty, as they may appear fresh after some weeks.

Spiral fractures are of great significance – those in an infant under 18 months are almost certainly the result of abuse. If a small child's limb is twisted accidentally, as when the foot is caught in a rail and the child falls over, the straining force will injure the weakest point, the epiphyseal/metaphyseal junction. To inflict a spiral fracture, force has to be applied directly to the bone. Thus, a fracture of the humerus is likely to have been caused by twisting at the elbow.

Periosteal reaction is seen where violence to a long bone stops just short of causing a fracture. Bleeding under the periosteum provokes calcification, seen radiologically as an extra line of opacity running alongside the affected length of bone. Such injuries have been seen in legs twisted against forcibly flexed knees.

Epiphyseal and metaphyseal fractures are seen as a disruption of the normal outline, sometimes with angulation and displacement. Found most commonly at the upper end of the tibia and the lower ends of the tibia and fibula, they indicate violence to the foot and ankle, and are of particular significance in babies as yet unable to walk.

More serious injuries may be encountered, resulting in the child's admission to hospital. If the forensic physician is assisting the paediatrician, he will find that careful notes of all accompanying lesser injuries will be very important in any subsequent court proceedings. Brain damage may exist in the absence of signs of external injury of the scalp, even when the skull is fractured. Significant marks may, however, be found on the trunk where the baby was held. If the head is hit against a smooth flat surface such as a wall, no mark may be left on the scalp. Severe shaking of a baby causes his loose head to flop backwards and forwards, producing brain and retinal haemorrhages. Examination of the fundi of small chidren is difficult, so an ophthalmological opinion may be necessary. Permanent loss of vision in such cases is possible.

Visceral damage may be caused and, here again, it is necessary to use any visible external mark to help understand the mechanism of injury.

Mistaken diagnoses

Errors in diagnosis must distress parents innocent of any ill-treatment. Where an independent third party is present, abuse is unlikely. Bizarre mishaps can have serious repercussions yet remain accidental. All the available evidence must be examined, and a case conference convened to review the whole matter. For example, in cases of Munchausen's syndrome by proxy (where the perpetrator repeatedly inflicts injury, then seeks medical attention for the child) action to safeguard the child may only be possible after several supposedly accidental occurrences.

The following points should be kept in mind when examining any case of physical abuse:

a) Calcium deficiency, abnormalities in copper metabolism, rickets, scurvy, severe anaemia and haemophilia must all be excluded by appropriate investigation.

b) Disorders of bone formation and 'brittle bones', although rare, must also be excluded routinely and a skeletal survey performed.

c) Pigment anomalies, Mongolian spots, birth marks and skin disorders must be identified and dealt with accordingly.

d) Blood extravasation seeping down tissue planes from lesser injury can simulate widespread bruising. An injury to the forehead may cause blood to appear in the upper eyelids or inner corners of the eye, so simulating direct injury to the eye.

e) Alopecia areata can be mistaken for hair pulling.

f) Lesions of impetigo, chickenpox and, more rarely, shingles or chilblains may be mistaken for cigarette burns. Unfortunately for the child, the reverse may also happen.

g) Burns involving contact with hot radiators and other heaters need careful investigation as accidental contact is not uncommon.

h) Accidental scalds from tipping pans or kettles usually produce secondary splashes in addition to the main injury.

i) In scalds received in the bath, clear areas on the soles of the feet could confirm that the child was standing up and turned the taps on himself.

j) Some fractures are more likely to be accidental: for instance, an impacted fracture of the upper end of the humerus is consistent with a fall on the point of the elbow.

k) The possibility of self-inflicted injuries in older children should be borne in mind.

l) In adolescents, striae running across the lumbar region have been mistaken for marks of beating (Davies 1985).

In all but a few incidents, careful consideration of the history, thorough and competent examination and the application of good forensic principles and practice when allied to a growing experience, will allow a firm opinion to be arrived at. If doubt remains, close supervision by the domiciliary team of general practitioner, health visitor and social workers should ensure the protection of the child and the early detection of any future incidents.

CHILD SEXUAL ABUSE

Child sexual abuse (CSA) is a difficult area where great skill and understanding are required. Examinations and assessments should only be carried out by doctors who have had in-depth training in this field and who continue their professional development in it, keeping abreast of world literature and attending lectures and training seminars. Where such experience is lacking, joint examinations, photographic or video recorded evidence, video conferencing and peer review may assist in obtaining the best evidence for court and avoid the need for repeated examinations of children.

Doctors asked to examine children who may have been abused are part of a multi-disciplinary team which must work together in the best interests of the child, respecting each other's skills and being open and honest in sharing concerns (Department of Health 1995). In many cases a full paediatric assessment is necessary, with a consultant paediatrician being part of the initial investigating team and having responsibility for continuing care for the child. The forensic medical officer's role is primarily, but not exclusively, to provide evidence for court proceedings but this must always be combined with a concern for the welfare of the child.

Medical evidence may be only a very small part of the picture and doctors must accept this. In some cases the doctor will be very much less important than the social worker, the clinical psychologist, the child's parents or even a neighbour; often what the doctor says will be of less significance than what the child has said.

Timing of the examination

Whereas child physical abuse usually presents as a medical emergency, CSA usually does not, the offences having occurred some time previously and only come to light later. Where there has been a recent sexual assault, for example a child abducted and raped by a stranger, the matter is one of extreme urgency and the examination must be conducted at the earliest possible moment to preserve forensic evidence, and to document injuries many of which may heal without trace. In many other cases, however, while there is no medical or forensic urgency, the child and his family are in a situation of great stress which may be alleviated to some extent by the calm professional approach of the doctor and by having the examination over and done with. Legal rules may impose time constraints if a suspect is in police custody. It may also be very important for the investigating officers to have information obtained in the medical examination before they interview a suspect. In other cases the examination can be scheduled for a time convenient to all concerned, particularly the child and his family.

Confidentiality

Sharing information with non-medical colleagues raises issues of confidentiality. The General Medical Council's advice[3] is that where a doctor believes that a patient may be the victim of abuse or neglect the patient's best medical interests will usually require the doctor to disclose information to an appropriate responsible person or statutory agency "in order to prevent further harm to the patient". This may be done "without the patient's consent, but only if you consider that the patient is unable to give consent ...".

Doctors who have examined children should attend case conferences or provide a report wherever possible. This may raise difficulties when the parents are present and doctors are reluctant to share their information. It may be appropriate to seek advice from one's defence organisation before attending and to discuss concerns beforehand with whoever chairs the conference.

Consent to examination

Consent is covered in detail in chapter 3, but there are special considerations with regard to juveniles. Although it is not always necessary in law, the consent of the child, as well as the parent, should be obtained. A young child may not be able to give truly informed consent to an investigation of this nature, with all its possible consequences such as disruption of the family or imprisonment of the perpetrator, but the child must agree to be examined and no child should be forcibly examined. The only exception would be a crying toddler who might be held firmly on the mother's knee during a genital inspection.

Consent to examination is normally given by the person having parental responsibility under the terms of the Children Act 1989, usually the parent (see also page 137 for the position in Scotland). For a child in the care of the local authority this responsibility rests with the authority and consent is given by the

---

3. GMC booklet on Confidentiality 1995 §11.

social worker. It is rare now for a child to be a Ward of Court but no Ward of Court may be examined without leave of the Court; under the Children Act there may be a Prohibited Steps Order forbidding a medical examination.

A child may disclose sexual abuse by a parent and wish to be examined without parental consent. Usually the local authority seeks an Emergency Protection Order which confers on it the power to give consent for examination, but exceptionally the examination may need to be conducted before this step can be taken. In such circumstances the doctor should consider very carefully, using the criteria established in *Gillick v West Norfolk and Wisbech Area Health Authority and ano.* (1986) AC 112; [1986] 1WLR 224, whether the child is of sufficient age and understanding to consent to what is proposed, consulting with the police officers and social workers involved and documenting very carefully and fully the factors which have been taken into account in reaching a decision. The doctor must establish clearly before conducting any examination who is able to give valid consent.

Refusal to be examined

A teenage girl sometimes refuses to be examined for reasons of embarrassment, or because she is all too aware of the consequences for the family of what may be found. Having considered all the circumstances, especially that the child is in a safe environment and protected from further abuse, the doctor may deem it better not to persist in attempts to carry out the examination.

When a child is apprehensive, refusing to be examined, she must not be forced: she may agree to a limited examination. Ask her permission to do no more than look. If you promise not to go further you must stick by that promise.

Sometimes it is right to defer the examination, and carry it out successfully at another time. For example, it is unkind to press a girl who is menstruating unless the matter is urgent.

Obtaining information

The doctor should obtain details of the alleged offence from the police officer and social worker and make full notes, ideally on a special proforma which includes body charts on which to record the findings, but the format of notes varies across the country.

Where a child is seen in hospital the forensic examiner should also make notes in the hospital file, signing and dating them and adding a contact telephone number. Where notes are made both in the doctor's own notes and the hospital records it is imperative that both accounts should contain the same information, though not necessarily in identical form, bearing in mind that in the event of court proceedings, hospital records as well as forensic notes may be disclosed to the defence; minor discrepancies, omissions or inaccuracies can be used to discredit the doctor's evidence.

The child should not be interviewed in depth about the allegations because of the strict rules about the way such interviews are conducted, set down in the Memorandum of Good Practice on Video Recorded Interviews with Child Witnesses in Criminal Proceedings (Home Office 1992) but the doctor should have some knowledge of how a child who may have been sexually abused is interviewed. This is clearly and succinctly described by Jones (1992).

In England and Wales, interviewing must be conducted by trained police officers and social workers, and is normally video recorded. If it came to the notice of a court that the child had been questioned in detail by the doctor, it is possible that the child's evidence would be regarded as contaminated and might be inadmissible.

In most cases, therefore, it is appropriate not to question the child at all about the allegations. If questions are asked they must not be leading, that is to say suggesting the answer, but must be non-directional. The questions put, as well as the answers received, should be recorded in the notes; for example it is acceptable to say to a child, "Oh this looks sore, do you know what made it sore?" but not to ask, "Did your uncle rub you with his penis and make it sore?"

Sometimes children are seen with an allegedly accidental genital injury, but where medical personnel, perhaps in the A&E department, consider that abuse is a possibility. In this type of case a proper history of the allegation should be taken from the carers and also from the child. If the child is able to give a clear and detailed account of an accidental injury which is consistent with the findings, then the matter may be resolved at an early stage, perhaps without police or social services involvement.

Introduction to the child

After introducing yourself by name to the child and accompanying persons and explaining who you are and why you have been called in, obtain consent, ideally but not essentially written, to examination and to disclosure of reports.

Explain what is to happen, invite the co-operation of the child, allow older children to decide who will also be in the medical room, if anyone, and give reassurance that the child will be able to know what is going on and will be able to ask the doctor to stop if he or she is becoming distressed.

A general medical and social history should be taken from the child and accompanying carer, with particular note being made of any medical condition which may cause abnormalities which might be confused with signs of abuse. A careful bowel history is essential if there is any question of anal abuse. Behavioural problems are common in abused children with changes in behaviour such as recent onset of a tendency to cling, not wanting to be with a particular adult, bedwetting or soiling being particularly important. In older girls the menstrual history should be recorded, noting whether tampons are used for menstrual hygiene.

The medical examination

The medical examination must be tailored to the individual case and carried out with the greatest care and sensitivity. A child who has been indecently touched by a family member, but not physically hurt, should never be subjected to an intrusive medical examination which may well be perceived by the child as more abusive and traumatic than the alleged offences. At the same time, an examination which fails to reveal evidence which is present is also detrimental to the welfare of the child.

It is a matter for the individual doctor to assess, on the facts of the case, what procedures should be carried out, remembering that actions may have to be justified in court under cross-examination. Where there has been a recent or serious sexual assault the procedures and techniques described in chapter 11 may be more appropriate, taking into account differences between the adults considered there and children.

The examination should be taken at the child's pace and not rushed. The doctor should talk to the child throughout. Weighing and measuring helps the child to settle down and to perceive the examination as an ordinary encounter with a doctor. The findings should be checked on the Tanner growth charts[4] and the percentiles recorded. Failure to thrive and dips in the normal growth pattern are commonly associated with abuse of all types.

A full general examination should then be done looking for classic signs of abuse such as a torn frenulum of the upper lip, bruises of different ages and bite marks as described in the first section of this chapter. Injuries thought to be bite marks should be photographed, and the advice of a forensic odontologist sought.

The genital examination in girls

(see figure 11 – external features)

In a small child, particularly when only a careful visual inspection is to be carried out, it is often appropriate to do this with the child sitting on the mother's knee, the mother gently holding the child's legs apart, or with the child lying prone over the mother's knee and the doctor examining from behind.

---

4. Obtainable from Castlemead Publications, Welwyn Garden City, UK.

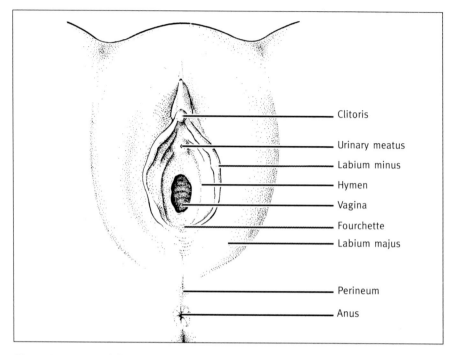

- Clitoris
- Urinary meatus
- Labium minus
- Hymen
- Vagina
- Fourchette
- Labium majus
- Perineum
- Anus

Figure 11 – General features of external genitalia in the female child

In older children the usual technique is for the child to be examined lying supine on the medical couch with her knees flexed and separated - the frog position. With the child in this position, the labia may be gently separated by the examiner's fingers (labial separation) or traction exerted in a forward and downward position on the labia majora by the examiner gently grasping the labia between thumb and forefinger (labial traction).

The genital area can also be examined thoroughly with the child in the knee–chest position, that is crouched on the examination couch with the small of the back arched downwards, knees flexed under the chest and bottom in the air. In this position the important posterior edge of the hymen can often be seen more clearly than when the child is lying supine on the couch, so rendering unnecessary the use of a Glaister's globe (see below) or moistened swab.

Ideally each child should be examined both in the frog position and the knee–chest position, but children should be offered the choice. Some examiners used to consider that the knee-chest position was possibly abusive in itself, but many children prefer to be examined in this position because they then do not have to look at the examiner or see what he or she is doing.

A magnifying light, optical loupes, or a colposcope with a standard measuring device and camera enable a thorough examination to be done, and make possible a permanent record of the findings. The vulval structures, labia majora, labia minora, clitoris, urethra and posterior fourchette (Fig. 11) should all be carefully inspected for bruises, scratches, or petechiae in recent cases and scars in late cases.

In many children, when the genitalia are examined in different positions, the edge of the hymen will have been clearly visualised without the need for any kind of intrusive examination, but in some cases it is helpful to use a probe – a Glaister's globe. These are glass or plastic rods with a diameter of 0.6 cm, having a globe at one end varying in size from 1 to 2.5 cm. They can be gently inserted behind the hymen so as to display its edges over the glass. In this way apparent folds and indentations often smooth out and small clefts and tears can be more easily identified. Glass rods used in this way, with explanation and demonstration to the child, are much less traumatic than using moistened cotton wool swabs which often cause pain in a very delicate area. It is important to spend some time inspecting the hymen before coming to any conclusion about it and to record the apparent size of its orifice in the antero-posterior and lateral diameters when first seen, with labial separation and traction if used. Diameters are usually larger when the child is in the knee/chest position.

If swabs have to be taken for forensic purposes or to carry out tests for sexually transmitted diseases, it is helpful to show the child an unused swab, in some cases to allow the child to use the swab herself and keep control, and certainly to be allowed to halt the proceedings if distressed.

In most cases where indecent acts are alleged it is not necessary, after the above procedures, to insert any object into the vagina. Where there is an allegation of full sexual intercourse or findings such as a completely torn hymen have been visualised, it is appropriate to carry out a gentle digital examination of the vagina to establish whether the hymenal ring is completely disrupted; whether the vagina can admit an object the size of an erect penis, and whether its walls are small and rugose as in the virginal state or smoothed and enlarged indicating that sexual intercourse or penetration by a penis-sized object has occurred on more than a very few occasions (Mant 1984). Where the vagina has been fully penetrated by a penis-sized object, the feeling of the introitus is characteristic: the finger can be pressed against the lateral wall of the pelvis without meeting resistance. Where this has not occurred, the hymenal ring can be felt against the finger.

In older girls, it may be appropriate to carry out a full gynaecological examination, including the insertion of a speculum to inspect the cervix, and a bimanual examination to check for signs of pregnancy; a pregnancy test may also be indicated.

The genital examination in boys

Genital injury in boys who have been indecently assaulted is rare, but the penis and testicles should be carefully inspected for signs of bruising, tears of the frenulum and "love bites" or signs of sucking. It is important to bear in mind that the child's penis may have been sucked and that saliva may persist on the skin for up to a week. Swabs moistened with sterile water should therefore be taken from the shaft of the penis and under the foreskin around the frenulum.

The anal area

The anus should be inspected in every case, with the child in the left lateral position or in the knee–chest position. The position used in the examination should be noted.

The buttocks should be gently separated without using traction and the anal orifice observed for about 30 seconds to see if it dilates. Slight twitchiness or dilatation of the external sphincter is probably of no significance, and anal dilatation in the presence of stool in the rectum is regarded by most experienced examiners as unlikely to be a sign of abuse. The size of the dilatation in milli metres should be recorded, making a note whether it is present initially on separating the buttocks and whether it is repeated. If stool is present re-examination after the bowels have been moved is essential.

The anal folds should be regular and symmetrical around the anal opening but there is often a redundant anterior fold, particularly in boys, which can be confused with a skin tag or healed fissure. A midline raphe extending backwards from the scrotum is normal and should not be confused with signs of injury.

Prominent veins are sometimes claimed (Hobbs *et al* 1993) as significant pointers to abuse. However, they often come up during the examination as the child tenses and relaxes his muscles and were noted in 52% of apparently unabused children after 2 minutes in the knee-chest position (McCann *et al* 1990b). Venous congestion has been confused with bruising which is commonly present shortly after buggery but which persists for a few days only.

If no abnormality is seen on careful inspection of the anus it is appropriate to do no more. However, if there is an allegation of anal abuse, a finger should gently be placed against the anal orifice to test its tone. A very good estimate of anal tone can be obtained in this way without a full digital examination, but in a few cases a digital examination should be done, the subject being asked to squeeze the examining finger to test the anal tone. It is important to remember, however, that this procedure relies on a subjective assessment by the examiner based on experience and may be unreliable.

Sexually transmitted diseases

In many cases, tests for sexually transmitted diseases are not done. Where the allegation is of indecent touching and a careful and thorough visual inspection has found no sign of injury or inflammation, the examination becomes much more intrusive if such tests are done and the likelihood in such cases of finding an infection is low (Estreich & Forster 1992). Siegel *et al* (1995) confirmed the low incidence in pre-pubertal girls (8 of 249 girls had a discharge) but concluded that girls of Tanner stage 3 had a sufficiently high incidence of asymptomatic infection to be tested as a routine; they also required follow-up for papilloma virus. If the child can easily tolerate the procedures, if there are any genital symptoms, or the parents or child are particularly worried, tests may be taken either by the forensic examiner or the paediatrician after any forensic tests have been obtained. Any samples for sexually transmitted diseases should be correctly gathered, the swabs placed in appropriate transport media and sent to the hospital laboratory. Small wire per-nasal swabs are are sometimes better tolerated. If ano-genital warts are seen the advice of a virologist should be sought on whether typing should be done and contacts examined.

Occasionally a parent will ask to have the child tested for HIV. It is not appropriate for the forensic medical examiner to do this, but the parents might be referred for appropriate counselling.

Reassurance

Finally, after the examination, and with the child dressed, the doctor should take some time to talk to both child and parent about the examination and its results. The sexually abused child often believes that serious physical damage has been done, even when no penetration has occurred, and the doctor can assist greatly in the process of recovery by assuring the child that all is well. Even where minor abnormalities have been found, it is possible to give strong reassurance that in a short time everything will be back to normal and nothing which may have happened will affect whether the child can grow up to marry and have babies if that is what she wants. Boys also need reassurance that they have not been permanently damaged.

It is important to emphasise and reinforce what other professionals will have said to the child: that whatever has happened is not the child's fault. A few minutes spent on this task at the end of the examination is of enormous benefit to both the child and the family.

A careful and thorough medical examination carried out with skill and sensitivity in the way described has a direct and important therapeutic effect, helping to begin the process of recovery and to minimise the long-term consequences of abuse.

Significant findings

Before describing findings and the conclusions to be drawn from them, it is worthwhile setting out a few general considerations.

Most published work (see, for example, the review by Bays & Chadwick 1993) confirms that no medical evidence will be found in around 70% of children where sexual abuse is alleged, for two reasons: (a) that the intention has not been to hurt the child physically, and (b) the offences may have occurred some time earlier.

Slight injuries heal in days. Bruises, splits and abrasions usually leave no sign. The fourchette is only likely to scar if there has been repeated slight splitting.

A prepubertal child may make an honest mistake and genuinely believe that full sexual intercourse has occurred if a penis has been pushed against the vulval tissues. The prepubertal child experiences pain in these tissues if they are touched, as they are both delicate and sensitive.

It is important that a doctor preparing a report for court make these points, because non-medical people tend to assume that there would certainly have been physical signs had the allegation been true.

It is difficult to differentiate the normal from the abnormal. Research (for example, McCann *et al* 1990 a and b), particularly in the United States, has demonstrated much greater variations in the normal than was previously believed. For instance, the view put forward in the 1980s that 0.4 cm was the upper limit of normal of the hymenal orifice in a non-abused child has been shown by careful study of apparently unabused children to be incorrect; a rough working guide to this diameter would be 1mm per year of age.

Excessive claims are made for the value of medical evidence. Doctors must guard against trying to fit the evidence to the case. This type of behaviour has all too frequently led to medical evidence being discredited in court. It can, however, be difficult to say to the investigating police officer and social worker that one cannot find any medical evidence. The doctor may feel that he or she is letting the child down, but it is very much worse for the child and does not assist the cause of justice if the medical evidence is later discredited.

A great many articles are being published at the present time on the medical findings in child sexual abuse. Many of them are anecdotal and of dubious scientific worth, there being no control studies or statistical analysis. Minute variations in genital anatomy, the incidence of which in the unabused population has not been established, are sometimes used to support a diagnosis which may have been reached on equally shaky evidence from other sources. These articles are often quoted in court, and it is imperative for any doctor giving evidence to have read the original articles very critically.

In turning to the medical examination, the questions to be answered are:

- If you saw these findings in a child where there was no allegation or suspicion of abuse, would you consider abuse to be a likely cause?

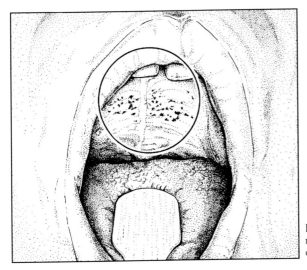

Figure 12 — Petechiae on roof of mouth following oral intercourse

- Do these findings occur commonly in unabused children?
- What is the mechanism of causation if the findings are due to abuse?

General injuries

These are unusual except in cases of stranger rape, but bruises, particularly on the lower face or grip marks on the arms and legs or over the pelvis may be seen. Inside the mouth a torn frenulum, bruising inside the cheeks where the face has been gripped or patchy petechial haemorrhages on the roof of the mouth caused by forceful insertion of a penis may be observed (fig. 12). Such petechiae occur in only a small proportion of cases (10% of the author's cases seen within 48 hours of the alleged offence) and persist for a day or two only. They can also occur in upper respiratory infections and be caused by sucking hard sweets. "Love bites" caused by sucking and tongue pressure are occasionally seen, but are unusual in children. Care should be taken not to misinterpret signs caused by friction from clothing or skin abnormalities as evidence of abuse.

The vulval area

Any patchy or general redness of the genitalia caused by rubbing and fondling is unlikely to persist for more than a few hours, but if very vigorous rubbing has occurred swelling and some bruising may persist for a few days. The skin over the clitoris may be reddened and swollen, but the clitoris itself does not enlarge as a result of fingering or masturbation. In some children the clitoris is naturally very large.

Intercrural intercourse or vulvar coitus usually leaves no clinical sign, though there may be redness or, less commonly, slight splits of the posterior

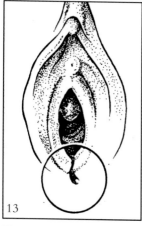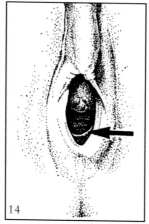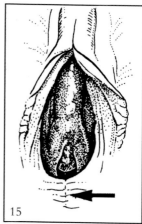

Figure 13 – Bleeding at the fourchette

Figure 14 – Prominent vestibule — the edge of the hymen (arrowed) is obscured by labial tissue

Figure 15 – Atrophic vuvlitis with adhesion (arrowed)

fourchette (fig. 13); occasionally petechiae may be seen around the urethra. With repeated injury the posterior fourchette may develop an irregular thickened scar which must be carefully distinguished from a normal mid-line raphe.

Flattening and wrinkling of the labia majora has sometimes been ascribed to abuse but there is such individual variation that these signs should not be relied on. Tramline redness on the inner aspects of the labia majora is a non-specific finding common in abused and non-abused children.

In some children the vestibule inside the labia minora is prominent and some-times, with or without labial adhesions, may form a complete ellipse which has occasionally been mistaken for the hymenal orifice (fig. 14).

Labial adhesions are common; some are congenital and others are associated with atrophic vulvitis (fig. 15). It has been theorised that rubbing may cause superficial trauma to the edges of the labia, allowing them to stick together. They are not reliable as a sign of abuse but extensive adhesions in an older child might provide weak support for a clear account by the child. Many children have bands of tissue running across the periurethral and perihymenal area. These are normal and are not to be mistaken for adhesions.

It has been recognised in recent years, particularly as a result of examinations of large numbers of children not thought to have been abused, that there is much more variation in the character of the hymen than was previously thought (McCann *et al* 1990 a and b). Hymens may be crescentic, the commonest type, where the membrane appears deficient anteriorly, with notches or clefts at the 11 and 1 o'clock positions, towards the front of the child, which may be equal in size or more prominent on one side than the other (fig. 16). Care must be taken not to confuse such findings with hymenal tears. Annular hymens with a round or oval opening are less common; fimbriated, septate and cribriform hymens are even less common (fig. 17). An imperforate hymen is rare and no child has been described as having a congenitally absent hymen. In the newborn and up to the age of 3 or even 4 years the hymen is often fleshy and fimbriated. From then until the onset of puberty it is usually a thin, delicate, almost translucent, membrane with a width of tissue of at least 4mm at the posterior aspect, at the 6 o'clock position. During pubertal development the hymen changes dramatically and becomes thickened, often with a fimbriated or wavy edge. It can be extremely difficult, particularly in the child going through puberty, to distinguish natural fimbriation from tears, unless the tear extends the full width of the membrane.

A few years ago much emphasis was placed on the apparent size of the hymenal orifice, though no account appeared to have been taken of the variations in the same child from minute to minute nor the variations with position and examination technique. Four millimetres in the transverse diameter was said to be strongly correlated with sexual abuse, but the consensus is now that 1 mm per year of age is a more reasonable guide to this measurement, and that a finding in excess of 1 cm in a prepubertal child occurs more commonly in abused girls (Royal College of Physicians 1991[5]).

Much more attention is now paid to the width of the hymenal membrane at its midline attachment along the posterior rim of the introitus. Figure 18 shows

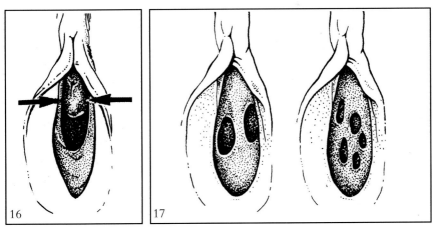

Figure 16 – Recesses on either side of the buttress (arrowed) are usually a develop-mental variation which disappears at puberty

Figure 17 – Congenital variations of the hymen include septate and cribiform types. Hymenal tissue is probably never absent at birth.

5. A new edition is in preparation.

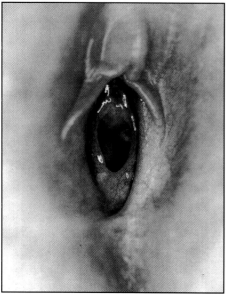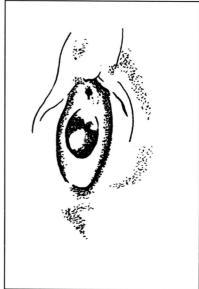

Figure 18 – An intact, broad crescentic hymen in a four year old

an intact, broad crescentic hymen in a four year old. Whatever the penetrating object (penis, finger or instrument) tears usually occur here because the hymen lies suspended across a potential space, whereas anteriorly the periurethral tissues buttress the hymen. Any object passing through the hymenal orifice, which is larger than its original opening, will cause a "V" shaped cleft or clefts. There may be one deep tear at the 6 o'clock position or a number of tears most commonly in the posterior half of the membrane. With healing, over a period of months, "V" shaped tears become rounded off to leave a "U" shaped defect (McCann 1993). In prepubertal children who have been penetrated by an adult penis, the posterior tear of the hymen may extend into the area of the fourchette, leaving a character-istic, deep "U" shaped defect (fig. 19), but other than this, it is impossible to tell in a girl who has gone through puberty whether any tears of the hymen have been caused before or after puberty. There is no reliable evidence that tears of the hymen sustained before puberty impair its natural development under the influence of oestrogens.

A study of hymenal findings (Kerns *et al* 1992) in over 1,000 girls showed that anterior concavities in the hymen did not change with age, indicating that they were congenital, whereas posterior and lateral concavities in the hymen and attenuation (a reduction in the width of hymenal tissue present between the attached and free border of the membrane) increased in frequency with age, consistent with features that are acquired. Tears in the anterior part of the hymen may have been caused by penetration, but it is unsafe to ascribe them to this cause

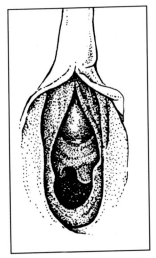 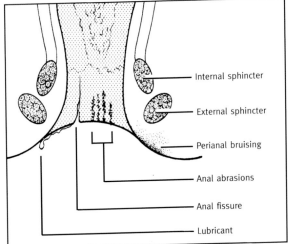

Figure 19 – Bumps on the edge of the hymen mark the origin of an old tear

Figure 20 – Cross section of anus and lower rectum: some of the possible signs in recent penetration

unless they are seen in the acute stage when they can be shown to be obviously traumatic.

Bays & Chadwick (1993) after reviewing 36 clinical studies and 19 other papers, proposed that a markedly enlarged hymenal opening for age with associated findings of hymen disruption including absent hymen, hymenal remnants, healed transections or scars in the absence of an adequate accidental or surgical explanation, would be diagnostic of sexual abuse, as would be the presence of spermatozoa or pregnancy. Positive tests for syphilis or gonorrhoea were regarded as strongly correlated but trichomonas, chlamydia and herpes slightly less so. There is still much uncertainty about the significance of ano-genital warts, only some of the many types of which are transmitted sexually. Vertical transmission from the mother during childbirth accounts for some cases but in many the origin is never established.

The anal area

In the anal area there is rarely any incontrovertible medical evidence unless the examination is conducted within hours or days of the alleged offence. An anus recently forcibly penetrated may be gaping open with one or more fresh fissures either in the mid-line or radiating out like the spokes of a wheel from the anal margin. The fissures may or may not be bleeding. Bruising and fissures may be seen inside the anal canal. Such lesions heal in days, usually leaving no sign though fissures may heal with the formation of a scar or skin tag. Smoothing and thickening of the anal skin, with loss of anal folds and reduction of anal sphincter tone, may occur with repeated penetration over long periods of time – months or years rather than weeks – but in many cases where such acts have occurred medical signs are absent. (See figs 20 and 21.)

Differential diagnosis

Accidental straddle injury is common (74 of 87 girls presenting with genital injury in the 1993 study by Pierce & Robson). There is usually a clear history of injury, the genital findings are usually of bruising which is anterior to the hymen, most often on one side in the fold between the clitoris and labia (fig. 22). Accidental trauma is a common cause of vulval or vaginal bleeding in children and 'splits' injuries may damage the posterior fourchette. Prolapse of the urethra is an unusual but not rare cause of vulval bleeding in girls of mixed race.

Findings often described as associated with sexual abuse may have other causes, including bacterial vaginosis, labial adhesions and posterior fourchette friability. Findings which are unlikely to be due to abuse include Candida albicans, dermatitis, small labial adhesions or more extensive labial adhesions in girls in nappies, erythema, periurethral bands, lymphoid follicles in the fossa navicularis, midline avascular areas in the fossa navicularis or posterior fourchette and urethral dilatation, small hymenal mounds, projections or septal remnants, concavities of the hymen that are anterior and intravaginal ridges and rugae behind a normal hymen.

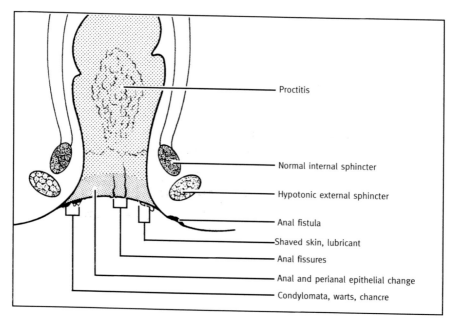

Figure 21 – Some signs of chronic anal abuse

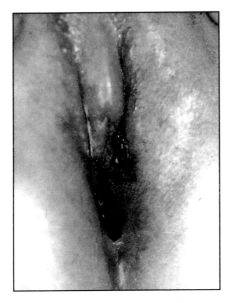
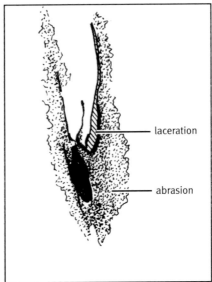

Figure 22 – There is a longitudinal laceration in the sulcus to the left of the prepuce of the clitoris

Vulvitis is common in childhood, usually caused by lack of hygiene and particularly by wiping the genital and anal areas from back to front. Non-specific vulvitis due to low oestrogen status is also common and there may be friability of the fourchette and labial adhesions.

Vulvitis may follow an episode of respiratory infection. Monilia may appear after the use of antibiotics; threadworms are a common cause of vulval irritation and vulvovaginitis; lichen sclerosus et atrophicus is rare, but has on a number of occasions been mistaken for sexual abuse. Foreign bodies in the vagina, although uncommon, should be remembered as a cause of a profuse green, perhaps blood-stained, vaginal discharge.

It is important to remember that a child suffering from any of these conditions might also have been the subject of sexual abuse.

THE CHILDREN ACT 1989

When this Act came into force in October 1991 it made radical changes to the law in England and Wales relating to children. There is emphasis on parental responsibility and on the rights of the child. The welfare of the child is considered to be paramount.

A number of new Orders were created which may concern the forensic medical examiner; these are:

The emergency protection order

This is a short-term order which enables a child to be made safe when he might otherwise suffer harm. Anyone may apply for an order but it is usually the local authority which does so. It lasts for eight days and may be extended for a further seven days. It transfers parental responsibility to the applicant. Its importance to the forensic clinician relates to consent for medical examination.

EMERGENCY PROTECTION ORDER (E.P.O.)	
Duration	8 days. Renewable once with good reason for 7 days
Applicant	Anyone
Apply to	Magistrates
Purpose	(a) Prevent significant harm (b) Investigate
Parental responsibility	Yes. (Limited to immediate matters)

Police protection order

A child may be taken into police protection under such an order; this does not transfer parental responsibility, though usually the local authority will take over the care of the child and decide whether an Emergency Protection Order should be sought.

POLICE PROTECTION ORDER (P.P.O.)	
Duration	72 hours. Not renewable
Applicant	Police officer. Has power without application to magistrates
Purpose	Prevent significant harm
Parental responsibility	No. Designated Officer takes case

Child assessment order

This assists the local authority with its investigative duty where there are concerns about a child. The court may direct what kind of assessment is to take place, but does not authorise an assessment or examination which the child itself refuses to undergo. It does not transfer parental responsibility to the local authority.

ASSESSMENT ORDER	
Duration	7 days or less. Not renewable
Applicant	Local Authority or NSPCC
Apply to	Magistrates
Parental Responsibility	No
Purpose	Non-urgent medical, social work or other investigation

Note: Parent may appeal against the application.
Court may grant E.P.O. instead, if it thinks this more appropriate

CHILD PROTECTION PROCEDURES IN SCOTLAND[6]

The Social Work (Scotland) Act 1968 brought a different perspective to working with children. Gone were juvenile courts: children who were themselves delinquent became subject to procedures no less applicable to children in need. Central to this system is the Reporter to the Children's Panel.

The reporter

Formerly appointed by the local authority, reporters now form part of a national service (Local Government etc (Scotland) Act 1994; Children (Scotland) Act 1995) headed by the Principal Reporter. The reporter's functions are part administrative, part investigative, part quasi-judicial. He acts as the central clearing agency, considering reports from the police, social workers, teachers, indeed anyone with an interest in the welfare of a child. To paraphrase the Social Work Act, anyone with a reasonable cause to believe that a child needs compulsory measures of care may give information to the reporter.

When considering reports on a child he must satisfy himself that he has grounds to refer the child to the children's hearing (see below) and that he could substantiate these grounds before a sheriff. He must also satisfy himself that the child concerned is in need of compulsory measures of supervision (whether remaining at home, with foster parents or in an institution) as set out in s52 of the Children (Scotland) Act. The section lists examples, some from other Acts, of conditions giving rise to the need for compulsory supervision; these include moral danger or criminal association, lack of parental control or care, commission of offences, misuse of drugs or alcohol. Supervision means protection, guidance, treatment or control of the child.

---

6. Contributed by WDS McLay.

If he cannot be satisfied on these two counts, he must either take no further action or refer the case to the local authority with a view to their making arrangements for advice, guidance and assistance. It must be emphasised that the reporter's view is not swayed by supposed criminality on the child's part: the sole criterion is the need of that child.

When conduct would have constituted an offence had the perpetrator been older, the police will report the case to the reporter rather than to the fiscal, unless the offence is a serious one or adults are accused of the same matter. In general, however, a child under 16 does not appear in court as an accused.

A child who has been abused is seen to be vulnerable. Both fiscal and reporter, then, have distinct functions, the former as prosecutor, the latter as protector, but they will consult together, bearing always in mind the best interests of the victim.

Children's hearings

In each local authority area lay people constituting a Panel receive training to fit them to take part in a hearing, most often as one of three, the sexes always being mixed. Efforts are made, too, to ensure that Panel members come from varied social backgrounds but, as in other largely voluntary fields, the older and more leisured must be available to participate to a greater degree.

Hearings are conducted in private, the child being accompanied by parents, unless there is a good reason (an obvious cause of absence exists when one parent is accused of abusing the child and has been remanded in custody). Proceedings involving children may not be disclosed in newspapers or elsewhere. The reporter intimates to the hearing the grounds on which he is referring the child. If these grounds are not accepted by the child and his parent the hearing must be adjourned forthwith (see below).

If the hearing proceeds, the aim is to secure the co-operation of the whole family for the better care of the child. Where a hearing concludes that compulsory measures of care are indicated, the options are supervision at home or removal from the home. When the Social Work (Scotland) Act first came into force high hopes were entertained, but the reality is that too few places are available whether in local authority or voluntary social work premises. There has been an expansion of fostering on a short-term basis.

Proof hearings

To reduce the seeming intimidation of proceedings, parents and children are not legally represented at a children's hearing, nor need the reporter and his deputes be legally qualified. Disputed grounds of referral are taken before a sheriff whose duty it is to decide whether the grounds are adequate. At this stage, legal representation is allowed (the child in care being represented by the reporter) and medical witnesses will often find themselves closely questioned if the case turns on evidence of, for example, sexual abuse. Because the sheriff is exercising civil powers, the standard of proof is not the 'beyond reasonable doubt' familiar in the criminal courts, but the lesser 'balance of probabilities'.

For the sake of children who appear at such a proof, formality is reduced to a minimum. The sheriff sits on the bench, but police officers do not wear uniform if they have to give evidence, nor are gowns and wigs to be seen. Evidence is given on oath or affirmation, as in any other court.

When he has heard all the evidence, the sheriff determines only the adequacy of the reporter's grounds of referral. If he considers them inadequate, the referral is discharged. If he is satisfied, the initiative returns to the children's hearing. On one occasion, the Court of Session has used its power to order what was, in effect, a further proof to be heard. Section 85 of the Children (Scotland) Act now allows the sheriff to review the proceedings (if the grounds were held adequate) in the light of new evidence that could not have been available at the original proof.

Place of safety

Police officers have powers under s61(5) of the Children (Scotland) Act 1995 to remove any child in need of emergency care to a place of safety (such as a police station or hospital). Social workers require the authorisation of a justice before whom they must appear (s61(2)). Authorisation may require any person to produce the child (s61(3)). A place of safety authorisation should be exhibited to clinical staff if the child is to be kept in hospital, and has equal effect when the child is transferred to other premises, for example to a specialist unit. The staff of the place of safety must know the terms and consequences of the authorisation as well as the action they ought to take in the face of any attempt to remove the child.

A justice's authorisation is granted only when it is not practicable to seek a child protection order (s57) from a sheriff and depends upon the same grounds, namely neglect or significant harm, actual or potential to the child. In general, the order ceases when adequate arrangements have been made by the reporter, the children's hearing and the local authority for the care and protection of the child.

The order may allow the transfer of parental rights to the applicant (the local authority or other person). The order may overcome refusal of parents to permit operation or blood transfusion, or confer authority on a doctor to examine the child for evidence of sexual abuse. The question of consent for such an examination is a difficult one but the Act (s90) does not prejudice a child's capacity under s2(4) of the Age of Legal Capacity (Scotland) Act 1991 to consent to (or refuse consent to) surgical, medical or dental procedures or treatment. For police surgeons, the importance is that consent to examine must be obtained from the child 'with capacity' (certainly of twelve years or older) despite any warrant to examine given under ss66, 69 and 70 of the Children (Scotland) Act.

A parent has the responsibility, as defined by s1 of the Children (Scotland) Act, to safeguard and promote the child's health, development and welfare; 'direction' is provided up to the age of sixteen, and 'guidance' up to eighteen. Mothers always possess the rights necessary to perform these responsibilities as does the father if married at or after the time of conception. Parental rights and responsibilities may be transferred by court order to the local authority (s11).

Case conferences

Personnel from the various agencies - these include social workers, teachers, clinical psychologist, hospital staff, police, general practitioner, health visitor, police surgeon - have an opportunity to pool knowledge, to discuss future management and, most significantly, to place a child on the 'at risk' register. Attenders at the conference should be limited to those with a personal professional interest, for they can easily become unwieldy. Police officers may find themselves in a difficult position if any criminal record of parents is to be discussed, or some other investigation cannot be revealed. Parents may be invited to attend part, or even all, the proceedings, but this must inevitably inhibit the exchange of views. They must, of course, be advised of the outcome. General practitioners often complain that the conference is arranged for a time when they are at a busy surgery, but a good deal of flexibility ought to be practised, and those who cannot attend should not hesitate to send a written report. The chair is usually taken by a senior social work administrator, and confidential minutes are kept.

Case discussions are held at the early stages of an investigation, to allow the agencies to decide upon a common approach, to agree to set procedures and to arrange for medical examinations. Follow-up conferences are held as required, for example, whenever a decision of major significance in the management of the child is proposed by one of the agencies. These are attended by a narrower spectrum of personnel. Only such a conference may decide to remove a child's name from the register.

Child Protection Register

The register is designed to assist the agencies which have child care responsibilities by listing those children who have been the subject of abuse or neglect, or are thought to be at risk of such abuse. The register should help in diagnosis and is a source of statistical data. It is maintained by social work departments, and may be consulted by staff of the relevant agencies, at any hour of the day or night. Local government reorganisation in early 1996, with consequent break up of established social work departments, must have an effect upon the service provided for children, but the result can only be awaited.

References

Bays J, Chadwick D 1993 Medical diagnosis of the sexually abused child. *Child Abuse & Neglect* **17**: 91-110.

Davies H de la H. 1985 Adolescent lumbar striae mistaken for non-accidental injury. *The Police Surgeon* **27**: 72-76.

Department of Health, British Medical Association and the Conference of Medical Royal Colleges 1995 Child Protection: Medical Responsibilities. (Addendum to Working Together under the Children Act 1989) Department of Health, London.

Estreich S, Forster GE 1992 Sexually transmitted diseases in children *Genito-Urinary Medicine* **68**: 2-8.

Hobbs CJ, Hanks HGI, Wynne JM. 1993 *Child Abuse and Neglect – a clinician's handbook.* Churchill Livingstone, Edinburgh

Home Office and Department of Health 1992 *Memorandum of Good Practice on Video Recorded Interviews of Child Witnesses in Criminal Proceedings.* HMSO, London

Jones DPH 1992 *Interviewing the Sexually Abused Child* 4th Ed. Gaskell/Royal College of Psychiatrists.

Kerns DL, Ritter ML, Thomas RG 1992 Concave hymenal variations in suspected child abuse victims *Pediatrics* **90**(2): 265-272.

Mant K 1984 *Taylor's Principles and Practice of Medical Jurisprudence* Ed. Churchill Livingstone, Edinburgh p78.

McCann J The medical evaluation of the sexually abused girl. Workshop at World Police Medical Officers'/Association of Police Surgeons Conference, Harrogate, September 1993.

McCann J, Voris J, Simon M, Wells R 1990a Comparison of genital examination techniques in prepubertal girls. *Pediatrics* **85**(2):182-7.

McCann J, Wells R, Simon M, Voris J, 1990b Genital findings in prepubertal girls selected for nonabuse: a descriptive study. *Pediatrics* **86**(3): 428-39.

Pierce AM, Robson WJ 1993 Genital injury in girls – accidental or not? *Pediatric Surgery International* 1993: **8**; 239-243.

Royal College of Physicians 1991 *Physical Signs of Sexual Abuse in Children.* RCP Publications, London

Siegel RM, Schubert CJ, Myers PA, Shapiro RA 1995 Prevalence of sexually transmitted diseases in children and adolescents in Cincinnati. *Pediatrics* **96**(6): 1090-1094.

8

INJURY

J Crane

The accurate description and interpretation of injuries is one of the most important functions of the forensic physician. Marks of violence may be found on the victim of an assault, either physical or sexual, on a child suspected of having been abused, on a police officer arresting a violent suspect, on a prisoner alleging ill-treatment whilst in custody, or on a body found dead in suspicious circumstances. The doctor asked to carry out an examination in such cases must be able to record injuries accurately, be aware of their medico-legal significance and be able to give a useful opinion as to how they may have been caused.

DESCRIBING WOUNDS

The examination should preferably be made in good light; in practice however, conditions may be less than ideal, for example, when called out at night, in the rain, to examine a dead body in a dark entry. Under such circumstances a powerful torch or flood lighting of the scene may be required. A few basic items of equipment are also essential: a hand-lens (or better still, an illuminated magnifier), a ruler with clear metric markings, a tape measure and a pair of calipers. Body charts, such as those available from the Association of Police Surgeons for copying, are invaluable for recording injuries. A portable ultra-violet torch may help to highlight faint bruises. In cases of serious assault or when injuries have distinctive characteristics of patterning, it is essential that the wounds are photographed with a suitable scale included beside the wound. Self-adhesive tape incorporating both imperial and metric graduations are readily available for this purpose.

The important points to consider in describing a wound are the nature of the injury, its age, its size and shape, and its location. When examining the living, injured areas need to be palpated to discern swelling and tenderness.

Nature of the injury

Under the Offences Against the Person Act 1861 a 'wound' requires the integrity of the body surface to be breached, however superficially or minutely. As this obviously excludes bruising and internal injury it is unrealistic in a medical sense. In legal terms, however, there is the definition of 'causing serious bodily harm' which covers any injury to any tissue or organ. Local reaction to injury also includes erythema and oedema which, on occasions, may be the only indication of the application of violence. Thermal damage also occurs locally as a response to chemical and electrical burns and due to the application of dry heat. Scalds are due to the application of moist heat. In spite of the confusing assortment of names used by doctors and others it is essential that for medico-legal purposes, forensic physicians, like forensic pathologists, use a standardised nomenclature when describing wounds. The classification which should be used is:

1. Bruises – often called 'contusions'
2. Abrasions - known as scratches or grazes
3. Lacerations - sometimes known as cuts or tears
4. Incisions - colloquially called slashes
5. Stab wounds - sometimes known as penetrating wounds.

It must, of course, be recognised that a variety of types of wounds may co-exist following a single traumatic incident. Furthermore, a single wound may show characteristics of different types: a bruised abrasion or an abrasion within which is a laceration.

Age

Injuries inflicted just before examination or indeed shortly before death show no sign of healing; this process (and eventual resolution) provides some guidance as to the age of the wound, but the many variables – such as site, force applied, amount of tissue damage, infection, treatment – all make judgements difficult. Bruises often become more prominent some hours or even days after infliction because of diffusion of blood closer to the skin surface. Bruises resolve over a variable period, ranging from days to weeks. The larger the bruise the longer it will take to disappear. Reddish-blue, blue or purplish-black bruises are almost certainly recent. As the extravasated red cells are destroyed, the ageing bruise goes through variable colour changes of bluish-green, greenish-yellow and brown. Estimating the age of non-recent bruises is one of the most contentious areas of forensic medicine. It must be clearly understood that it is impossible to age a bruise precisely; if asked to do so in court, a medical witness would be prudent to state that a bruise undergoing these colour changes is obviously not recent.

During life, an abrasion remains moist until it forms a scab, which consists of hardened exudate. The time taken for this process varies mainly with its depth, but also with any disturbance to which the surface is subjected, for instance, across a joint. The scab organises over a period of days up to a couple of weeks, before detaching, leaving a pink, usually intact surface. The colour gradually fades, unless the lesion is extensive, develops keloid or becomes very scarred. After death, an unscabbed abrasion dries and has a parchment-like brown colour. Abrasions caused after death tend to have a hard, yellow, translucent appearance and are devoid of any colour change at the periphery.

A laceration, or any wound healing by secondary intention, is associated with scab formation and eventual scarring, both taking days or weeks to develop. An incision, the edges of which are apposed, heals within a few days. The wound's colour, as with a bruise, may help in assessing the age of the lesion.

Size and shape

Size is determined with the aid of a ruler or a pair of calipers and **must** now be measured on the metric scale (not compared with items such as eggs and oranges). Since measurements given in imperial units may be easier for a jury to understand, it is acceptable to include the equivalent size in inches after that given in millimetres or centimetres. The shape of the wound should also be noted: simple terms such as circular, triangular, V-shaped or crescentic best express this characteristic, and can easily be demonstrated on the appropriate body chart. Wounds also have depth, but it is often not possible to estimate this clinically, nor to see the base. This may have significance, as in distinguishing lacerations or incised wounds of the scalp, and in identifying and recovering foreign (trace) material.

Position

Firstly the general location should be noted – for example, on the right upper limb, face or scalp. Then the precise location should be determined using fixed anatomical landmarks, such as 'on the scalp, three centimetres above and one centimetre behind the outer opening of the left ear' or 'on the inner aspect of the right upper arm, five centimetres above the medial epicondyle of the humerus'. On the neck, landmarks such as the prominence of the thyroid cartilage and the sterno-cleidomastoid muscles are useful, while on the trunk, the nipples, umbilicus and bony prominence of the pelvis can be used as points of reference. Technical anatomical terms are useful in reports for putting the site of the injury beyond doubt, but these must be explained in language suitable for a lay audience when giving oral evidence or a written statement. Simple anatomical diagrams and body charts are invaluable for locating the site of an injury.

TYPES OF INJURY

Transient lesions

Friction and irritants applied to the skin often cause transient erythema, sometimes accompanied by swelling. The skin over a weal may or may not be reddened. In susceptible individuals, a light touch causes a histamine reaction, seen as dermatographia. On the face, neck, upper chest and arms and behind the ears, patchy reddening which persists for a time varying from minutes to several hours, may be seen in some sensitive individuals, as a response to fear or embarrassment. It diminishes on digital pressure and must not be confused with bruising. Simple pressure from tight clothing may also cause erythema.

Red marks outlining an apparent injury, for example the mark of a hand on a slapped face or the buttock of a child, should be photographed without delay as such images may fade within an hour or so of infliction.

Reddening on the genital area, for example within the vulva, cannot be attributed to trauma with any certainty. It must not be taken as unequivocal evidence of forceful acts of intercourse unless there are other signs such as bruising and abrasion. In very young girls, where the diaphanous lining of the vestibule is transparent, redness is the normal colour. Mild vulvitis, too, is a common cause of redness.

Bruises

A bruise is due to the application of blunt force. The blow ruptures small blood vessels beneath the intact skin surface and blood escapes to infiltrate the surrounding tissues under the pumping action of the heart (see fig. 1). It follows that established bruising is only produced during life; postmortem wounds are not associated with any significant bruising as there is no internal pressure in the small vessels which have been ruptured.

Pinhead-sized haemorrhages within the skin, usually termed petechiae, may be produced by mechanical trauma as in reproducing the texture of clothing, but may also be produced by sucking (as in love bites) and are often seen on the serous membranes and conjunctivae as well as the skin as a result of congestion, possibly associated with mechanical asphyxia. Purpura are seen in those with a haemorrhagic tendency and in the elderly and tend to be larger and less regular in outline. Larger blotchy areas of haemorrhage within the skin are often referred to as ecchymoses but the medical witness needs to exercise care in the use of the term lest he or she becomes embroiled in problems of definition in the witness box. When blood collects within a mass beneath the skin, rather than being diffused within the tissues, it forms a haematoma. Bruising must not be confused with naevi or Campbell de Morgan spots. Also, innocent striae running transversely

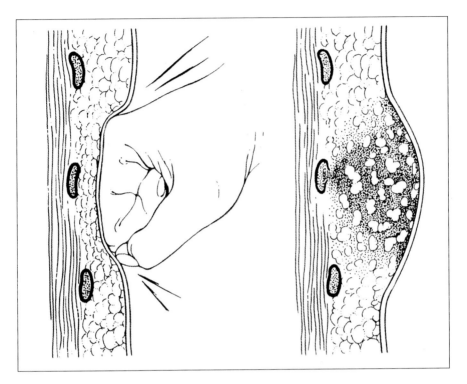

Figure 1 – Bruising

across the lower back of adolescents have been mistaken for injuries caused by beating. Finally, cyanosis is also a cause of blue discoloration in the skin which may be a source of confusion.

The initial site of a bruise corresponds with the point of impact but, if the victim lives, its boundaries are likely to exceed the original area of contact. Thus one cannot state that a bruise, 6 cm in diameter, was caused by an object of similar dimensions.

The extension of bruising can also mislead as to the actual site of the injury. Since a bruise is a simple mechanical permeation of the tissue spaces by fluid blood, its extension may be affected by gravity. Bruising of the thigh could result from a blow on the hip and facial bruising from an injury to the scalp. Difficulty arises when a bruise, as it extends, tracks along tissue planes from an invisible to a visible situation. Bruising of this kind may not become apparent externally for some time and then at a point well removed from the site of the original injury. This delay in the appearance of bruising is of considerable significance since lack of positive findings at an initial examination is not inconsistent with positive findings at an examination 24 or 48 hours later. Therefore, in many cases of assault, it may be essential to conduct a further examination a day or so later.

The size of a bruise is not necessarily related to the severity of the blow. In the living, a small bruise usually indicates no more than a slight blow, whereas a small bruise on a dead body may result from a violent blow if death occurred soon after the injury was inflicted. In contradistinction, a minor knock may produce a large bruise in the very young, the elderly, alcoholics or those with a compromised peripheral circulation. Bruising which seems inconsistent with the violence inflicted should lead one to exclude the possibility of a bleeding diathesis. Much depends on the general health of the individual and the condition and resilience of the skin, factors to be taken into account when recording findings made on general examination.

Some areas of the body bruise more readily than others, and this depends, among other things, on their blood supply and the density of the supporting tissues. Where there is an underlying bony surface and the tissues are lax, such as the facial area, a relatively light blow may produce considerable puffy bruising, particularly around the eyes. The scalp is a tissue which bruises more readily than it appears to; bruising there is easily detected at postmortem examination when the scalp is reflected but in the living, scalp bruising frequently goes undetected.

Sometimes a bruise has a pattern which may indicate the agent responsible. This is particularly so when death occurs soon after the injury is sustained, the pattern remaining sufficiently clear for diagnosis. In the living, this may become obscured as the area of bruising tends to extend and merge with others. Despite this, it may still be possible to make out such features as the links of a dog chain or the ridges on the patterned sole of a shoe. Beating with a rod often leaves a patterned bruise consisting of an area of central pallor outlined by two narrow parallel bands of bruising ('tramline bruising'). Perhaps the commonest pattern of bruising is that composed of petechial haemorrhages which reproduce the texture of clothing. This may occur if a person is struck a violent blow on a clothed area of the body or if the clothing is grabbed and twisted over the skin. Another type of patterning occasionally seen is the streaky linear purple bruising on the neck, wrists or ankles caused by the application of a ligature.

Other bruises of particular medico-legal significance are the small circular or oval bruises, usually about one to two centimetres in diameter, characteristic of fingertip pressure from either grabbing with the hand or prodding with the fingers. They are often seen on the limbs in cases of child abuse when the child is forcibly gripped by the arms or legs and shaken, or on the abdomen when the victim is poked and prodded. Similar bruises from the fingertips may be seen on the neck in manual strangulation and are then usually associated with other signs of asphyxia.

When sexual assault is alleged, the presence of bruising on the victim may help to corroborate the complaint and give some indication of how much violence was used. Moreover, bruising found elsewhere than about the genitalia gives some indication of how the attack was conducted, for example, bruising on the back could be in keeping with the complainant having been pinned to the ground. Grip marks or 'defence' injuries may be present on the upper arms and forearms while bruising on the thighs and inner sides of the knees may occur as the victim's legs are forcibly pulled apart. Bruising of the mouth and lips is frequently caused when the assailant places a hand over the face to keep the victim quiet. Also in cases of sexual assault, discrete areas of bruising – 'love bites' – may be found on the neck, breasts and other parts of the body.

Abrasions

An abrasion is an injury involving only the outer layers of the skin; that is, it does not penetrate the full thickness of the epidermis. From a clinical standpoint it is of little importance but to the pathologist or police surgeon, however, an abrasion is valuable in that, unlike a bruise, it always indicates the precise point of impact. In theory the abrasion does not bleed as blood vessels are confined to the dermis. Nevertheless, because of the corrugations of the dermal papillae, many abrasions do extend into the corium and thus bleeding will occur.

The abrasion may have a linear arrangement and close examination may show ruffling of the superficial epidermis to one end, indicating the direction of travel of the opposing surface (see fig. 2) Thus a tangential blow could be shown to have been horizontal or vertical, or it may be possible to infer that a body had been dragged over a rough surface. Trace material will often adhere to abraded skin and should be preserved. Multiple scratches running in different planes may corroborate a history of being pulled through bushes and trace vegetation may provide further confirmation.

The patterning of abrasions is clearer than that of bruises because abrasions, once inflicted, do not extend or gravitate. In manual strangulation small, crescentic marks caused by fingernails, although causing little in terms of injury, may be the

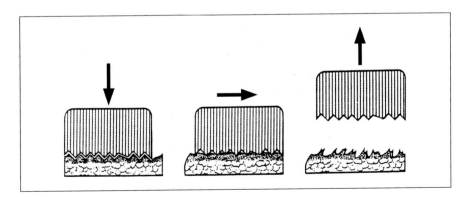

Figure 2 – Abrasion

only external feature by which one can prove that a hand has gripped the neck. In addition the victim of strangulation, whether manual or by a ligature, may attempt to tear away the assailant's fingers or the ligature and leave linear vertical abrasions on the skin. Similarly a victim resisting a sexual or other attack may rake her nails down the assailant's face leaving linear parallel abrasions on the cheeks. Biting may also abrade the skin in a way which not only clearly demonstrates the mechanism but may also assist in the identification of the assailant (see chapter 15).

Lacerations

Whenever blunt force splits the full thickness of the skin the wound is called a laceration. These wounds are often inflicted during assaults when the victim is struck with a stick, bottle, stone, hammer or pistol butt. They can also be sustained in falls and road traffic accidents.

Lacerations have characteristic features (see fig. 3). They are ragged wounds with irregular division of the tissue planes. They tend to gape because of the pull of elastic and muscular tissues. Their margins are often bruised and abraded and these are important diagnostic features which must be looked for with a hand-lens if necessary. Blood vessels, nerves and delicate tissue bridges may be exposed in the depth of the wound which might be soiled by, for instance, grit, dirt or particles

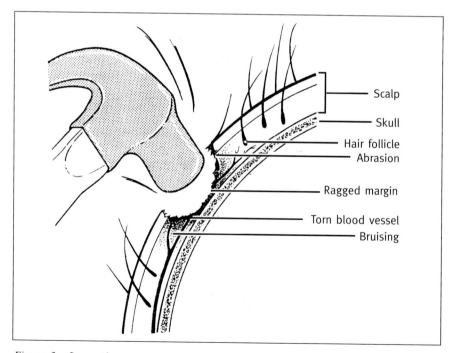

Figure 3 – Laceration

of glass. Occasionally, the margins are shelved or flaps of skin are produced by a shearing blow, the direction of which can then be deduced. Laceration of skin overlying bone may split the skin so cleanly as to simulate an incision; this is particularly so on the scalp, face or shin but close examination of the wound together with the history of how the injury came to be sustained should clarify the situation.

The shape of a laceration may indicate the agent responsible. For example, blows to the scalp inflicted with the circular head of a hammer or the spherical knob of a poker could cause crescentic lacerations; when the face of the weapon is square or rectangular, as the butt of an axe, its corners will produce a three-legged laceration.

Lacerations may be inflicted after death but the distinction from antemortem wounds is usually not difficult because of the absence of antemortem abrasions or bruising of the margins.

Lacerations are rarely self-inflicted because they cause pain. The suicide or attempted suicide victim is more likely to inflict incised wounds.

Incisions

These wounds are caused by sharp cutting instruments and their infliction in criminal circumstances implies intent. They are frequently caused by bladed weapons such as knives and razors, but sharp slivers of glass, the sharp edges of tin cans and sharp tools are examples of objects which may be used accidentally or criminally. Axes, hatchets and the like, though capable of cutting, usually produce lacerations when they are blunt or wielded so that a glancing blow is struck. Glass is another material often responsible for irregular lacerated wounds.

An incision is usually longer than its depth (see fig. 4). The margins tend to be straight, unbruised and without abrasion. The deeper tissues are cut in the same plane, blood vessels and nerves are cleanly divided and bleeding is often profuse. When they cross Langer's cleavage lines of the skin, the wounds tend to gape as elastic tissue contracts, and when caused by a slash with a blade, are deeper at their origin and shallower at the end from which the blade is withdrawn. These wounds are rarely soiled. When the skin is lax, as on the wrist and neck, it may crease as the blade is drawn over it, causing notching of the wound. A blunt weapon can cause a similar appearance.

When incised wounds are inflicted in an attack, the usual target is the victim's head and neck. When the attacker has a sexual motive, injury and mutilation of the breasts and genitalia may be seen (particularly in homicidal cases). Incisions to the fingers and forearms may be as a result of a defensive gesture by the victim as described below.

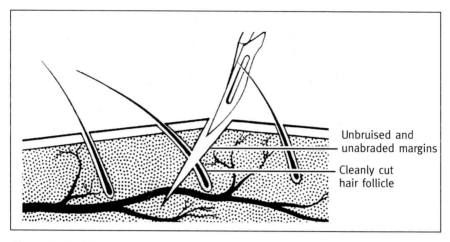

Unbruised and unabraded margins

Cleanly cut hair follicle

Figure 4 – Incision

Incised wounds, found in suicide or attempted suicide, are often multiple and parallel, most of them being tentative and superficial, and are usually located on the front of the forearm or wrist or on the front and sides of the neck.

Stab wounds

The typical feature of these penetrating wounds is a depth greater than their width or length. The list of instruments is endless, including knives, scissors, screwdrivers and pokers. Stabbing can cause serious penetrating injuries to deeper structures which may lead to rapid death, usually from haemorrhage or occasionally air embolism. Delayed deaths from infection, pulmonary embolism or other complications may also occur. Occasionally, a stab wound track perforates a limb, and the blade of the weapon extends to injure another structure.

Some stab wounds are accidental, as occur from time to time in butchers' shops, some are suicidal (although this is not common), but in the majority of cases infliction is deliberate by another party and in such circumstances may be associated with the presence of defence injuries to the arms and hands.

The appearance of the wound in the skin will vary depending on the weapon responsible. The double-edged blade of a dagger tends to produce an elliptical wound with sharp edges and clean-cut ends, whereas a stab wound from a single-edged blade such as a kitchen knife may cause squaring-off or fish-tailing of one extremity of the wound caused by the non-cutting back of the blade (see fig. 5). When blunt weapons are used, for example a pair of scissors, the wound will be more rounded with bruising surrounding its margins. Wounds caused by scissors can also sometimes have a cross shape caused by the blade screws or rivets. The blade of a weapon which is partially withdrawn and then

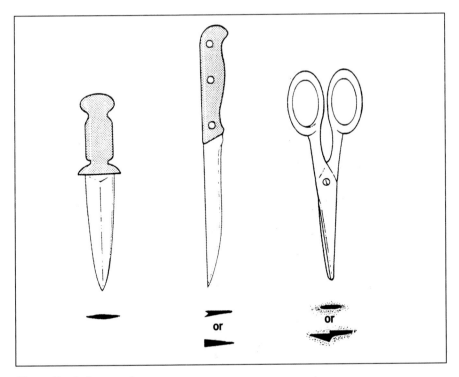

Figure 5 – Stab wounds

re-introduced at a slightly different angle, may give the stab wound a notched appearance.

It is important to remember that the external dimensions of a stab wound are a poor guide to the width of the knife blade. The skin tends to retract after the blade of the weapon is withdrawn, causing the length of the wound to shorten while its width increases. Moreover, the blade of the weapon may not have been introduced and withdrawn perpendicular to the skin surface and, as a result, the wound may be considerably longer than the actual width of the blade.

DEFENCE WOUNDS

The natural response to attack by an assailant, with or without a weapon, is to shield oneself with raised arms. In consequence, deflected blows are received usually on the extensor and ulnar surfaces of the forearms and hands. These may take the form of bruises, abrasions or lacerations. In the course of an assault there is a great deal of movement and defence injuries should be sought in less familiar sites. A victim lying on the ground curls up to protect the face and the front of the trunk from kicking feet, so that other surfaces of the limbs are liable to defensive bruising.

If the assailant is armed with a sharp instrument, such as a knife or razor, bruises and lacerations are replaced by incised wounds. In a struggle the victim will often try to wrest the weapon from the assailant, sustaining injuries in the process. If the blade of the weapon is grasped in the hand, incisions are to be expected on the palm and the palmar surfaces of the fingers and between the fingers.

SELF-MUTILATION

Self-inflicted injuries may be seen in a variety of circumstances but they tend to fall into three broad categories. Firstly, there are those individuals attempting to commit suicide or who, in desperation, are making a cry for help. Injuries in this group are often multiple, parallel, superficial linear incisions, mostly of a tentative nature. The preferred sites are the forearms (both flexor and extensor aspects), the front surfaces of the wrists and occasionally on the neck. Old linear scars in these areas suggest previous similar attempts. Inexpertly executed tattoos are not an uncommon form of self-mutilation, carrying the dangers of infection, especially when the needles used are contaminated with hepatitis B or C virus or HIV.

The second group comprises individuals who allege that they have been assaulted by a third party; the motive is often malicious, directed against an individual, but may be for financial gain. An example of the former is a young woman, jilted by her boyfriend, who concocts a story that she has been sexually assaulted and deliberately injures herself to give support to her story. Such wounds are of a trivial nature, consisting for the most part of linear abrasions and superficial incisions. Common characteristics are that such wounds tend to be found in groups, with roughly parallel orientation and with each wound having much the same depth throughout its length. There is usually no significant bruising and the wounds tend to be located on those areas of the body easily accessible to the victim, that is, on the face, on the front of the trunk, on the arms and on the fronts of the legs. The clothing is often deliberately and extensively torn, soiled or disarranged. The whole picture is incompatible with a real struggle, where a more random infliction is to be expected in type, site and severity of injury. When confronted, the complainant often admits how he or she came by the wounds.

In the third situation which is encountered by the forensic physician, a prisoner intentionally injures himself and then alleges that he has been assaulted by the police while in custody. A thorough and meticulous examination in these cases is essential since the medical evidence may go a long way in corroborating or refuting the allegations. As already discussed, the injuries are commonly multiple abrasions and occasionally incisions but the determined prisoner will inflict serious damage on himself, including bruises and head injuries, by using items and materials within his cell. The prudent doctor should examine the cell for agents which could have been used as weapons. In one case a prisoner with multiple linear abrasions on his legs made an allegation that he had been assaulted by the police. The wounds were self-inflicted and were found to have been made by the bristles of a toilet brush. Infliction of injuries on a willing 'victim' by others, for example a cell mate, has been known in an attempt to throw suspicion on the police.

Cigarette burns may also be self-inflicted but are less common since the subject anticipates that they will be painful. Bruising, which is also painful to sustain, is also infrequently seen and therefore if present, should raise suspicions that the prisoner's allegations might not be without foundation. Psychotic patients are capable of inflicting bizarre and painful injuries upon themselves which do not conform to the patterns outlined. Any injuries, self-inflicted or otherwise, found on a prisoner must be carefully documented and preferably also photographed. Suspected terrorists and those with a previous history of complaints against the police should be examined on detention, before and after interview and before release from custody.

FIREARM WOUNDS

Some basic knowledge of ballistics is essential for a proper understanding of wounds caused by firearms. There are essentially two types of weapon, smooth bore and rifled (see fig. 6)

Smooth bore weapons

Shotguns are the commonest type of smooth bore weapons and are typified by having a smooth barrel lining. They are commonly used in agricultural activities and by sportsmen and may be either single or double-barrelled. The usual barrel is from 66 to 81 centimetres (26 to 32 inches) in length, but criminals frequently shorten this ('sawn-off shotgun') to aid concealment and give a wider spread of

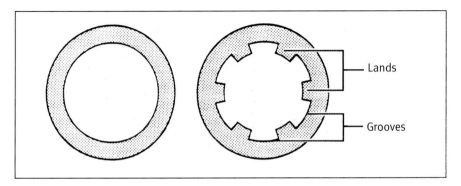

Figure 6 – Smooth bore (left) and rifled (right) gun barrels in cross section

shot. In double-barrelled weapons, the right barrel is usually a true cylinder but the diameter of the left barrel narrows towards the muzzle: this is called 'the choke'. Choking of the barrel helps to keep the shot together over a longer distance. The bore or gauge of a shotgun is determined by the number of solid balls of lead, each with the diameter of the barrel, that can be prepared from one pound of lead. Thus if 12 balls can be made from one pound of lead, the weapon is of 12-bore. In the 12-bore shotgun the diameter of the unchoked barrel is 19 mm (0.73 inches).

Shotgun ammunition consists of a cardboard or plastic cartridge case with a brass base containing primer. Inside the main part of the cartridge is a layer of powder, one or more felt or card wads and a mass of pellets (lead shot of variable size).

Rifled weapons

These are characterised by a number of parallel but spiral lands (projecting ridges) and grooves (depressed spaces between the lands) on the interior of the barrel from the breech to the muzzle. This rifling causes the bullet to spin, thus imparting gyroscopic steadiness to its flight. The rifling also leaves characteristic scratches, rifling marks, unique to that weapon, on the bullet.

There are three common types of rifled weapons; the rifle, revolver and pistol. The rifle is a long-barrelled shoulder weapon which may be capable of firing bullets with muzzle velocities of 450–1500 metres/second. Examples include the Armalite and the SA80 military rifle. Most military weapons are 'automatic' which means that the weapon will continue to fire while the trigger is depressed until the magazine is empty and thus is capable of discharging many rounds within seconds. The revolver, which has a low muzzle velocity of the order of 150 metres/second, is a short-barrelled rifled weapon with its ammunition held in a metal drum which rotates each time the trigger is released. The spent cartridge case is retained within the cylinder after firing. In the self-loading pistol, often called 'semi-automatic' or erroneously 'automatic', the ammunition is held in a metal clip-type magazine under the breech. Each time the trigger is pulled the bullet in the breech is fired and the spent cartridge automatically ejected. At the same time, a spring mechanism pushes the next live cartridge into the breech ready to be fired. The muzzle velocity of pistols may be between 300 and 360 metres/second.

Shotgun wounds

When a shotgun is discharged, the lead pellets emerge together en masse, then gradually diverge in a cone-shape as the distance from the weapon increases. The pellets are accompanied by particles of unburnt powder, flame, smoke, gases, wads and cards. A number of different factors affect the appearance of the entrance wound on the body but probably the most important of these is the range of fire. Both the estimated range of fire and the site of the wound are crucial factors in determining whether the wound was self-inflicted or not.

Contact wounds are caused by the muzzle of the weapon being held against the skin. This usually leaves a circular or oval entrance wound depending on whether the muzzle was perpendicular or not to the skin surface. The margins of the wound are usually clean-cut although they may be bruised or abraded due to so-called "recoil" impact of the muzzle. In the case of a double-barrelled weapon the circular abraded imprint of the non-firing muzzle may be clearly seen adjacent to the contact wound. The wound margins and the tissues within the base of the wound are usually blackened by smoke and there may even be charring of the wound margins or singeing of the skin hairs by flame. Because the shot and gases are contained within the wound there is often severe disruption of the underlying tissues and the gas forced into the wound may cause the tissues along its track to turn pink from carbon monoxide. The severity of the injuries associated with these contact wounds is dramatically demonstrated in wounds to the head where there is often gross mutilation with bursting ruptures of the scalp and face, multiple explosive fractures of the skull and extrusion or partial extrusion of the underlying brain. Most contact wounds of the head are suicidal in nature with the temple regions, the mouth and under the chin being the common sites. In these types of head wounds, fragments of scalp, skull and brain tissue may be dispersed over a wide area. The pellets and wads may or may not be retained within the fragmented skull.

At close range, with the muzzle up to 15 cm (6 inches) from the body, the entrance wound is still usually round or oval with fairly clean-cut margins. The clothing or skin may show slight burning from the flame and there may be blackening by smoke and unburnt powder. Blackening due to smoke is rarely seen beyond about 20 to 40 cm, while punctate abrasion or "tattooing" from unburnt powder usually only extends to about a metre or so. The wads and cards travel a relatively short distance, rarely being found beyond 2 metres.

Up to about a metre the pellets tend to travel as a compact mass and thus usually cause a single circular hole although at the upper end of this range the edges of the wound will be crenated and scalloped. With increasing range of fire, from about 1 to 3 metres, the pellets start to scatter and cause variable numbers of satellite pellet holes surrounding a larger central hole. Longer distances reveal a greater scatter of pellets. At long ranges, over about 8 to 10 metres there is no main entrance wound, only 'peppering' of the skin from individual pellets (see fig. 7).

As a rough rule of thumb, which is often incorrect, burning and singeing occurs over the first 15 cm (6 inches), soot staining can be seen for the first 40 cm (15 inches) and a single large hole persists for at least 1 metre (3 feet).

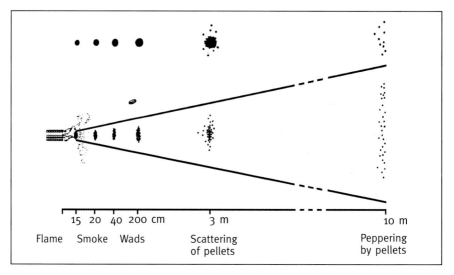

Figure 7 – Dispersal of shot from a shotgun

Rifled weapon wounds

Entrance bullet wounds tend to be neat round holes ranging from about 3 to 10 mm. diameter. The wound margin is usually fairly smooth and bordered by an even zone of creamy-pink abrasion. This collar of abrasion will be eccentric and the entrance hole more oval if the bullet strikes the skin at an angle (see fig. 8). If there is thick bone immediately subjacent to the skin, particularly with close range wounds to the head, the entrance wound may appear atypical with irregular ragged margins. This is because the underlying bone resists the entry of gases which accumulate under the skin and blow back causing subsidiary tears in the wound margins, giving rise to a stellate or irregular lacerated appearance.

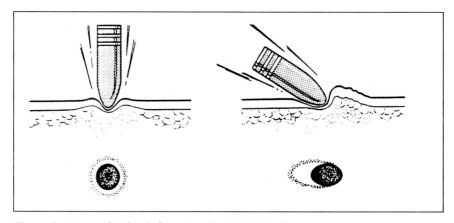

Figure 8 – Perpendicular (left) and angled (right) bullet penetration

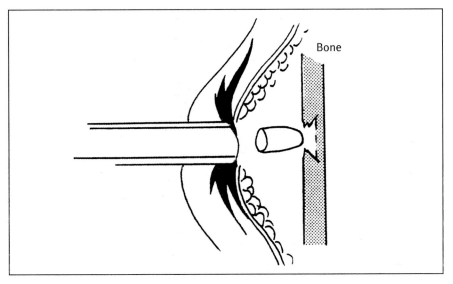

Figure 9 – Stellate close-range bullet wound due to underlying bone

Careful examination of such wounds however should reveal evidence of burning of the wound margins, blackening in the base of the wound and possibly the imprint of the muzzle on the skin surface (see fig. 9). Atypical entrance wounds are also found when bullets have ricocheted, struck an intermediate target, or have fragmented before striking the skin.

In contact wounds, the entrance hole may be bordered by the imprint of the muzzle. The margin may be charred and parchmented by flame and the surrounding skin may be pink in colour due to the effects of carbon monoxide in the underlying tissues. Punctate discharge abrasion and soot soiling are usually absent but the subcutaneous tissues within the depth of the wound are usually soiled. In close range wounds, singeing due to flame is rarely seen beyond about 15 cm (6 inches) with sooty soiling extending to about 30 cm (12 inches). Punctate discharge abrasion, which may be particularly heavy with revolver ammunition, is often present with ranges up to about 60 cm (24 inches).

Exit bullet wounds tend to be larger than the corresponding entrance wounds and usually consist of irregular lacerations or lacerated holes with everted, unbruised and unabraded margins. There are exceptions, however, and one must not be too dogmatic in the interpretation of bullet injuries, particularly when there are multiple wounds on the body. Remember that close range wounds may not show the typical features associated with flame, smoke and discharge particles if clothing or other material is interposed between the skin surface and the muzzle of the weapon. Care must also be taken when cleaning bullet wounds to remove blood and debris as smoke soiling of the wound margins or surrounding skin can easily be wiped away.

It is inadvisable to express an opinion on the calibre of a bullet based on the size of the entrance wound, nor is it possible to state confidently, from the appearance of an entrance wound, whether the bullet was fired from a rifle or a pistol. The differentiation between high and low velocity wounds is best determined by an assessment of the internal damage, although, as a rule to thumb, a large ragged exit wound is more consistent with the high velocity of a rifle bullet than that of a pistol or revolver.

TORTURE

Regrettably, abuse of human rights is so widespread throughout the world that reference must be made to it in this book. As far as the forensic physician is concerned, torture is seen in two main contexts: firstly, that perpetrated by criminal and terrorist groups and secondly, that carried out, or allegedly carried out, by the police or other security force personnel during the detention and interrogation of prisoners and suspects.

Torture is a sinister and abhorrent weapon of terrorist groups and, in Northern Ireland, has been used by various paramilitary groups, to instil fear and division in the community. The victims are usually members of their own organisation who are suspected of giving information to the police or to a rival group, members of rival organisations and occasionally captured members of the security forces. Often the torture occurs during interrogation and usually ends with the victim being shot. The victim is usually bound and the wrists and ankles bear the pale streaky bruises and abrasions caused by ligatures. "Beating up" is fairly standard with extensive bruises and abrasions to the face and body. The typical picture is of black eyes, fractures of the nose and jaws and displacement of the teeth. Burning with a cigarette causes discrete circular, yellow (in the dead) parchmented burns while more severe burns may be caused by branding with a hot poker. Patterned injuries due to being struck with the butt of a rifle or pistol may be seen, while incisions and stab wounds are inflicted by knives. It is not uncommon for a finger or the lobule of the ear to be amputated. Finally, the victim may be hooded and taken to a deserted spot, made to kneel on the ground and then shot, at close range, through the back of the head, possibly with a coup de grace on the face. It has been the experience in Northern Ireland that, in some instances, the beating has been so severe that death by shooting must have come as a merciful relief.

Doctors who have access to prisoners in custody have an onerous responsibility to ensure that they are properly treated during detention and interrogation. The Tokyo Declaration of 1975 defines torture 'as the deliberate, systematic or wanton infliction of physical or mental suffering by one or more persons acting alone or on the orders of any authority, to force another person to yield information, to make a confession, or for any other reason'. The Declaration also lays down guidelines for doctors when faced with cases or suspected cases of torture. The methods employed during interrogation range from apparent physical abuse to the more subtle use of threats and intimidation. Hooding, prolonged standing, the use of continuous high-pitched sound have all been used and subsequently condemned, as have attempts to disorientate the prisoner by offering food at erratic times, frequently waking the person up after short intervals of sleep and by burning a light in the cell twenty-four hours per day. A doctor, charged with the responsibility of caring for prisoners, particularly in interrogation units, must satisfy himself that such methods are not employed.

Actual physical abuse is thankfully less frequently seen and can be prevented, as in Northern Ireland, by regular medical examinations which would otherwise bring to light evidence of assault whilst in custody. However, methods of physical assault may be employed which, on casual examination, may leave no apparent marks of violence. These include vigorous hair-pulling (detected by scalp tenderness and areas of recent balding) face-slapping (detected by redness, tenderness and swelling) and blows to the side of the head such as by the arm of the interrogator. Both vigorous face slapping and blows to the head may result in perforation of the eardrum and therefore it is imperative to examine the ears carefully during routine examination. Blows to the abdomen may not leave any apparent mark, but just occasionally the faint petechial impression of the clothing may be seen on the skin of the abdominal wall. Pinching, squeezing and blows to the testes have been employed and the scrotal skin must be carefully examined for bruising or other marks. The underlying testes may be swollen and tender. Doctors do not normally inspect the soles of the feet, but it has been known for prisoners to be repeatedly struck here with a baton. In all cases of suspected or alleged ill-treatment of prisoners it is essential that the doctor carries out a methodical and detailed 'head to toe' examination. All injuries and marks must be accurately recorded and photographed and the appropriate authorities informed immediately.

INVESTIGATION OF SUSPICIOUS DEATH

The forensic medical examiner is often one of the first 'experts' to attend the scene of a suspicious death and once his preliminary function of confirming that death has taken place he should ensure, as far as possible, that no further disturbance of the scene takes place until the other appropriate investigators (see chapter 13) have arrived. Calls to scenes frequently occur at unusual hours, and the forensic physician must ensure that he has appropriate equipment and clothing ready to hand; often the items required may not be easy to locate at 3 o'clock in the morning. The wearing of protective disposable overalls and overshoes should be mandatory at all scenes and it goes without saying that such garments must be changed if the doctor is subsequently asked to examine a suspect in the case.

There is an unfortunate tendency for some doctors to take 'control' of the scene and to undertake inappropriate procedures which should best be left to the pathologist, for example, the taking of liver temperatures. The scene is the responsibility of the investigating police officer and the doctor must be prepared to accept his instructions regarding the approach to the body and how much or how little he is expected to do. Certainly it is essential to avoid the unnecessary touching of objects, particularly possible weapons, and to refrain from smoking or leaving any objects or debris behind. Disturbance of the body should be kept to a minimum and the clothing should not be unnecessarily dishevelled or removed even though this may mean that some injuries, for example, those on the back of the body, are not seen. A more detailed examination of the body will be undertaken by the pathologist at a later stage and the full extent of the injuries can then be assessed.

In summary, the main functions of the forensic medical examiner are to observe the scene, to confirm that death has taken place, to ensure that trace evidence is not removed or destroyed from the body or its surroundings, to offer an opinion as to the possible nature, as opposed to the cause of death and, where necessary, to assist and supervise the removal of the body from the scene. In addition, the taking of detailed contemporaneous notes, possibly complemented by clear line diagrams, will ensure that if the doctor is subsequently required to make a statement or attend court about the case he has sufficient documentation to refresh his memory.

Further reading

Forensic Pathology (Edward Arnold 1991) by Professor Bernard Knight, provides a detailed description of wounds and their interpretation.

Forensic Medicine – An Illustrated Reference 1995 (Chapman and Hall Medical) edited by J. K. Mason and *Colour Atlas of Wounds and Wounding* (MTP Press Ltd., 1986) by G. A. Gresham both illustrate the appearances of the various types of injuries encountered in forensic medical practice.

9

SUBSTANCE MISUSE

M Stark, G Norfolk

INTRODUCTION

Substance misuse is a major and growing problem often resulting in drug-related criminal activity. Forensic physicians are seeing an increasing number of substance misusers in the setting of a police station (Stark 1994). These misusers may be intoxicated, withdrawing or dependent on alcohol or drugs. The police may request a medical assessment regarding fitness for detention, fitness to be interviewed, mental state examination, a comprehensive examination to assess a person's ability to drive a motor vehicle as well as intimate searches for drugs.

On arrest, some substance misusers will, for a variety of reasons, attempt to hide their misuse from the authorities and it is, therefore, most important that an examining forensic physician should make a conscious effort to look for any indication of substance misuse or dependence. A sympathetic approach from the doctor is more likely to result in disclosure and a reliable history from the detainee, who should be reassured that effective treatment will be given where necessary and that the overriding consideration of the doctor is the clinical safety and wellbeing of the detainee.

CRIMINALITY AND DRUG USE

The relationship between crime and drug use is very complex. Drug-related crime encompasses any criminal activity which is committed either to fund the purchase of drugs or as a consequence of drug misuse (*Tackling Drugs Together* 1995). Examples include acquisitive crimes, such as shop-lifting or burglary; offences under the various acts established to control the possession, distribution and consumption of drugs, such as the Pharmacy Act 1933, Medicines Act 1968 and the Misuse of Drugs Act 1971, and criminal acts carried out by persons in an abnormal mental state due to drug intoxication or withdrawal, such as assault or damage to property.

DRUG LAWS

Two main statutes regulate the availability of drugs in the United Kingdom: the Misuse of Drugs Act 1971 and the Medicines Act 1968. The Medicines Act 1968 governs the manufacture and supply of medicinal products and divides drugs into prescription only medicines (POM) which must be prescribed by a doctor, a dentist or in exceptional circumstances another health professional; pharmacy medicines (PM) sold under the supervision of a pharmacist from a pharmacy; general sale list medicines (GSL) which can be sold from any premises without supervision or advice from a doctor or pharmacist.

The Misuse of Drugs Act 1971 aims to prevent the unauthorised use of drugs which are likely to be misused and are capable of having harmful effects sufficient to constitute a social problem. It is also the way the UK fulfils its obligation to control drugs in accordance with international agreements. The drugs are divided into various classes for penalty purposes (see table 1). Regulations made under the Act divide controlled drugs into schedules that take account of the needs of medical practice (see table 2).

DEFINITIONS

A drug is "any substance, other than those required for the maintenance of normal health, that, when taken into the living organism may modify one or more of its functions" (WHO definition).

MISUSE OF DRUGS ACT 1971		
PENALTY PURPOSES		
	Class A	major natural and synthetic opiates
		cocaine
		LSD
		injectable amphetamines
		cannabinol
	Class B	oral amphetamines
		cannabis plant material and resin
		codeine, dihydrocodeine
		certain barbiturates
	Class C	benzodiazepines
		methaqualone

Table 1

MISUSE OF DRUGS REGULATIONS 1985	
CONTROL PURPOSES	
Schedule 1	Prohibited drugs except with Home Office authority e.g cannabis, LSD, raw opium, ecstasy
Schedule 2	Full controlled drug requirements in relation to prescribing, safe custody, keeping of registers e.g diamorphine, pethidine, cocaine
Schedule 3	Barbiturates, meprobamate, pentazocine
Schedule 4	Benzodiazepines
Schedule 5	Preparations containing small amounts of controlled drugs

Table 2

Drug misuse has been defined as "any taking of a drug which harms or threatens to harm the physical and mental health or social well-being of an individual, of other individuals, or of society at large, or which is illegal" (Royal College of Psychiatrists 1987). Drug misuse can occur in the absence of dependence which is defined as "a state, psychic and sometimes also physical, resulting from the interaction between a living organism and a drug, characterised by behavioural and other responses that always include a compulsion to take the drug on a continuous or periodic basis in order to experience its psychic effects and sometimes to avoid discomfort of its absence. Tolerance may or may not be present" (WHO definition). Drug dependence can occur without drug misuse but it is more common for both to occur together. It is important to note that for drug dependence to exist psychological dependence must be present but that physical dependence may not necessarily occur. Tolerance occurs when increased doses are required to produce the same effect and will only be maintained if the drug is taken regularly and in sufficient doses.

GENERAL PRINCIPLES

A careful and well documented history and examination are required to look for objective signs of intoxication, dependence or withdrawal. Often more than one drug is misused; this may be a combination of prescribed and illicit substances as well as alcohol. The prescribed dose of a drug may not necessarily indicate accurately the true amount taken per day; some may be sold and perhaps other drugs taken as well. For each drug, an estimate of the average quantity taken each day, the frequency of use, time of the last dose, amount used in the past 24 hours as well as the route of administration should be noted. The effect of a particular drug on an individual varies and the severity of withdrawal, for example, is influenced by psychological factors.

SPECIFIC DRUGS
(classified by their most characteristic pharmacological effect)

Drugs that stimulate the nervous system

These drugs, which include amphetamine, khat and cocaine, result in euphoria, increased energy and alertness with loss of appetite. Aggressive behaviour and confused thinking may occur resulting in exhaustion and sleep. The heart rate, blood pressure and respiratory rate may be increased and associated with dry mouth, sweating, dilated pupils and hyperactive reflexes. Hallucinations, delusions, paranoia may occur as well as fits, coma and death.

Stimulants such as amphetamines, cocaine and ecstasy can cause psychological dependence but do not produce a major physical withdrawal syndrome. However, there may be insomnia and a severe depression which will require that the detainee is closely supervised whilst in custody and may need pharmacological treatment.

Amphetamine is the most popular stimulant and may be taken intravenously, orally or sniffed (snorted). The clinical effects come on quickly and can last several hours.

Khat (catha edulis) is chewed for its stimulant effect and the main component is cathinone so the effects produced are similar to those seen with amphetamine. Khat is legally sold in the United Kingdom.

Cocaine hydrochloride can be sniffed or injected; effects peak within 15 to 40 minutes. By injection, there is an intense rush or high within 1 to 2 minutes whereas, when sniffed, the drug absorption is slow with no rush. Crack (freebase cocaine) is produced when cocaine hydrochloride is dissolved in water and heated with a chemical reagent such as baking soda to free the cocaine alkaloid base from the salt. It is usually smoked and is a powerful central nervous system stimulant reaching the brain within seconds. The euphoric effects wear off very quickly and therefore have to be quickly repeated. Larger doses or a "binge" may result in anxiety and panic leading to paranoia. A dangerous combination of cocaine and heroin taken by injection is known as a "speedball".

Ecstasy (3,4, methylene-dioxymethamphetamine - MDMA) is a stimulant with hallucinogenic properties. A moderate dose of 75-100 mg produces effects within 20-60 minutes. In addition to the general effects of stimulants described above, trismus (spasm of the muscles of mastication) and bruxism (grinding of teeth) may be noted. Other effects have been reported including catatonic stupor and hyponatraemia, pneumomediastinum, paranoid psychosis, liver and renal problems, hyperpyrexia, disseminated intravascular coagulation, rhabdomyolysis and death.

The Advisory Council on the Misuse of Drugs (Home Office 1994) has stressed the importance of freely available cold water and the provision of rest facilities in a cool environment at raves where ecstasy may be misused.

Anabolic steroids may be used by athletes or body builders and taken orally or by injection. Effects include mood swings with an increase in aggressive behaviour, psychiatric problems such as depression and paranoia, rarely hepatitis and liver tumours and HIV from sharing injecting equipment.

Alkyl nitrites "poppers", such as amyl nitrite, are used as euphoric relaxants and as an aid to anal intercourse. The effects of inhalation of the vapour are almost instantaneous with headache, dizziness and flushing. Excessive use may result in methaemoglobinaemia.

Drugs that alter perceptual function

LSD (D-lysergic acid diethylamide) in a dose of 110-150 micrograms results in a "trip" usually after 30-60 minutes, peaking after 2 to 6 hours and fading out after 12 hours. The effects depend very much on the individual and the circumstances, with the same user having a bad or good "trip" on different occasions or even within the same trip, so friendly reassurance can help until the drug has worn off. Visual effects such as intensified colours and distorted shapes occur, but true visual hallucinations are rare; there may be distortions of hearing. Other physical effects may be mild but include slight pupil dilatation. In the recovery stage of an LSD experience there may also be apprehension and distraction that is not immediately obvious to onlookers and, therefore, a detainee's fitness to be interviewed may be affected. The forensic physician should advise the police accordingly.

Cannabis is the most popular illicit drug. When smoked, effects occur within a few minutes and last up to one hour with low doses, two to three hours with higher doses. If it is ingested, it may take an hour or more to have an effect which can last 12 hours or more. The effects include drowsiness, giggling, euphoria, tachycardia, red eyes, dilated pupils, loss of co-ordination and an ataxic gait.

Hallucinogenic mushrooms or "magic mushrooms" contain psilocybin and psilocin and are taken orally, raw or cooked to enhance potency.

Drugs that depress the nervous system

Depression of the nervous system results in sedation and relief of anxiety, but because of disinhibition may initially result in euphoria, excitation and risk taking. Physical effects include disorientation, drowsiness, slurred speech, nystagmus, loss of co-ordination, ataxia, coma and death and there may be delusions and hallucinations. At high doses cerebral depression may occur, so these drugs are more dangerous when taken with other cerebral depressants such as alcohol.

CLINICAL FORENSIC MEDICINE

Volatile substance misuse is the deliberate inhalation of a volatile substance to achieve a change in mental state. The many substances which can be misused include fuel gases such as butane, petrol, aerosol propellants, glues and adhesives containing toluene and cleaning agents such as trichlorethylene. These substances can result in a mixture of sedative, anaesthetic and hallucinogenic effects.

Death can occur from a variety of mechanisms including anoxia, vagal inhibition (if the larynx is stimulated directly), respiratory depression, cardiac dysrhythmias, trauma as well as unexplained sudden death either during exposure or in the hours after. These substances should be discontinued abruptly. There is no physical withdrawal syndrome.

Ketamine is an anaesthetic agent which can be taken intranasally, orally or intravenously. Effects start within 30 seconds or so if used intravenously and 20 minutes if taken orally and can last for 3 hours. Users can experience a cocaine-like "rush" with psychological dissociation.

Gammahydroxybutyrate (GHB or GBH) is an anaesthetic with primarily sedative properties. Clinical effects start within 10 minutes.

Benzodiazepines are increasingly misused, particularly when the drug of first choice, for example heroin, is not available. The withdrawal syndrome from benzodiazepines includes the major complications of fits and psychosis. In addition anxiety symptoms, such as sweating, insomnia, headache, tremor, nausea and disordered perceptions, such as feelings of unreality, abnormal bodily sensations and hypersensitivity to stimuli may be seen. Treatment of benzodiazepine withdrawal should be with a long acting drug such as chlordiazepoxide or diazepam to prevent the medical complications of withdrawal.

Barbiturates are particularly dangerous drugs when taken in overdose and cause a physical and psychological dependence. They have limited therapeutic uses now and have largely been replaced by the benzodiazepines but may still occasionally be encountered in forensic practice.

Opiates

Opiate intoxication results in a feeling of well-being. There may be euphoria or the misuser may seem distant and drowsy with an inability to concentrate. The pupils will be small or pin-point with a sluggish reaction to light. Severe intoxication can result in respiratory depression and death. Tolerance develops to the analgesic and respiratory depressive actions of opiates, but not the action on the pupil or the bowel, so that a dependent individual usually displays a typically constricted pupil and suffers from constipation.

The start of the abstinence syndrome will depend on the opioid used. For example, heroin withdrawal will usually start within 8 hours, progress to a peak and then gradually improve over 48–72 hours, whereas withdrawal from methadone may lead to a longer abstinence syndrome. The misuser may experience sweating, lachrymation, rhinorrhea, yawning, a feeling of going hot and cold, anorexia, abdominal cramps, nausea, vomiting, diarrhoea, tremor, restlessness, insomnia and generalised aches and weakness. On examination there may be dilated pupils, gooseflesh, an increase of pulse rate and blood pressure, and hyperactive bowel sounds.

TREATMENT OF OPIATE WITHDRAWAL

Symptomatic treatment may be helpful for a number of detainees. Paracetamol and the non-steroidal anti-inflammatory drugs, such as ibuprofen, may be useful for generalised aches and pains. Other drugs may be used for specific problems: loperamide (imodium), diphenoxylate and atropine (Lomotil) for abdominal cramps and diarrhoea; promethazine, which has antiemetic and sedative properties or metoclopramide for nausea and vomiting; thioridazine may be useful for anxiety but should be avoided if there is any history of fits; benzodiazepines are useful for the treatment of anxiety and insomnia in this controlled environment. Lofexidine can also be used to alleviate withdrawal symptoms and is less sedative and hypotensive than clonidine which requires strict monitoring of blood pressure and is therefore not suitable for use in police stations.

Substitution treatment includes methadone, dihydrocodeine or codeine. Methadone has a long duration of action (24–36 hours) and, therefore, can be given once a day. Dihydrocodeine or codeine may be suitable for the less severely opiate dependent not controlled with symptomatic medication. If the detainee is receiving opiates as part of a detoxification programme this prescription should be continued once the presence of intoxication by other drugs has been excluded. The detainee may be carrying prescribed and accurately labelled medication on arrest or the details may be verified with the local clinic or chemist. If there is concern about the dose, for example a very large dose (methadone 100 mg), the dose can easily be split and the detainee reviewed at each stage. Otherwise, treatment should be given after a full assessment of the detainee. It may be necessary to review the detainee after a period of time to establish whether there are signs of withdrawal.

Sudden cessation of opioid use in a dependent pregnant women may be life-threatening to the fetus and special care should be taken to ensure that a pregnant women continues any prescribed medication and that treatment is instigated promptly to alleviate withdrawal.

The assessment of fitness to interview is of the utmost importance; mild opiate withdrawal may not affect a detainee's fitness with respect to an interview, but in more severe cases the detainee may require treatment prior to being interviewed.

The distinction between intoxication and dependence must be made as this will affect treatment. A person may be intoxicated without being dependent or dependent without being intoxicated. In the latter case medical treatment may be required to permit a detainee to achieve a stable state and be fit for questioning (see fig.1).

HARM MINIMISATION

Harm minimisation aims to reduce the damage from drug misuse. Many substance misusers have little or no contact with doctors and the forensic physician should use this opportunity to advise the substance misuser on minimising the harm from continued substance misuse, for example on injecting behaviour, the availability of hepatitis B vaccination and HIV awareness, as well

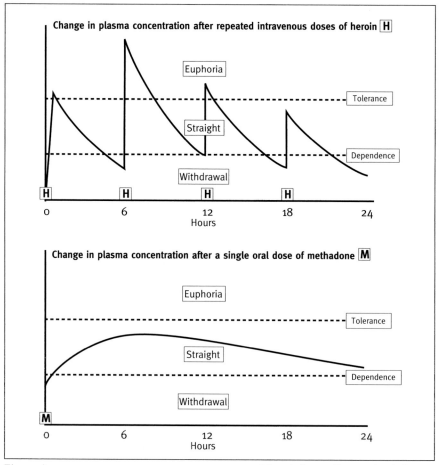

Figure 1   *Schematic diagram of heroin and methadone use.*
                                                        Reproduced from Ghodse 1995

MEDICAL COMPLICATIONS OF DRUG MISUSE

Self-neglect, malnutrition, dental decay

Complication of injection
- intra-arterial may cause vascular damage resulting in gangrene
- intravenous superficial thrombophlebitis, deep vein thrombosis, pulmonary embolism; post thrombotic complications such as limb swelling and ulcers

Inhalation of certain drugs may precipitate asthma or bronchitis; pneumothorax, pneumomediastinum, vomiting with inhalation and asphyxiation

Infection
- at the injection site may result in cellulitis and abscess formation
- septicaemia and infective endocarditis
- increased risk of tuberculosis
- hepatitis and HIV

Acute and chronic liver disease

Kidney problems and amyloidosis

Psychiatric complications

Overdose and death

Table 3

as supplying information about the local agencies involved in counselling and treatment. Treatment may be needed for the medical complications of substance misuse (see table 3). All detainees should be seen as a potential infectious risk, but the police should not be informed of a detainee's HIV status as this would be a breach of patient confidentiality.

OVERDOSE

Naloxone is an opioid antagonist used to reverse the effects of intoxication. If naloxone is used then observation in hospital is required as most misused opioids have a longer half-life than naloxone. It can be given by the intramuscular route as it may be difficult initially to establish intravenous access. This has the advantage that there is slower absorption from the intramuscular site, so providing a slightly longer duration of action.

MENTAL HEALTH ACT

Drug misuse and dependence are explicitly excluded as grounds for compulsory admission under the Mental Health Act 1983. However, the mental state of detainees may occasionally be such as to require assessment in hospital in the interests of their own health or for the safety of others. Chronic misuse of stimulants or cannabis may give rise to a psychotic state.

In the absence of mental disorder, substance misuse in itself, is not an indication for an appropriate adult (see p108) to be called.

CONCEALMENT

Drugs may be concealed in the ears, mouth, nose, vagina or rectum. They may be systematically ingested or packed in order to smuggle drugs into the country or hide drugs from the authorities - body packers or "mules". Occasionally they may be swallowed just prior to arrest - body stuffers or swallowers.

Intimate searches in England and Wales are governed by section 55 of the Police and Criminal Evidence Act 1984. In Scotland, where in the interests of justice and to obtain evidence it is necessary to carry out an intimate search, it must only take place under the authority of a sheriff's warrant. The searches should take place in properly equipped medical room, not a police station, by a registered medical practitioner or registered nurse. Occasionally concealed packages may be at risk of rupture and full resuscitation facilities must be available.

The search should only be performed if the detainee gives full informed consent (British Medical Association 1994) and the appropriate police superintendent's authorisation is given. Furthermore, such a search can legally only be performed for Class A drugs, such as heroin or cocaine, which therefore excludes cannabis and amphetamines, commonly concealed substances. If the detainee refuses to be searched the forensic physician may have to arrange admission and observation in hospital.

NOTIFICATION

A doctor has a statutory duty to send specified details of persons whom they consider or have reasonable grounds to suspect to be addicted to a number of controlled drugs (see table 4) to the Chief Medical Officer at the Home Office. This information has to be sent within seven days. A person is to be regarded as being addicted to a drug if he has, as a result of a repeated administration, become so dependent on the drug that he has an overpowering desire for the administration of it to be continued (Misuse of Drugs Regulations 1973). This statutory duty applies whether or not treatment has been prescribed to the person and is exempt from the rules of confidentiality. Local Drug Misuse Databases have now been established to gather information on a greater range of drugs. Usually the completion of a single form allows the doctor to report to the Database and fulfil the statutory duty.

CONTROLLED DRUGS REQUIRING NOTIFICATION	
cocaine	methadone
dextromoramide	morphine
diamorphine (heroin)	opium
dipipanone	oxycodone
hydrocodone	pethidine
hydromorphone	phenazocine
levorphanol	piritramide

Table 4

ALCOHOL

The substance

An alcohol is any substance which contains a hydroxyl group attached to a carbon atom, and many thousands of these substances are known to chemists. Although there is no legal definition of alcohol, the term is generally assumed to relate to one specific alcohol, namely ethanol.

Ethanol is produced by the fermentation of sugar by yeast, a process that stops at an alcohol concentration of about 15% by volume, because of the death of the yeast. Thus, three main types of liquor can be drunk: those produced by fermentation alone, such as beers, cider and wine; those made by distillation (spirits); and those wines that have been fortified with spirits, such as sherry and port. The strength of such drinks is generally referred to as a percentage of alcohol volume for volume (v/v). Therefore, 100 ml of a drink with a strength of 10 % alcohol v/v, will contain 10 ml of alcohol, or approximately 10 grams. (As alcohol is lighter than water the actual weight will be slightly less than this.) Increasingly, consumers are being encouraged to measure the amount of alcohol they drink in terms of units. One unit of alcohol contains 8 grams of pure spirit and is equivalent to approximately one half pint of beer, a glass of wine or a single pub measure of spirits.

Metabolism

Alcohol is absorbed in the stomach and duodenum. The rate of absorption is fastest in the duodenum, so any condition that causes the drink to enter the upper small intestine more quickly than normal, such as a gastrectomy, will lead to more rapid absorption and an earlier, higher peak blood alcohol level. As soon as alcohol enters the bloodstream mechanisms for its removal come into action.

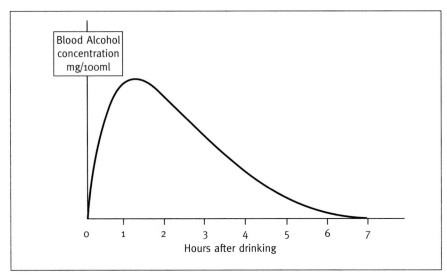

Figure 2 – Blood alcohol curve

The overall rate of elimination is practically constant, and much less than the rate of absorption. These facts give rise to the well known blood alcohol curve (see fig. 2). The blood alcohol usually peaks between 30 and 60 minutes after drinking, although the range may be anything from 20 minutes to 3 hours. Any factor that affects the rate of absorption will also affect the peak blood alcohol concentration, as the faster alcohol is absorbed the less time there is for elimination and the higher the peak.

Various factors may influence the shape of the blood alcohol curve and these include:

Sex and weight. – The blood-alcohol level reached after the consumption of a given amount of alcohol will depend on the weight and sex of the drinker. The smaller the body throughout which the alcohol is distributed, the less water it contains, and the higher therefore the alcohol concentration in this water. As women are proportionally fatter than men, and fat contains less water than other body tissues, the blood alcohol level will be approximately 20 per cent higher in a woman who drinks the same quantity of alcohol as a man of the same weight. It is for this reason that safe drinking limits are always lower for women than men.

The duration of drinking. – If alcohol is consumed slowly it may be eliminated almost as quickly as it is absorbed, giving rise to much lower peak alcohol concentrations.

The nature of the drink consumed. – Alcohol absorption is maximal from drinks of 20 per cent strength. Below this level the dilution in a larger volume delays mucosal transfer, whilst stronger spirits irritate the gastric mucosa and delay gastric opening, thereby slowing down absorption. Absorption is also delayed by the presence of soluble nutrients in the drink. This applies particularly to beers, which contain a lot of carbohydrates. Thus, drinking beer can lead to a peak alcohol concentration one hour later and 25 per cent lower than that achieved by drinking the same amount of alcohol as spirits.

Food in the stomach. – A full meal before drinking can reduce the peak by as much as 50 per cent, although the effect is much less marked when drinking beer, because this is absorbed so slowly anyway.

Physiological factors and genetic variation.– Factors such as stomach wall permeability, the blood supply to the alimentary tract and the rate of gastric emptying will vary from person to person, and from time to time in the same drinker. All of these will have a bearing on the shape of the blood alcohol curve.

The rate of elimination. – About 90 per cent of absorbed alcohol is oxidised by the liver in a reaction catalysed by alcohol dehydrogenase. The remainder is excreted unchanged, mainly in urine but also in the sweat and breath. The rate of elimination has been determined experimentally. Although it may vary between 10 to 25 mg/100 ml blood/hour, the average rate is 15 mg/100 ml/hour, which is equivalent to one unit of alcohol per hour in a 70 kilogram male. Habituation to alcohol is the single most important factor affecting the rate of elimination, with chronic alcoholics having facilitated liver enzyme systems and rates of 20 mg/100 ml/hour or higher.

The effects

Alcohol is a central nervous system depressant. Its apparent stimulatory effects are due to the fact that it acts first on the so-called higher centres of the brain which govern inhibition. In addition, the slight anaesthetic action may make the drinker less aware of depression or fatigue. There is a large variation in the susceptibility of drinkers to the effects of alcohol. Young persons, or those unused to drinking, will be affected by much lower levels of blood alcohol than the average, whereas alcoholics show tremendous tolerance to the effects. Table 5 indicates the effects that may be caused by a given blood alcohol concentration, but should be seen only as a rough guide. Acute hypoglycaemia occasionally complicates severe intoxication and must be excluded in all cases of coma.

Most recorded fatalities due to alcohol intoxication have a blood alcohol level above 400 mg/100 ml blood. If the level is below 350 other complicating factors are almost certainly present, most commonly an interaction between the alcohol and other drugs that have also been ingested. In particular, the doctor needs to be aware of the likelihood of respiratory depression in those combining alcohol with chlormethiazole, a drug that is frequently prescribed to alcoholics to alleviate withdrawal symptoms.

EFFECTS OF ALCOHOL		
BLOOD ALCOHOL mg/100 ml	STAGE OF INFLUENCE	EFFECTS
Under 50	Sobriety	No obvious effect but subject may be more talkative with a sense of well-being.
50–100	Euphoria	Slurred speech, bravado, some loss of concentration and sensory perception.
100–150	Excitement	Emotional instability. Marked loss of concentration. Poor sensory perception.
150–200	Drunkenness	Disorientation, mental confusion and dizziness. Decreased pain sense, impaired balance and slurred speech.
200–300	Stupor	General inertia, approaching paralysis. Marked lack of response to stimuli. Vomiting, incontinence of urine and faeces.
300–450	Coma	Coma and anaesthesia. Depressed or abolished reflexes.
Over 450	Death	Probable death from respiratory paralysis.

Table 5 – Effects of alcohol

Clinical signs of intoxication include slurred speech, suffused conjunctivae, dilated pupils with a sluggish response to light, lateral nystagmus, ataxia and loss of co-ordination, a pulse rate that is both rapid and full, and warm, dry, flushed skin. No one clinical sign is diagnostic of intoxication; a combination of these signs and the overall clinical picture suggests the diagnosis.

ALCOHOL AND CRIME

Drunkenness alone is not a criminal offence, yet being drunk may lead to some public danger, so bringing the offender within the criminal law. The most obvious of these is driving a motor vehicle, which is dealt with elsewhere (see page 225). Other offences include for example, being drunk and incapable, being drunk in charge of a child, and being drunk in charge of a horse-drawn vehicle. In these cases drunkenness is usually diagnosed by a police officer.

Of greater concern than these relatively minor offences is the observed association between alcohol and a variety of other types of crime. Although studies have failed to show a direct causal relationship between alcohol and crime, those working within the criminal justice system all recognise alcohol as a significant problem. The British Medical Association estimates that alcohol is associated with 60 to 70 per cent of homicides (one third of victims being intoxicated at the time of death), 75 per cent of stabbings, 70 per cent of beatings, and 50 per cent of fights or domestic violence (British Medical Association 1989). Figures such as these have led to calls for a more concerted and coherent response to alcohol-related crime (All Party Group on Alcohol Misuse 1995).

ALCOHOL WITHDRAWAL

Many alcoholics develop symptoms of withdrawal when in custody. The severity of the alcohol withdrawal symptoms will depend mainly on the amount and duration of alcohol intake, although other factors, such as concurrent withdrawal from other drugs like benzodiazepines, may contribute to the clinical picture. Withdrawal symptoms have been classified in many different ways, but it is now customary to recognise two distinct clinical presentations.

Uncomplicated alcohol withdrawal. – This is the most frequent and benign type, usually occurring some 12-48 hours after reduction in alcohol intake, although it can begin as early as 6 hours after drinking has stopped. The essential features are a coarse tremor of the hands, tongue and eyelids in association with at least one of the following:

a) nausea and vomiting

b) malaise and weakness

c) autonomic hyperactivity (raised blood pressure, tachycardia and sweating)

d) anxiety, depressed mood and irritability

e) transient hallucinations and illusions

f) headache and insomnia

The severity of these symptoms depends mainly on the degree of the alcohol problem, and they will be seen most commonly in those who have been in custody for over 24 hours. If symptoms are mild it is quite safe to recommend simple observation, but significant tremor and agitation will usually require sedation. The drugs of choice are the benzodiazepines, which will not only treat alcohol withdrawal symptoms but will also prevent later complications. The starting dosages of benzodiazepines depend on the severity of the withdrawal but generally 20 mg of chlordiazepoxide, or 10 mg of diazepam, both given four times a day, will be appropriate. Although chlormethiazole is widely used for the treatment of alcohol withdrawal in a hospital setting, the risk of giving a lethal overdose, particularly when taken in conjunction with alcohol, makes it unsuitable for use in custody.

Alcohol withdrawal delirium. – Traditionally referred to as delirium tremens, this withdrawal state typically begins 72 to 96 hours after the last drink, and so is uncommon within the normal span of detention in police custody. The hallmark is profound disorientation and confusion often accompanied by terrifying hallucinations – usually visual – but any sensory modality can be affected. Manifestations include diarrhoea, dilated pupils, fever, tachycardia and hypertension. The condition is associated with a mortality rate of about 5 per cent, and once diagnosed, the detainee with delirium requires urgent hospitalisation.

Complications of alcohol withdrawal

Several complications of alcohol withdrawal have been recognised and may be encountered in alcoholics held in police custody.

Withdrawal seizures. – Seizures in withdrawal are typically single and generalised. If they occur, they most commonly develop between 6 and 48 hours after drinking has stopped. Contrary to common belief, these seizures are rarely life threatening, their importance being as a prognostic sign of more serious withdrawal complications; about one third of these patients will develop delirium tremens unless preventive measures are taken. For this reason hospitalisation is often appropriate.

Wernicke's encephalopathy. – This is an acute, potentially reversible neurological disorder which is thought to be caused by a deficiency of thiamine and is often secondary to chronic alcohol abuse. Features include disturbance of consciousness (ranging from mild confusion to coma), ophthalmoplegia, nystagmus and ataxia. The disorder has a high mortality and can lead to death within 24 hours. If untreated it can progress to a more chronic condition known as Korsakoff's psychosis.

Korsakoff's psychosis. – This usually presents as impairment of short-term memory with inability to learn new information and compensatory confabulation.

Alcoholic hallucinosis. – This is a feature of severe alcoholism and results in vivid and persistent hallucinations developing shortly (usually within 48 hours) after cessation of or reduction in alcohol intake. The hallucinations may be auditory or visual and their content is usually unpleasant and disturbing. The disorder may last several weeks or months and the experience is quite different from the fleeting and disorganised hallucinations that occur with uncomplicated alcohol withdrawal and delirium tremens.

Cardiac dysrhythmias. – The frequency of tachyrhythmias in alcohol withdrawal is high, probably because of high adrenergic nervous system activity. Sudden deaths in alcohol withdrawal are most likely due to such dysrhythmias. Adequate sedation will play a part in preventing such unwanted occurrences happening in police custody.

References

All Party Group on Alcohol Misuse 1995 *Alcohol and Crime: Breaking the Link*. Alcohol Concern, London.

British Medical Association 1994 *Guidelines for Doctors asked to Perform Intimate Body Searches*. BMA, London.

British Medical Association 1989 *Alcohol & Accidents*. BMA, London.

Home Office 1994 *Drug Misusers and the Criminal Justice System Part II Police Drug Misusers and the Community Report by the Advisory Council on the Misuse of Drugs*. HMSO, London.

Misuse of Drugs (Notification and Supply to Addicts) Regulations 1973.

Royal College of Psychiatrists 1987 *Drug Scenes*. A Report on Drugs and Drug Dependence by the Royal College of Psychiatrists, London.

Stark MM 1994 Management of drug misusers in police custody. *Journal of the Royal Society of Medicine* **87:**584-587.

Tackling Drugs Together - A Strategy for England 1995-98. 1995 HMSO, London.

Further reading

British Medical Association 1954 *The Recognition of Intoxication*. BMA, London.

Chick J, Cantwell (Eds) 1994 Seminars in Alcohol and Drug Misuse. Royal College of Psychiatrists, London.

Department of Health, Scottish Office Home and Health Department, Welsh Office 1991 Substance Misuse Detainees in Police Custody – Guidelines on Clinical Management. HMSO, London.

Department of Health, Scottish Office Home and Health Department, Welsh Office 1994 Subatance Misuse and Detainees in Police Custody – Guidelines for Clinical Management. HMSO, London.

Ghodse H. 1995 *Drugs and Addictive Behaviour – A Guide to Treatment*. Blackwell Science

Institute for the Study of Drug Dependence 1993 *Drug Notes Series*. ISDD, London.

Paton A. (Ed) 1994 *ABC of Alcohol*. BMJ Publishing Group, London

Wallis HJ, Brownlie AR 1985 *Drink, Drugs & Driving*. Sweet & Maxwell, London.

10

PSYCHIATRIC DISORDER

V Evans, J Baird

INTRODUCTION

The psychiatric conditions found in people who have been taken into police custody are no different from those which may be present within the general population. This is an obvious statement, because detainees are merely members of the public, but it is intended to emphasise that the clinical assessment should, wherever possible, be as it would be elsewhere in a more normal setting. It is the range of options thereafter and the recommendations which can be made which differ from practice in the community and it is at this stage that criminal justice considerations arise and have to be taken into account.

As in every other area of clinical forensic medicine, it is of paramount importance to keep clear, comprehensive, legible, contemporaneous notes.

Clinical assessment includes an interview and an examination of the mental state, together with an attempt to gather such background information as may be readily available and required. In addition, the circumstance of the arrest may include details of clinical relevance, and previous convictions may also be helpful in showing a pattern of deteriorating social functioning or a previous psychiatric disposal. A relative or friend may act as an informant.

A police cell is not always an easy place in which to make a precise diagnosis, except when a condition is very florid. When examining a detainee, the task is not necessarily to make a precise diagnosis, but rather to determine those cases where a committal to hospital should be arranged and in certain circumstances those cases in which the person is not fit for interview. As a result of recommendations made in the Reed Report (1992) in England and Wales, referral to a locally based Mentally Disordered Offenders Panel or its equivalent may need to be considered and police surgeons should be familiar with the schemes operating in their area.

An abnormal mental state may be due to a functional psychosis, to substance misuse, to an abnormal metabolic state such as hypoglycaemia, or it may be due to other less common problems such as learning disability, organic brain disease or head injury. In many cases, when the mental state appears abnormal the effects of stress, anxiety, fear or anger may coexist with intoxication of some kind, and assessment can be difficult because behaviour may be bizarre. Further difficulty in assessment may result from some of the extreme effects of intoxication following ingestion of certain illicit drugs such as hallucinogenics and stimulants. This is dealt with in chapter 9.

As in other branches of medicine, the police surgeon should be alert to the unusual or less obvious presentation of mental disorder. This may range from the elderly person with dementia found wandering along the motorway to the shoplifter with undiagnosed depression.

The bulk of mental state assessments carried out by a police surgeon will not be in response to requests for specific assessment under the provisions of the Mental Health Acts but as an integral part of their routine assessment of Fitness to Detain or Interview. Whenever previously unsuspected mental illness or learning disability is diagnosed or suspected this should be drawn to the attention of the custody officer so that this can be given due consideration.

EXAMINATION OF THE MENTAL STATE

This is the central activity in assessment and without it a valid opinion cannot be expressed. Information from all other sources, although important, is supportive.

In examining the mental state every aspect of the person's behaviour, demeanour and appearance while in the presence of the clinician should be observed. The more consistent the clinician is in style and approach, the more significant are any variations on the part of the detainee. The clinician's own reactions towards the detainee, whether they be sympathy, apprehension, confusion, despondency or attraction should also be noted objectively.

The general arrangements for the interview should be as clinical as possible. The detainee and the doctor should both be seated. Careful consideration should be given in each case to the presence of a police officer in the examination room, but in any case it is prudent to ask an officer to wait outside the door or nearby.

A professional and clinical approach is often very effective in calming an agitated, fearful or aggressive detainee; in all circumstances the interview should begin with an introduction by the doctor and a brief explanation as to what will happen and why. Thereafter, personal details should be checked, an account of recent circumstances and details concerning previous treatment, substance misuse, previous offending and anything else of relevance noted. The underlying purpose is to gain some knowledge of who the person is, where he is from, how he has been living and whether there has been contact with mental health services. During the course of this structured interview, which need last no more than a few minutes, the doctor will simultaneously have been observing the appearance, speech pattern and mood of the detainee, together with the form and content of his thinking. Some initial impression of intelligence will also have been gained from his use of vocabulary and capacity for self expression. Specific questions can be asked at a later stage about perceptual disorders, if there seems any reason to do so. An enquiry can be made in the form, 'Sometimes, when people are under pressure or feel unwell, they are troubled by noises or voices which seem strange or unpleasant; has this ever happened to you?' When there is doubt about orientation, simple questions can be asked; when there is doubt about intellectual level or literacy simple mental arithmetic, particularly subtraction involving a one digit number taken away from a two digit number, can be used as a test and a simple test of reading can also be given. Adult illiteracy is more common than learning disability and detainees who are illiterate may try to conceal that fact through shame or embarrassment. By the end of the examination, the doctor should have a view of the degree of mental disorder, if any, which is present.

CLINICAL SYNDROMES

Functional psychosis (schizophrenia or manic depressive psychosis) is the most common and the most important mental disorder which will be encountered in detainees who exhibit major mental disorder. Symptoms may be either positive or negative. Positive psychotic symptoms, be they hallucination, disorder of the form or content of thought, or primary abnormality of mood, are all features which are alien to normal human experience. None of us throughout our lives could expect to experience the sensation of hearing voices inside our head talking about us. None of us can expect to form the fixed unshakeable belief that other people can hear what we are thinking and can insert thoughts into our head. None of us can expect to have the experience of our thought process suddenly stopping and continuing on a completely different topic in a way which leaves us feeling that our thinking is not under our own control. None of us can expect to feel so despondent that we believe that we are responsible for all the evil in the world or so elated that we want to follow our mission to save everyone in the world because we are the son of God.

All these are merely random examples of positive psychotic symptoms, none of which will always be present, the nature of the abnormality in the mental state varying considerably. Questions should always be sufficiently open to allow the detainee to describe his or her own experience. The only consistent feature is that the psychotic phenomena will be alien to normal experience.

The negative symptoms are the various forms of deficit which are caused by functional psychiatric illness, particularly schizophrenia: loss of drive, energy and ambition together with blunting of personality and judgement. The person can seem shallow, facile and empty or may seem dour, unresponsive and inaccessible.

The pattern of mental illness will often show itself in a person's life history; when attempting to determine whether or not a person is ill, it should be remembered that illness begins at a certain time, and that the effect of mental illness is very often the cause not only of a deterioration in a person's behaviour but also the cause of a marked social decline. A story of having led an uneventful life during school years and having been in employment until the late teens or early 20's, which is the age when schizophrenia often develops, declining socially, losing contact with family and drifting, should raise suspicions of mental illness. This is particularly so if the person himself does not appear to be aware of the significance of the marked social slide.

While many patients with mental illness use that diagnostic term about themselves and use clinical terms to describe their symptoms, others never gain insight nor use such terminology.

Schizophrenia usually develops in early adult life and while some patients make a full recovery, others never do; after an acute episode of illness they are left with life long negative features such as lack of volition, apathy, impaired judgement and a rather shallow personality. Paranoid schizophrenia develops later in life and symptoms can remain encapsulated without the same global deterioration.

Manic depressive illness is characterised by recurrent episodes of illness where the predominant abnormality is an abnormality of mood, either elation or depression.

There are two practical areas in which difficulties can arise and mistakes can be made in forensic practice. Firstly, there is the relationship between substance misuse and mental illness. While it is true that drugs can cause psychotic symptomatology, these tend to be short lived and the history can give a clue to the cause. Very often, while the positive symptomatology including hallucinations and delusions may be present, the negative symptomatology of a mental illness will not be present. It is very important to keep in mind that mentally ill people who have not been adequately treated by mental health services very frequently ingest illicit drugs or alcohol in order to try to gain relief from their distressing mental illness or as part of their deteriorating lifestyle. When the person presents, therefore, there will be the features of illness, but there may also be a history of substance misuse. It is very important to take a careful history and not to dismiss such individuals as having 'merely' a drug or alcohol problem.

Secondly, there is the matter of simulation - the belief that a detainee may pretend to be ill when he is not. This is much less common than is sometimes believed.

Certain mentally disordered people who are "hard to like" and demanding, or who are inconsistent in their symptoms may be suspected of malingering and simulating. As in other branches of medicine, the manner in which an ill person behaves is a product not just of the illness but also of his underlying personality and the kind of person he is. Patients can distort or exaggerate their symptoms, but true simulation is very uncommon. Acceptance of the latter as the explanation of the positive signs and symptoms in a detainee should only be considered with great caution and after very careful assessment over a lengthy period.

It is in the matter of disposal that criminal justice factors must be considered. Illness on its own does not necessarily require committal to hospital or diversion from the criminal justice system: each case must be considered on its merits. If a hospital bed is required and the detainee is facing serious charges then the bed must be in a hospital which offers adequate security. Each police surgeon should have a working knowledge of the range of services in his own area and how these may be accessed.

Great care should be exercised in determining whether or not a person who is mentally ill or mentally handicapped can be interviewed by the police and/or is fit to be charged. Such persons should only be interviewed if their responses to the interview are not affected by their mental disorder. They must be capable of understanding their rights, including the implications of the caution and their right to request the presence of a lawyer and be able to instruct the latter. In England and Wales, the custody officer should be informed of the presence of any mental disorder so that the attendance of an Appropriate Adult may be secured if this has not already been done. There is no comparable scheme in operation at present in Scotland.

ASSESSMENT OF SUICIDE RISK

This is a crucial part of the police surgeon's task. There will always be some successful suicides in police custody which could not be predicted, but consideration of the following factors in every case should alert the examining doctor to the possibility of suicide risk and hence to the need for extra vigilance on the part of the custody staff or even to the need for admission to hospital.

Such factors include in general: a history of mental illness, alcohol or drug abuse; experience of sexual or child abuse; recent bereavement or relationship break-up; financial problems; previous suicidal behaviour; history of suicide in the family; family pressures; social isolation; and access to lethal means.

Special additional factors pertinent to detention in police custody include the nature of the offence - in particular, offences of violence, sex, arson or a domestic (in its widest possible sense) offence; feelings of guilt; first time in custody; worries about children or other family concerns; withdrawal from drugs or alcohol.

THE MENTAL HEALTH ACT 1983

This legislation applies in England and Wales whether the process is civil or criminal. All police surgeons should have access to a copy of this Act and be familiar with the contents of the Code of Practice published by the Department of Health and the Welsh Office.

It is important to remember that the Act specifically excludes promiscuity or other immoral conduct, sexual deviancy or dependence on alcohol or drugs alone as reasons for compulsory admission under the Act. Where "mental disorder" as defined in the Act is also present the provisions of the Act are applicable.

The sections of the Act most frequently encountered by police surgeons are:

Section 2 (MHA 1983):
Compulsory Admission to Hospital for Assessment
Grounds: That the patient

a) is suffering from a mental disorder of such a nature or degree which warrants the detention of the patient in a hospital for assessment (or for assessment followed by medical treatment) for at least a limited period; *and*

b) ought to be so detained in the interests of his own health or safety or with a view to the protection of other persons.

Recommendations: two medical recommendations – ideally one doctor to be s12 approved (see below) and to have had previous acquaintance with the patient.

Application: Approved Social Worker (ASW) or nearest relative.

Duration: not more than 28 days.

Note: the most commonly used section of the Act.

Section 3 (MHA 1983):
Compulsory Admission to Hospital for Treatment
Grounds: that the patient

a) is suffering from mental illness, severe mental impairment, psychopathic disorder or mental impairment and his mental disorder is of a nature or degree which makes it appropriate for him to receive medical treatment in a hospital; *and*

b) in the case of psychopathic disorder or mental impairment, such treatment is likely to alleviate or prevent a deterioration of his condition; *and*

c) it is necessary for the health or safety of the patient or for the protection of other persons that he should receive such treatment and it cannot be provided unless he is detained under this section.

Recommendations: two medical recommendations – ideally at least one doctor to be s12 approved (see below) and one doctor to have had previous acquaintance with the patient. Usually one of the doctors will be the consultant psychiatrist under whose care the patient is to be admitted.

Application: ASW or nearest relative. If the nearest relative objects, the application cannot proceed.

Duration: a period not exceeding 6 months in the first instance.

Note: this Section of the MHA 1983 is more rarely used by police surgeons. Usually the patient will have been in hospital where a firm diagnosis has been made: subsequent non-compliance with treatment has then led to relapse.

Section 4 (MHA 1983):

Compulsory Admission for Assessment in an Emergency

Grounds:

a) as for section 2; *and*

b) the matter is of urgent necessity and there is not enough time to get a second medical recommendation. To be satisfied that an emergency has arisen there must be evidence of:

– the existence of a significant risk of mental or physical harm to the patient or others; *and/or*

– the danger of serious harm to property; *and/or*

– the need for physical restraint of the patient.

Recommendations: one medical recommendation.

Application: approved social worker.

Duration: up to 72 hours.

Note: this should hardly, if ever, be used, and never for "administrative convenience".

Section 136 (MHA 1983):

The police power to remove to a Place of Safety

Grounds: the person whom the constable removes must be in a place to which the public have access and must appear to the constable to be suffering from mental disorder and to be in immediate need of care and control.

Purpose: to enable a mental health assessment as soon as practicable by a doctor and an ASW. Once the assessment is complete, unless the outcome is to arrange compulsory admission under the appropriate section of the MHA, the detainee must be released.

Duration: up to 72 hours.

Note: the extent to which this power is used varies throughout the country. The involvement of the police surgeon in assessments under the provisions of this section largely depends on whether or not the usual place of safety is the police station.

Section 135: MHA 1983

This gives a named police constable authority to enter and search premises specified on a warrant issued by a Justice of the Peace subsequent to information laid on oath by an ASW, in order to remove to a place of safety for assessment where there is reasonable cause to suspect that a person suffering from mental disorder – (a) has been, or is being, ill-treated, neglected, or kept otherwise than under proper control ... or (b) being unable to care for himself, is living alone in any such place.... Such entry is usually undertaken in the presence of the ASW and a doctor.

Duration: maximum 72 hours.

Other provisions of the Act: police surgeon involvement may be sought from time to time – referral to the Act itself and to the Codes of Practice is to be recommended in such instances.

Part III of the Act refers to patients concerned in criminal proceedings or under sentence. Powers under these sections of the Act are usually exercised by the courts or within the prison system and therefore police surgeons will not normally be involved.

Section 12 approval refers to s12(2) of the Act, by which a practitioner may be approved .... by the Secretary of State as having special experience in the diagnosis or treatment of mental disorder ...

At present only a few police surgeons are so approved. However, those with the requisite experience are recommended to apply for approval, as in most areas the majority of acute mental health assessments involve police surgeons.

Summary of options following mental health assessment

These are not mutually exclusive:

1. Where the problem is a social one, refer to Social Services.

2. If organic pathology is suspected, take appropriate remedial action. Consider referral or admission to local district hospital.

3. Voluntary admission to psychiatric facility.

4. Compulsory admission to hospital under the appropriate section of the

Mental Health Act 1983. This must never be undertaken lightly as it may be that the length of detention in hospital is a greater deprivation of liberty than a court could or would impose for the misdemeanour that has brought the offender to police attention.

5. Release of detainee back into the community (i) after assessment under s136 MHA 1983 or (ii) on police bail with referral to Mentally Disordered Offenders Panel (or local equivalent). In all cases due consideration must be given to and, where appropriate arrangements made for, continuity of care in the community setting, be these medical or social or a combination of the two.

6. Where the detainee is considered fit to detain and interview but mental disorder is present or suspected, the involvement of an appropriate adult should be advised in writing.

7. Where a serious offence has been committed, or the local psychiatric facility has refused the patient admission because of a diagnosis of personality disorder or psychopathy, several questions need to be answered:

a) is the patient's psychiatric state so bad that it puts him or others at risk and he cannot be managed in police custody? - consider admission to a Regional Secure Unit. This is usually a lengthy business and will involve initial assessment as for s2 MHA 1983, involving the district psychiatric team, before making an emergency request for assessment by the duty forensic psychiatrist and his team.

b) can the patient be safely managed in police custody and is he fit to go before the court? If the answer is "yes", then the best course is to let the court make an appropriate disposal. Sometimes it is helpful to the court in their deliberations with regard to this initial disposal to have a short hand-written report from the doctor stating his opinion.

ARRANGEMENTS IN SCOTLAND

The clinical problems encountered by police surgeons working in Scotland are, of course, exactly the same as in England and Wales, but there are certain differences in practice which arise for one of two reasons. Firstly, legislation differs and, secondly, the organisation of services is affected by the relatively greater number of hospital beds in Scotland at the present time and that, since the country is smaller, it is more likely that professionals from different disciplines will know one another. It is less likely, therefore, that mentally disordered offenders will get 'lost in the system'. Transfer from prison both before and after conviction is easier to arrange than in England and Wales and a mentally disordered offender who has not been diverted to a hospital by a police surgeon could still be admitted to a hospital from prison not long thereafter, were this deemed necessary.

The legislation which applies to mentally disordered offenders in Scotland is the Mental Health (Scotland) Act 1984 and the Criminal Procedure (Scotland) Act 1975. The Notes for Guidance prepared by the Scottish Office and the Code of Practice prepared by the Mental Welfare Commission for Scotland are also commended. In 1996, the Criminal Procedure (Scotland) Act 1995 replaced the 1975 Act.

The most frequently encountered sections are as follows:

Section 24 MH(S)A 1984:

Emergency Committal to Hospital

All that is required is for any registered medical practitioner to confirm that he has examined the patient that day, that the patient suffers from a mental disorder and that it is urgently necessary for the patient's own protection or for the protection of others that he be admitted to hospital. The consent of a relative or an approved social worker should be obtained whenever possible; if this is not possible, the reasons for not obtaining consent should be stated, whereupon the certificate will nevertheless be valid. A bed must be obtained in the patient's catchment area hospital and once he is admitted he may be detained for up to 72 hours. In Scotland this is the most frequently used provision for compulsory admission. It may be used from a police station if a person has been conveyed there but is not to be charged.

Section 117 MH(S)A 1984:

This gives authority to a mental health officer (that is, an approved social worker) to request entry to any premises where there are reasonable grounds for believing that a person within, who is suffering from mental disorder, is either being ill-treated or neglected in some way or being unable to care for himself is either living alone or is uncared for. If entry is refused, a court may give a named police officer authority to use force, if necessary to gain entry, and to remove, if it seems proper to do so, the mentally disordered person and convey him or her to hospital for detention for up to 72 hours.

Section 118 MH(S)A 1984:

This permits a constable who finds in a public place a person who appears to him to be suffering from mental disorder and to be in need of care or control, to be removed by the officer to a hospital where he may be detained for up to 72 hours. The use of this provision in Scotland varies considerably from area to area, the pattern largely being determined by the willingness of different hospitals to accept patients brought by the police in this way.

Section 52 CP(S)A 1995:

Under this section, remand orders are made by a court when a person has been charged with an offence and is appearing in court on the first or second occasion. The remand to hospital can be made by the court on the basis of a written statement by a medical practitioner that the accused person appears to be suffering from mental disorder and that a hospital is available for his admission and is suitable for his detention. In practice, either the police surgeon or, more frequently now, an on-call psychiatrist examines the accused person and provides a short hand-written report for the court. The availability of an on-call psychiatry service to police cells and the court varies from one part of Scotland to the next. When the charges are serious or potentially serious, admission to a psychiatric hospital should be arranged by a psychiatrist who has examined the patient himself.

★   ★   ★   ★   ★

Many accused persons who are remanded in custody return to court after seven days; in the intervening period, if mental disorder could be present, they will have been examined by a psychiatrist at the request of the procurator fiscal. The role of the police surgeon in the remand process tends to be confined to persons facing less serious charges in areas where no on-call psychiatrist is available to attend at a police station.

MENS REA, THE M'NAGHTEN RULES AND DIMINISHED RESPONSIBILITY

It is useful to have some knowledge of these legal concepts. A crime is considered to have two components: the actus reus (guilty act) and the mens rea (the state of mind required for the crime to have been committed). If either is missing no crime has been committed. Rarely, there may be cases where, on the basis of the evidence, it appears that persons did commit a crime, but at the time of doing so, their actions were not under their control: that is, mens rea was absent. This could arise in the post-ictal state, with the person in a state of automatism.

The case of Daniel M'Naghten is now largely of historical interest. In 1843, Daniel M'Naghten attempted to assassinate the then prime minister, Sir Robert Peel, killing by mistake the prime minister's private secretary. Very detailed psychiatric evidence presented at his trial showed that, at the time of the offence, he was suffering from a paranoid psychosis and acting on delusional beliefs. As a result, he was acquitted on the grounds of insanity and committed for the rest of his life to a psychiatric hospital. There followed a preparation of guidelines by the judges of the day which have become known as the M'Naghten rules.

In summary, they state that every man is assumed to be sane until proved otherwise. Even insanity on its own does not excuse a man from punishment, but it is only if he did not know the nature and quality of the act which he was doing or if he did not know that what he was doing was wrong that he could be acquitted. These are very rigorous tests and could exclude even those very severely ill if their disorder of thinking is either not accessible or is unstable and liable to constant change.

Diminished responsibility applies only when a person faces a charge of murder. In such cases, if a court is satisfied, after considering psychiatric evidence, that the person was of diminished responsibility at the time of the offence, the charge of manslaughter (culpable homicide in Scotland) is substituted for that of murder. The basis on which a psychiatrist, after careful assessment, would form an opinion that a defendant was of diminished responsibility would be reasonable grounds for believing that, at the time of the offence, the person was suffering from a mental disorder which was of a nature (although not necessarily of a degree) which could have warranted compulsory detention in a hospital in terms of civil mental health legislation. The effect of this difference is that whereas in the case of a person convicted of murder the court has no discretion in terms of sentence and the sentence of life imprisonment must be imposed, the court has wide discretion in the sentencing of a person convicted of manslaughter.

Further reading

Code of Practice: Mental Health Act 1983. London: HMSO 1993 and the Act itself.

Codes of Practice: Police and Criminal Evidence Act 1984. London: HMSO 1995.

Bluglass RS, Bowden P (Eds) 1990 *Principles of Forensic Psychiatry* Edinburgh: Churchill Livingstone.

Chiswick, Cope (Ed) 1995 *Seminars in Forensic Psychiatry* London: Gaskell.

Katia Herbst K, Gunn J (Ed) 1991 *The Mentally Disordered Offender* ed. London: Butterworth Heinemann 1991 Sections 1, 2, 5 and 6.

Mental Health (Scotland) Act 1984. *Notes on the Act* and *Code of Practice*. HMSO Scotland.

Review of health and social services for mentally disordered offenders and other requiring similar services. London: HMSO 1992 Cm 2088 (The Reed Report).

11

ADULT SEXUAL OFFENCES AND RELATED MATTERS

J Howitt, D Rogers

INTRODUCTION

Sexual offences constitute 10% of reported violent crime in England and Wales (Home Office 1995). The forensic medical examiner plays a fundamental role in their investigation. The first, and major, part of this chapter is designed to guide doctors through the complex forensic assessment of an adult sexual offence and to help them with the interpretation of the medical findings. The second part of the chapter deals with the medico-legal aspects of pregnancy and sexual variations.

DEFINITIONS

Rape

Under English law 'A man commits rape if he has sexual intercourse with another person (whether vaginal or anal) who at the time of the intercourse does not consent to it, and at the time he knows that the person does not consent to the intercourse or is reckless as to whether that person consents to it' (Sexual Offences Act [SOA] 1956 as amended by the Criminal Justice and Public Order Act [CJPOA] 1994). The SOA 1956 also states that '...intercourse shall be deemed complete upon *proof of penetration* only' and there is no requirement '...to prove completion of the intercourse by the emission of seed...'. Case law has determined that if the penis was 'within the labia...(no matter how little) ...that will be sufficient to constitute a penetration' (*Lines* 1844 1.C. and K. 393). In Scotland, rape is a crime at common law. It consists of the carnal knowledge of a female by a male against her will.

Buggery

Buggery is traditionally interpreted as anal intercourse but it also relates to vaginal intercourse, by a woman or a man, with an animal. Buggery between two males, or a man and woman, with consent is not an offence if both parties have reached 18 years of age and the act takes place in private. If buggery occurs without consent a rape will have been committed (SOA 1956 as amended by CJPOA 1994). In Scotland, the term *sodomy* is used.

Gross indecency between males

The SOA 1956 (as amended by the Sexual Offences Act 1967 and CJPOA 1994) says that 'It is an offence for a man to commit an act of gross indecency with another man...'. This offence does not apply if the acts are conducted in private between only two males who have reached 18 years of age. 'Gross indecency' is not defined but the charge will usually relate to acts of masturbation and oral-genital contact although it is not necessary for there to have been contact between the individuals (Smith & Hogan 1988).

Indecent assault

English law simply states that it is an offence '...for a person to make an indecent assault on a woman (or a man)' (SOA 1956). The law has not attempted to define what constitutes 'indecency' and cases rest on whether the event appears indecent to the reasonable observer; again there need not be contact between the involved parties (Smith & Hogan 1988).

Indecent exposure

Indecent exposure is defined under the Vagrancy Act 1824 in which it states '...every person wilfully, openly, lewdly and obscenely exposing his person with intent to insult any female...shall be deemed a rogue and vagabond...'. As case law has determined the term 'person' in this context to mean penis (*Evans v Ewels* 1972 2 All ER 22 1 WLR 671) the exposure of any other part of a man's body (for example, his bottom) does not amount to an indecent exposure. Whatever parts of her body a female chooses to expose, albeit with intent to insult, she cannot be charged with indecent exposure under this act but she could be guilty of an offence at common law.

The complainant (complainer in Scotland)

The complainant is usually the person alleging that a crime has taken place although crimes can be reported by a third party. Not all allegations of sexual assault will come to the attention of the police. Complainants, who may be male or female, should, when possible, be able to choose the sex of the doctor called to examine them. In this chapter, the complainant will be referred to by the female pronoun.

The examining doctor

In order to give a valid interpretation of the medical findings in complainants of sexual assault, the examining doctor needs to be experienced in general clinical forensic medicine and should also be familiar with the range of normal genital and anal findings among the adult population.

Calls to these cases should be dealt with expeditiously to avoid loss of forensic evidence. Furthermore, delay is likely to add to the distress of the complainant. Such patients must be handled sympathetically and should never be made to feel that their complaint has been doubted, however implausible the allegation.

Clear and comprehensive contemporary notes are essential. Information obtained should be recorded immediately (or as soon as practically possible during the physical phase of the examination). Subsequent to the examination, the doctor will be required to provide a clear and detailed statement containing interpretation of any injuries (and other findings) and to present that evidence in court. It should always be remembered that the doctor's original notes may be demanded by a judge in open court and may be seen by other medical witnesses. Doctors must remain unbiased and independent during the examination and in the presentation of their evidence.

Police chaperone (Victim Liaison Officer)

When a complaint of serious sexual assault is reported to the police, in most police areas in the United Kingdom, a specially trained police officer (ideally of the same sex) will be allocated to the case. This officer's main role is to befriend the complainant and take a detailed statement (usually deferred for at least 12 hours after the incident). In addition, the chaperone can undertake a number of other tasks to improve the comfort of the complainant and facilitate the examination. These include:

Before the examination:
- Arrange a change of clothing
- Obtain saliva, urine samples and mouth swabs (as their exhibits[1])
- Summarise the allegation for the examining doctor

During the examination:
- Collect (as their exhibits) significant clothing and the paper sheet on which the complainant has stood during examination[2]
- Chaperone and assist the examining doctor

---

1. See 'Labelling' on page 269.
2. In some areas these are functions of the Scenes of Crime Officer (SOCO).

After the examination:

    – Assist the doctor in the labelling and sealing of forensic exhibits[2]

    – Transport all forensic exhibits[2]

    – Organise follow-up appointments

EXAMINATION FACILITIES

The health and immediate medical needs of the complainant should always be considered paramount; any urgent medical treatment must be given priority over any forensic examination. Ill and severely injured patients requiring hospitalisation can only be forensically examined after permission has been given by the responsible hospital doctor.

Most of these examinations will take place in specifically designated and equipped examination suites (see chapter 4). To prevent later allegations of cross contamination, it is vital to avoid all possible contact between complainant and the alleged assailant. Therefore, they should not be examined at the same venue nor by the same doctor. If this proves impossible, the doctor is advised to change clothing and clean the room between each examination. However, even with these precautions, allegations of cross-contamination would be difficult to refute.

HISTORY OF THE ALLEGATION

The history of the allegation is necessary to direct the medical examination and to identify which samples will be required. Details should be obtained, in private, from the chaperone (record name in notes) before the examination commences. This saves the patient having to recount the whole incident. Usually, only specific questions will need to be asked of the examinee to clarify the account and to help direct sample taking; for instance, were you kissed and, if so, where?

When information is requested of the complainant the doctor should record the actual responses made as accurately as possible, verbatim ideally, otherwise discrepancies between the doctor's record and the complainant's subsequent statement may be used to discredit the witness in court.

The information in table 1 should be carefully recorded, when applicable.

FORENSIC EXHIBITS

A sexual examination kit containing all the necessary sample bottles, swabs, exhibit bags, should be provided by the police (or SOCO). After consideration of the history of the incident, the doctor should decide what samples will be necessary and prepare for these in advance to avoid confusion during the examination (table 2).

THE INCIDENT

- Date / time period
- Location: inside / outside (weather wet / dry)
- Number of alleged assailants
- Drugs / alcohol involved with details
- Restraints / weapons and their use
- Injuries sustained by complainant (when, how and where on body)
- Injuries sustained by assailant(s) (e.g. was assailant scratched by complainant)
- Type and number of sexual act(s) / use of condoms / lubricants
- Relative positions during sexual acts
- Site(s) of ejaculation / kissing / sucking / licking / biting
- Bleeding per vaginum or anum: due to injury / menstruation
- Use and disposal of sanitary pads / tampons

SUBSEQUENT TO THE INCIDENT

Relevant to all recent allegations
- Manner of leaving the scene and resulting injuries
- Changed / washed clothing
- Bathed / showered
- Washed / brushed / combed hair
- Alcohol / drugs taken
- Medical treatment received

RELEVANT TO ALLEGATIONS OF ORAL INTERCOURSE

- Cleaned teeth / rinsed mouth
- Drank any fluid / ate food

RELEVANT TO ALLEGATIONS OF VAGINAL INTERCOURSE

- Consensual vaginal intercourse
- Contraception (particularly condoms) used
- Lubricants used
- Douched
- Vaginal bleeding / pain

RELEVANT TO ALLEGATIONS OF ANAL INTERCOURSE

- Consensual anal and/or vaginal intercourse
- Protection (condoms) used
- Lubricants used
- Anal bleeding / pain
- Bowel action

Table 1 – Details of allegation

Table 2

EXHIBIT	REASON FOR ANALYSIS	METHOD OF SAMPLING	PACKAGING / STORAGE
Hair	A – Comparison with other hairs***	A – 10 hairs cut close to roots from different locations on the head	Polythene Bag Refrigerate / Freeze*
	B – Analysis for spermatozoa, lubricants etc.	B – Cut hairs matted by secretion	Polythene Bag Refrigerate / Freeze*
	C – To identify foreign hairs and particles	C – Comb with standard or special comb ** if fine particles sought e.g. Balaclava was used	Polythene Bag Refrigerate / Freeze*
	D – DNA from hair root*** (not pubic)	D – 10-15 hairs plucked individually with fingers to preserve roots.	Polythene Bag Refrigerate / Freeze*
Saliva	Spermatozoa if oral penetration/ ejaculation	10 ml of saliva	Bottle / Freeze
Mouth swab	A – Spermatozoa	A – Rub around inside mouth, under tongue and gum margins (patient to use like toothbrush)	Plain swab no transport medium / Freeze
	B – DNA from buccal cells.	B – Rub firmly over buccal mucosa	Plain swab no transport medium / Freeze
Skin swab	e.g. possible saliva, lubricant, semen, blood, faeces	If stain moist, dry swab If stain dry, dampen swab with tap/distilled water*	Plain swab no transport medium / Freeze
Blood plain preservative-EDTA*	Blood grouping & DNA profile	5-10 ml* venous blood Antecubital fossa (ACF)	Bottle Refrigerate / Freeze*
Blood preservative- Na fluoride & K oxalate	Quantitative analysis for drugs and alcohol	5-10 ml* venous from ACF (if solvents suspected fill to top of bottle)	Bottle / Refrigerate
Urine preservative- Na fluoride	Quantitative analysis for drugs and alcohol	Passed into container first if necessary complainant sample does not need to be witnessed	Bottle / Refrigerate
Fingernails	If circumstances suggest trace evidence possible/ if fingernail broken at scene	Cut for debris and comparison/ scrapings for debris if nails very short	Polythene bag / Refrigerate

EXHIBIT	REASON FOR ANALYSIS	METHOD OF SAMPLING	PACKAGING / STORAGE
Sanitary towels / Tampons	If in situ during or worn after vaginal intercourse		Polythene bag / Freeze
Condoms	If used during intercourse	Secure end with freezer-clip or knot	Polythene bag / Freeze
Paper sheet***	To identify foreign particles	Stand examinee on this whilst undressing	Polythene bag / Cool room
Vulval swab	Vaginal intercourse / Cunnilingus ejaculation on perineum/ Lubricant	Rub dry swab over whole of vulval area	Plain swab no transport medium / Freeze
Low Internal Vaginal swab***	Vaginal intercourse/ Lubricant	Insert dry swab into low vagina	Plain swab no transport medium / Freeze
2 High Internal Vaginal swabs	Vaginal / Anal intercourse/ Lubricant	Taken using unlubricated speculum or sheathed swab	Plain swab no transport medium / Freeze
Endocervical swab	If vaginal intercourse more 48 hours before the examination	Taken using unlubricated speculum	Plain swab no transport medium / Freeze
Penile swab	Fellatio / Vaginal intercourse/ Anal intercourse / Lubricant	1 Swab shaft of penis and 2 Swab coronal sulcus & glans	Plain swab no transport medium / Freeze
External anal swab	Anal intercourse / Analingus/ Lubricant	Swab anal margin and surrounding skin	Plain swab no transport medium / Freeze
Internal Anal / Rectal swab	Anal intercourse / Analingus/ Lubricant	Take by passing an unlubricated proctoscope 1-2 cm into anal canal	Plain swab no transport medium / Freeze
Control Swab*	Requirement of some areas***	Uncontaminated skin swab / tap water swab/unused swab*	Plain swab no transport medium / Refrigerate
Foreign Matter	Identified on body	Remove whilst gloved or end of a swab on the	Polythene bag / Refrigerate

*Dependant on local lab. requirements   ** Available from SOCO   *** Not routine requirement from complainant in Metropolitan area

Table 2 *continued*

Doctors should not take any sample which they consider inappropriate since they may have to justify their actions in court. Furthermore, the examination should not be more intrusive than necessary. On occasions the complainant will have no recall of a particular incident or be reticent in describing exactly what happened (particularly the sexual acts). In these circumstances it may be appropriate to obtain samples from all body orifices, otherwise the opportunity for retrieval of significant forensic evidence is lost. Saliva and mouth swabs must be collected in all cases where fellatio (with or without ejaculation) is alleged; spermatozoa may persist up to 36 hours in the oral cavity even after drinking (Keating & Allard 1994).

Debris or foreign matter located anywhere on the body, including within an injury, should be collected as an exhibit. If stains on body surfaces are dry, the swab may be dampened with water (tap or distilled according to local laboratory requirements). Dry swabs are sufficient for moist areas. Swabs must be taken from any body surface or orifice which has been licked, kissed, bitten, sucked, ejaculated on or penetrated by a penis. The doctor (or chaperone) should also collect and exhibit sanitary towels or tampons in situ during or used after

---

ORAL INTERCOURSE

- Local oral disease e.g. gingivitis / herpes simplex
- Relevant systemic disease e.g. AIDS
- Medication: topical / systemic
- Oral surgery
- Recent dental intervention
- Last act of oral intercourse

VAGINAL INTERCOURSE

- Local disease e.g. vulvitis / discharge / lichen sclerosus
- Relevant systemic disease e.g. thyrotoxicosis
- Medication: topical / systemic
- Genital surgery
- Menstrual history / L.M.P / intermenstrual bleeding
- Tampon use (only relevant to sexually inexperienced)
- Obstetric history / current pregnancy
- Normal contraceptive practice
- Last act of vaginal sexual intercourse: lubricant or condom used

ANAL INTERCOURSE

- Local disease e.g. haemorrhoids / neoplasms
- Relevant systemic disease e.g. blood dyscrasias / neurological disturbance
- Medication: topical / systemic
- Ano-rectal surgery
- Normal bowel habit / last bowel action
- Previous experience of anal intercourse
- Last act of anal intercourse: lubricant or condom used

Table 3 – Medical history relevant to alleged incident

the incident. Before completion of the examination the doctor should always check that the necessary samples have been taken. The samples taken are the responsibility of the doctor who must ensure that they have been properly timed, bagged, labelled, signed, sealed and given the correct exhibit numbers (see chapter 13). It is important to document all relevant history on the appropriate laboratory form (which accompanies the samples) to assist in the interpretation of the forensic evidence. To ensure confirmation of security and continuity, samples are handed to the chaperone (another police officer or SOCO) who should sign each exhibit. The doctor must record to whom the exhibits were handed and may choose to obtain a (timed) signature on the original notes.

CONSENT

Consent for the examination and the obtaining of forensic samples should not be assumed. The process of, and reasons for, the whole examination must be carefully explained to the examinee who should be informed that there is no obligation to consent. Implications of the lack of confidentiality must be addressed, that is to say that information from the examination will be passed to the police and courts (and thereby possibly to the defendant). Only when the doctor is satisfied that the examinee has understood and has freely (without coercion) given permission for the examination (preferably written and witnessed) can informed consent be considered granted (see also chapter 3).

MEDICAL AND SEXUAL HISTORY

The main purpose of obtaining a medical history is to identify any behaviour or conditions which may lead the doctor to misinterpret the physical findings, for example menstrual bleeding. The medical and sexual history may also be relevant in determining contraindications to medication, for example emergency hormonal contraception. It is important to know whether previous sexual intercourse (vaginal or anal) has been experienced and if intercourse has taken place within the two weeks preceding the medical examination, but full details of previous sexual history is inappropriate. Spermatozoa may persist up to 10 days after vaginal intercourse (Wilson 1982) and up to 3 days after anal intercourse (Willott & Allard 1982). The doctor is unable to guarantee confidentiality, therefore only relevant medical history should be requested. This will depend on the sexual assault alleged (table 3).

PHYSICAL EXAMINATION

A sympathetic but professional approach by the doctor is essential. Time taken to establish a rapport before the examination commences gives the complainant the reassurance that the doctor will be understanding and sensitive. The doctor should inquire how the patient is feeling, both emotionally and physically, and to ask her to identify any areas of discomfort so that these can be examined in close detail. The complainant should be allowed to control the pace at which the examination proceeds and be assured that the procedure can be stopped at any time. Respect for the modesty of the examinee is essential. It should never be necessary for the patient to suffer the embarrassment of being naked; she should be covered as the examination progresses by an examination gown or sheet.

Demeanour and mental state

The demeanour and mental state of the patient should be assessed throughout the examination since such information may be required by the court. The use of drugs and/or alcohol may affect behaviour and, therefore, evidence of substance use and intoxication must be noted.

Clothing and jewellery

A note should be made of clothing and jewellery (if worn at the time of the incident) and an appraisal of the state of the clothing (was it torn, stained, wet, worn inside out?) made. Some forensic science laboratories recommend that the complainant undress on a paper sheet in order to collect foreign matter that may fall from the clothing as it is removed. Each item of relevant clothing and the paper sheet are exhibited separately.

General examination

The complainant may be unaware of some injuries resulting from the incident. Therefore, a methodical inspection of every body surface should be performed using a good light source and, where necessary, a magnifying lens. This inspection must include recessed areas such as those behind ears, axillae, breasts, and non-intimate body orifices such as inside lips and mouth, eardrums.

Every significant, or potentially significant, injury or lesion should be recorded precisely, noting shape, colour, degree of swelling, degree of blanching (assessed by digital compression and release), site (related to a fixed bony point), size, and degree of healing (if any). Each injury should be palpated to identify any induration or more severe underlying injury. Body charts or diagrams can be used to record the physical findings. In some instances the patient may indicate an area of discomfort which shows no external signs of trauma. To avoid such findings being dismissed as subjective or hearsay, the doctor is advised to distract the examinee and note facial and motor responses (grimaces, withdrawal) when the area is touched. The doctor may choose to return to the area later in the examination to validate the findings.

The height and weight should be measured, or a subjective assessment made if scales and measuring devices are unavailable. The dominant hand is relevant when considering the possibility that injuries are self-inflicted. Further general examination, perhaps recording blood pressure, may be relevant. The forensic samples can be taken as the examination proceeds. The length of the fingernails should be noted but they will only need to be cut (or, if very short, scraped) if there is visible debris and the complainant believes she scratched her assailant.

Examination of genitalia and anus

The extent of the examination and forensic sampling of these areas should be tailored to the alleged incident. The location of all abnormalities should be recorded with reference to an imaginary clock face represented by 12 o'clock at the mons pubis and 6 o'clock at the coccyx. All areas must be systematically examined, as detailed below, wearing disposable gloves. **To avoid destruction or contamination of evidence it is imperative that all trace evidence be retrieved before any examination is conducted.** The degree of physical sexual maturity should be recorded using Tanner Stages.

Common to all examinations

Position the patient – The lithotomy position (without stirrups) is most appropriate for the examination of female genitalia. Male genitalia are examined with the patient supine. The anal area is usually inspected with the patient in the left lateral position. The position used should be recorded.

Visualise the ano-genital area – The inner thighs and buttocks are carefully inspected for evidence of injury or possible stains. The genital area is then exposed by gently parting the labia or buttocks. Secretions or stains (blood, seminal fluid, faeces, foreign material) should be noted and swabbed specifically.

Pubic hair – Secretions seen amongst the pubic hairs must be cut and exhibited. Combing may reveal foreign bodies or loose hairs which must be exhibited. If control pubic hairs are required these can be cut close to the roots.

FEMALE GENITALIA

Forensic samples

Vulval swab – An external vaginal (in reality a vulval) swab should be taken by rubbing a swab over the labia and vestibule.

Low vaginal swab – A low vaginal swab, obtained by passing the swab into the vagina under direct vision avoiding contact with the external genitalia, is still required in most police areas. However, even when taken very carefully it is difficult to refute the accusation that in taking the swab contamination had been introduced; its value is therefore questionable.

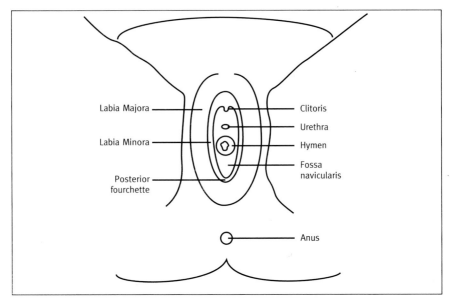

Figure 1 – Female genitalia

Removal of foreign bodies – Accessible tampons should first be removed and exhibited. A speculum of appropriate size is then inserted high into the vagina; this may be moistened only with warm tap or distilled water. No other lubricant should be used because they can interfere with the analysis of some forensic material. Care must be taken to avoid introducing contaminants from lower down in the vagina. When the speculum has been opened remaining vaginal foreign bodies are also carefully removed and exhibited.

High vaginal swab – With the speculum still in place two high vaginal swabs (HVS) should be taken from the vaginal fornices above the speculum avoiding contact with the side or the top of this instrument. HVS must also be taken when only anal intercourse is alleged as, although semen can be found in and around the anus following vaginal intercourse, it is not likely to be found in any significant amount in the high vagina after only anal intercourse (Keating & Allard 1994).

Glass sheathed swabs are sometimes used to obtain the HVS, particularly if a speculum cannot be tolerated. After taking the sample the attached glass sheath should be wiped clean, or air-dried, before both sheath and swab are replaced into the container. This prevents fluid on the outside of the glass sheath running down and contaminating the swab once it is in the container.

Endocervical swabs – If more than 48 hours have passed since the alleged incident one or two endocervical swabs should be taken in addition to the HVS, as spermatozoa remain longer in this area (Wilson 1982).

Inspection of the vagina

Inspection of the vaginal vault and cervix should then take place, facilitated by the speculum. Any evidence of discharge (amount and viscosity), bleeding (with source identified, perhaps the cervical os) and injuries should be recorded.

Inspection of the vulva

Close examination of the labia, clitoris, urethral opening, vestibule and posterior fourchette may now be undertaken, with any injuries or abnormalities noted. The appearance of the hymen (annular, crescentic, septate, remnants only) and the presence of congenital defects or clefts are recorded. The edge of the hymen must be carefully inspected. When the hymen is redundant, or fimbriated, a moistened swab can be used to tease out any folds in the tissue. If transection is identified a note should be made of whether it is complete, that is, extends to the vaginal wall, or incomplete. The degree of healing of the edges of the transection must also be recorded.

Bi-manual examination

Digital pelvic examination is sometimes indicated, after swabs have been taken, to localise pelvic tenderness or prior to prescribing emergency hormonal contraception. On occasions, when vaginal intercourse is alleged but it has not been possible to pass a speculum, a gentle digital assessment of the hymen should be undertaken to determine its elasticity. The dimensions of the hymenal opening are difficult to measure and are poor predictors of previous sexual activity. Parameters such as vaginal rugosity and length are impossible to determine accurately and, in the absence of baseline measurements, cannot be assigned any forensic significance.

MALE GENITALIA

Forensic samples

Penile swab – The skin of the shaft of the penis is rubbed with a swab.

Coronal sulcus – The foreskin (when present) is then retracted and a swab rubbed around the glans and coronal sulcus.

Inspection

Injuries or abnormalities of the foreskin, penile shaft, scrotal sacs or testes must be noted (including evidence of circumcision and vasectomy).

ANAL AREA

Forensic samples

External anal swab – If anal penetration is alleged an external anal swab is taken by rubbing a swab over the anal margin and the adjacent skin.

Internal anal/rectal swab – A disposable proctoscope, lubricated if necessary by warm water, is inserted one or two centimetres (distance passed should be noted) into the anal canal. The proctoscope obdurator is removed and an internal anal swab is taken from beyond the end of the proctoscope, taking care not to contaminate the swab from the sides of the instrument. Alternatively, a glass sheathed swab may be used to obtain this sample (see High Vaginal Swab).

Inspection of the anus and rectum

With the proctoscope still in place, any evidence of injury, blood or discharge within the anus or rectum should be noted and the source identified if possible.

Inspection of the anal margin

Abnormalities, such as gaping, swelling, reddening, lacerations (tears), fissures, warts, discharge, haemorrhoids, scars, thickening of the skin or flattening of the normally puckered anal verge margin must be noted. This is facilitated by using the fingers to stretch the skin gently, thereby smoothing out its folds.

Digital examination

A subjective estimation of the degree of anal tone should be made by digital examination of the anus.

SPECIAL TECHNIQUES

Semen and saliva may fluoresce under low output ultraviolet (UV) light (Wood's light) as may some lesions not apparent to the naked eye, but there are many false negative and positive results. Furthermore, injuries revealed by UV light are difficult to age. However, if the complainant was unconscious during the incident, or reluctant to detail what happened, the use of this light may show up possible semen or saliva, thereby indicating where to take swabs.

When the injuries are numerous or complex the doctor may advise that photographs are obtained. This is essential when there are dental imprints (see chapter 15). The doctor should be present if the genital or anal areas are to be photographed.

Colposcopes, which incorporate a light source and a magnifying lens, are being made more readily available to assist doctors in the assessment of the external genitalia. They also offer the facility of recording the genital findings using an attached video or still camera.

GENERAL INJURIES

The absence of injuries does not negate an allegation of sexual assault. There are many reasons why a complainant is uninjured; which include:

- submission of the victim may be achieved by emotional manipulation, fear of violence or death or by verbal threats;
- the force used, or the resistance offered, is insufficient to produce an injury;
- bruises may not become apparent for 48 hours following the assault and some bruises are never visible externally;
- a delay in reporting the incident will allow minor injuries to fade or heal.

When injuries are sustained, any type or combination of the injuries described in chapter 8 may be identified. Most of the injuries will be minor and will not require first aid, but even minor injuries may be forensically significant. When present, the potential causes of each injury or other finding must be considered, including the possibility that the injuries were self-inflicted or caused accidentally.

Although it is impossible to age an injury accurately, it should be possible for the doctor to form an opinion whether the appearance of the injury is consistent with it having been produced during the incident in the manner alleged, in other words whether the findings are consistent with the allegation made. The commonest extra-genital injuries and their mechanism of production in cases of sexual assault are described briefly below:

Reddening and abrasions

Reddening (blanching erythema) and abrasions are common but non-specific findings. However, features of these injuries may help to corroborate the history of the allegation; for example if the complainant describes being dragged across a surface such as carpet or brick wall, brush abrasions may be identified on the skin and foreign material may be found (which can be removed and exhibited) within an injury which will assist in identifying the location of the incident – in the examples given here, carpet fibre, brick dust.

Bruises

Bruises are also frequently identified. There may be features of the bruise which support the allegation. Bruises may be associated with lacerations when blunt trauma is inflicted close to underlying bone.

Petechial bruises/haemorrhages – In the living, petechial bruises are seen most commonly in two situations. Firstly, due to raised intravenous pressure, as seen, for example, on the face following manual strangulation. Secondly, patterned or diffuse petechial bruises may be identified anywhere on the body following blunt trauma or dragging of the skin which causes the small blood vessels to rupture. If the clothing is pulled over the skin there may be lines of petechiae from the clothing or finger-tips, or if a person falls upon a firm surface diffuse petechiae (which may match the weave of her clothing) may be produced. Patterned petechial bruises can also be caused by ligatures such as rope. In some instances petechiae have been described on the palate following non-consensual fellatio.

Confluent bruises – Bruises can be found anywhere if there has been a struggle between the parties or if the assailant has physically assaulted the complainant. In some instances the location or pattern of the bruising may be particularly significant; for example, clusters of circular or oval bruises, approximately 1cm in diameter which result from being gripped, and parallel (tram-line) bruises caused by stick-like objects such as base-ball bats. The ulnar borders of the arms and hands are the usual site for passive defence injuries produced as the complainant protects her head from blows.

Sucking and dragging the skin into the mouth can produce petechial bruises which may coalesce to form confluent bruises. These so-called 'love bites' are usually located on the neck and breasts but may be found elsewhere on the body (including the face). Aggressive bites may produce patterned bruises, often associated with abrasions and incisions (see chapter 15).

Incisions

Knives are the most common weapons carried by perpetrators of sexual assault although they are often just used as a threat. Minor incised wounds may be identified if the knife has been held against the skin (often seen on the neck) or if the tip of the knife has been used to taunt the complainant. Active defence wounds, caused as the complainant attempts to take the knife, may be found on the palms and the web spaces of the hands. The sharp edges of jewellery can produce minor incisions on the body.

On occasions there may be more serious incised or stab wounds resulting from a physical assault or a bid to escape.

GENITAL AND ANAL FINDINGS

Less than half of all complainants of sexual assault have injuries to the genital and anal areas. It is important for the examining doctor to be familiar with the reasons why injuries may not occur. These include:

- the alleged sexual act (such as rubbing, touching) was unlikely to result in injuries;

- sexually experienced;
- the natural elasticity of the post-pubertal female genitalia, including the hymen;
- the natural elasticity of the anus;
- the use of lubricants.

Any of the injuries detailed below may be identified following a sexual assault, although their precise forensic significance is limited by the lack of specific research into their relative prevalence following consensual and non-consensual intercourse. Some of the findings may have alternative non-sexual causes with which the doctor must be cognisant.

a) *Reddening* of the vulva, penis or anal margins, whether diffuse or localised, is a non-specific finding with a vast range of causative factors including consensual sexual intercourse. While it should be noted it cannot be assigned any forensic significance.

b) *Small lacerations or tears* (normally a few millimetres in length) of the vulva, foreskin, frenulum and anal margins may be produced by excessive stretching of the skin, with or without blunt impact trauma, or be related to general medical conditions, for example anal fissures in Crohn's disease. In the vulval area they are most commonly identified in the regions of the posterior fourchette and fossa navicularis. When located on the anal margin they are called 'fissures'. The lacerations may be single or multiple. They are seen more frequently when the skin is already inflamed or scarred, as around episiotomy scars.

These minor lacerations usually heal completely but if deep, or repeatedly traumatised, they may leave scarring, for example around the anal margin (although these may be concealed by the anal folds). Anal tags are said to be formed where anal fissures have healed. It is important not to confuse congenital variations, such as a linea vestibularis in the fossa navicularis, with scars.

c) *Genital or anal bruising* is indicative of trauma to that area if the skin is otherwise healthy. The pattern of the bruising may be very significant, for example when caused by teeth or blunt trauma through clothing. Bruising of the anal skin can be differentiated from prominent anal margin veins as the latter reduce if compressed.

d) *Abrasions* on the female genitalia (vulva, hymen and vagina), penis and anal margin are produced by the dragging of the skin or contact with rough objects such as fingernails.

e) *Incisions* on the genital or anal skin or mucosa are forensically significant as they are indicative of contact with sharp objects like jewellery. Incisions of the penile skin can be associated with sadomasochistic sexual gratification.

f) *Hymenal transections*. Fresh transections (lacerations, tears) of the hymen may be complete or incomplete depending on the original size of the hymenal opening, the size of the penetrating object and the elasticity of the tissues. When fresh, the edges of the transection may bleed but healing in this area is remarkably rapid. The presence of chronic or healed transections may be relevant if the extent of previous sexual activity is questioned. Significant transections of the hymen are usually located in the posterior half (3 o'clock to 9 o'clock). Transections of the posterior edge have been identified in post-pubertal females who deny sexual activity, but are seen much less frequently than amongst those who admit sexual activity (Emans *et al* 1994).

g) *Vaginal lacerations*. Lacerations within the vagina are rare findings, most commonly identified at the fornices. They are seen infrequently following consensual intercourse when there may be predisposing factors such as vaginal surgery or atrophic tissues (Smith *et al* 1983). Some lacerations will bleed extensively, requiring resuscitation and surgical intervention. It is extremely difficult to differentiate a laceration of the vagina from an incised wound as many of the features typically seen in a lacerated wound are difficult to identify in this area. Therefore, the differential diagnosis of a vaginal laceration would have to include causation by a sharp object such as glass.

h) *Deep anal lacerations*. Deep lacerations of the anal skin which extend into the anal canal are caused by significant dilatation of the anal skin and are rarely seen following consensual anal intercourse.

i) *Anal sphincter tone* may be unaffected following anal intercourse, held tightly closed or dilated. With repeated acts of anal intercourse contractibility of the sphincter may be diminished and reflex anal dilatation may be found. However, no reliable significance may be attributed to these findings.

j) *Anal skin texture* may alter (becoming thickened with flattening of the anal folds) if repeated anal penetration has occurred. It may also be associated with other medical conditions (pruritis ani, for example).

Penetrative sexual intercourse can only be reliably confirmed by the finding of semen in the high vaginal, cervical or internal anal swabs by the forensic science laboratory or if pregnancy ensues. It is usually not possible for the forensic physician to be specific that sexual intercourse has actually taken place. It should never be stated that the findings are consistent with rape.

SUBSEQUENT TO THE EXAMINATION

After completion of the examination procedure, the complainant should be offered the opportunity to bathe and wash her hair. This gives the doctor the time to complete notes and package the exhibits. It is important for the examining doctor to discuss findings with the investigation officer or chaperone. The following should be addressed:

— Medical Treatment

First aid treatment must be provided as necessary.

— Emergency Contraception

If relevant, emergency hormonal contraception (P.C.4) should be offered with verbal and written advice on administration. Referral for insertion of an intrauterine device (IUD) may be appropriate if 72 hours have elapsed since unprotected vaginal intercourse or if oestrogens are contraindicated.

— Sexually Transmitted Diseases (STD)

The complainant should be advised that screening for STDs is not usually conducted at the time of the forensic medical examination. The chaperone will organise a special appointment, on the advice of the doctor, for the complainant to be seen at an STD Clinic in 7 to 14 days after the alleged incident (see section on STDs below).

— Psychological consequences

Appropriate advice on support and counselling agencies (G.P., Victim Support, Survivors, social services) should be given in writing together with encouragement to seek emotional and practical support from a trusted friend or family member. The doctor should ask specifically whether or not the complainant wishes her own G.P. to be informed about the alleged incident.

THE PSYCHOLOGICAL CONSEQUENCES OF SEXUAL ASSAULT

The immediate and long term psychological sequelae experienced following a sexual assault will vary between individuals. However, patterns are now recognised which equate to the reactions following other extraordinarily stressful events like mass disasters, robbery and war.

Immediate phase

Only some of the complainants of sexual assault are emotionally expressive immediately following the incident (the stereotypical image of a person who has recently been sexually assaulted is a distraught, frightened individual) while others will dissociate themselves from the incident, appearing calm and controlled. Pre-existing or a past history of mental or physical illness or social problems may influence the initial behaviour of the complainant (Burgess & Holstrom 1974).

Heterosexual men are often very distressed that they had an erection and, on occasions, ejaculated during non-consensual anal intercourse. These responses can cause them to doubt their sexual orientation. They can be reassured by the knowledge that this is simply a physiological response and does not necessarily reflect sexual excitement.

Self-reproach is a common theme which can be addressed by the examining physician and advice given.

Long term response

The majority will experience an acute stress reaction in the weeks following sexual assault. The most common are listed in table 4. By definition, post-traumatic stress disorder cannot be diagnosed until symptoms persist for one month. Nevertheless, most women who report rape fulfil the other diagnostic criteria for post-traumatic stress disorder in the first week following the incident. Although many will recover fully, nearly half will continue to suffer from significant psychological problems three months after the assault (Rothbraum *et al* 1992).

The severity of the psychological disturbance appears to be unrelated to the particular sexual act(s) or degree of associated physical assault; complainants of attempted rape and acquaintance rape sometimes experience the most psychological trauma.

A consequence of these psychological sequelae is that the complainants of rape become frequent users of medical services for months, and often years, following the incident. Behavioural responses such as moving home, changing employment and not going out alone may also be found. The combination of

PSYCHOLOGICAL REACTIONS	SOMATIC SYMPTOMS
Intrusive thoughts	Sleep disturbances
Avoidance	Anorexia
Heightened arousal	Headaches
Numbing	Nausea
Poor concentration	Abdominal pain
Irritability	Genito-urinary discomfort
Fear	
Sexual dysfunction	
Depression	
Low esteem	
Suicidal ideation	

Table 4 – Recognised responses to sexual assault

behavioural, somatic and psychological reactions following a sexual assault have been termed 'The Rape Trauma Syndrome' (Burgess & Holstrom 1974).

SEXUALLY TRANSMITTED DISEASES

For many complainants of serious sexual offences, the initial physical and psychological trauma is superseded by the fear of acquiring human immunodeficiency virus (HIV). Fortunately, they can be reassured that the risk of contracting HIV during a sexual assault is believed to be extremely low; there is only one reported case in the United Kingdom of proven HIV transmission following a rape (Murphy 1990). Conversely, as many as a third of the complainants who are screened following such an incident, will be found to have one or more sexually transmitted diseases (STD) (Estreich et al 1990). The most frequently detected STD in these cases (excluding Candida albicans) are Neisseria gonorrhoeae (GC), Trichomonas vaginalis (TV), Chlamydia trachomatis (CT) and the human papilloma virus (HPV). All complainants of penetrative sexual assault must be encouraged by the examining doctor to attend an STD clinic, by a pre-arranged appointment, seven to fourteen days after the incident. The samples that are taken at the clinic will depend on the sites of penetration and the clinical signs.

The medico-legal significance of any detected STD depends on the timing of the sexual assault in relation to the incubation period for that organism. Some centres advocate performing STD screening simultaneously with the initial forensic assessment, but if a court orders disclosure of these results the revelation of a pre-existing infection may be used to imply promiscuity on the part of the complainant.

In the United Kingdom, broad-spectrum antibiotic prophylaxis is not routinely prescribed immediately after a sexual assault. Prophylaxis may be considered advisable if an intra-uterine contraceptive device is to be inserted (to prevent unwanted pregnancy) due to the risk of a pre-existing STD being transferred into the uterine cavity. Reasons cited against such prophylaxis are that the patient may perceive that there is no longer a risk of acquiring an STD, which will lessen the motivation to use barrier methods of contraception and to attend follow-up appointments, and there is the potential for exacerbating the feelings of 'dirtiness'.

Although the overall risk of acquiring hepatitis B virus following sexual assault is low, hepatitis B immunoglobulin (administered within 48 hours of the risk exposure) or an accelerated course of hepatitis B vaccine may be considered advisable if the alleged assailant(s) are known to be in a high risk group for carrying the disease. It is unlikely that even when the assailant is known to be HIV positive the complainant will be seen in time to receive the current 'prophylaxis' for HIV (Zidovudine) which should be administered within a few hours of the exposure. When relevant, the examining doctor should discuss these issues with a local STD consultant.

All complainants will be offered the opportunity to have serum stored so that should they be unfortunate enough to become sero-positive for hepatitis B, hepatitis C or HIV at subsequent testing, retrospective analysis can potentially relate seroconversion to the incident. Seroconversion may not only affect a judicial hearing but also the level of compensation awarded by the Criminal Injuries Compensation Board.

For medico-legal purposes, the detected organisms should be cultured (to minimise false positive results). With advance notice microbiology departments should be able to organise typing of some of the organisms (GC serotype, CT-immunotype). This specialist service provides potential for comparing with cultures taken from a defendant who consents to STD screening.

DEFENDANT (ALLEGED SUSPECT) EXAMINATIONS

Suspects in allegations of sexual assault should also be treated with respect and sensitivity. Sometimes examinations are requested to exclude the sexual partner of the complainant.

The examining doctor should ascertain from the investigating officer the essential details of the allegation and any significant findings following the examination of the complainant. It is important to note whether alcohol or drugs were involved and whether (and in what manner) the alleged assailant may have been injured. The police requirements (medical and forensic) should be established and the samples to be taken should be discussed. Samples may include blood (EDTA and clotted), saliva, urine, head and pubic hair, fingernails (cuttings or scrapings), penile swabs.

The examination should proceed in a similar manner to that described for the complainant after consent has been properly obtained. The Police and Criminal Evidence Act 1984 (PACE) requires that the defendant gives consent to the police for the obtaining of samples. Nonetheless, the doctor should obtain valid consent and advise the defendant not to incriminate himself (see chapter 4).

The exhibits should be bagged, labelled, signed and sealed in the presence of the detainee before being handed to the police officer (or SOCO) for signature. This action should reassure the defendant of the security of the samples.

The investigating officer should be informed of any injuries, abnormalities or any other concerns that the examination has brought to light. If there are symptoms or signs of sexually transmitted disease, the defendant should be advised to attend an STD clinic.

THE MEDICO-LEGAL IMPLICATIONS OF PREGNANCY

The medico-legal ramifications of pregnancy and the post-natal period are manifold and extend beyond the immediate brief of this chapter. However, the forensic medical examiner should be familiar with a number of issues discussed below.

Termination of pregnancy

The Offences Against the Person Act (OAPA) 1861 makes it a criminal offence to attempt, or achieve, a termination of a continuing pregnancy unless the strict requirements of the Human Fertilisation and Embryology Act (HFEA) 1990 are fulfilled; HFEA does not apply in Northern Ireland. Prior to the legislation allowing medical terminations (Abortion Act 1967) illegal abortions accounted for a significant proportion of maternal deaths (due to vagal inhibition, air embolus, primary haemorrhage, bowel perforations or secondary infections).

Except where there is a genuine medical emergency (when treatment is immediately necessary to save the life of the pregnant woman or to prevent grave permanent injury to her physical or mental health) two registered medical practitioners are required to certify that the decision to terminate is appropriate. All terminations must be notified to the Chief Medical Officer, Department of Health. The products of conception may be required for DNA profiling to determine paternity if the pregnancy resulted from a sexual assault.

Until the HFEA came into force, terminations were allowed only up to the 28th week of pregnancy. The HFEA reduced the limit to 24 weeks in cases where terminations were conducted because '... the continuance of the pregnancy would involve greater risk, greater than if the pregnancy were terminated, of injury to the physical or mental health of the pregnant woman (or any existing children in the family of the pregnant woman)'. However, in all other categories the upper limit for terminations was erased, which had the effect of nullifying the Infant Life (Preservation) Act 1929 (never applicable in Scotland) in cases conducted in accordance with HFEA. The Infant Life Preservation Act states that it is an offence to kill a child which was capable of being born alive: this crime is known as 'child destruction'.

Stillbirth

The decreased mortality of very premature infants was also recognised in the Stillbirth (Definition) Act 1992. This Act requires that all children delivered after 24 weeks gestation which show no sign of life be registered as stillbirths.

- Engorged lactating breasts
- Pink striae on the abdomen
- Enlarged uterus
- Fresh tears of the vulva, vagina or cervix
- Blood stained serous discharge (lochia) from the uterus

Table 5 – Signs of recent delivery

Concealment of birth

It is a civil offence to fail to notify the birth of a child. It is also a criminal offence under the OAPA for any person to dispose of the body of a dead child secretly, regardless of whether the child died before, during or after birth. In order to trace the mother, investigating officers may require a forensic medical examiner to state whether a suspected female shows signs of recent delivery (table 5). Furthermore, DNA of both the suspected mother and the dead child can be undertaken. Pathological assessment may assist in the determination of fetal age.

In Scotland, by the Concealment of Pregnancy Act 1809, a pregnant woman who conceals her being with child during the whole period of her pregnancy and does not call for nor make use of help or assistance at the birth, may be charged if the child is found dead or missing.

Infanticide

If it can be shown that a woman has caused the death of her child within a year of its birth, whether by wilful act or omission, she may be charged with murder or, if the balance of her mind can be shown to be disturbed because of the recent delivery or lactation, infanticide (Infanticide Act 1938). Infanticide is analogous to manslaughter in having the advantage of case dependent, not mandatory, sentencing. Proof that the child had a separate existence from its mother is fundamental to the charge of infanticide. However, there are very few signs that confirm a neonate had a separate existence; the most obvious are food in the stomach or separation of the stump of the umbilical cord.

PREMENSTRUAL SYNDROME

The diagnosis of PMS is dependent on a history of cyclical behavioural changes related to the post-ovulation period of the hormonal cycle. For the court to consider the diagnosis of PMS as mitigation there must be independent evidence that the condition predated the alleged offence. In some cases it may be appropriate for the forensic physician to note the date of the last menstrual period of a female detainee in case PMS is later proffered as a defence.

SEXUAL VARIATIONS

Normal sexuality is variously described as behaviour overtly approved of by society, statistically common or biologically desirable in the sense of leading to procreation (Faulk 1988). Sexual behaviour and gender identity disorders deviating from the norm are considered to be sexual variations or paraphilia (table 6).

Sexual variant behaviour may be illegal if it involves children, male homosexuals under 18 years, animals, sadism, exhibitionism or frotteurism. Unless combined with a recognised mental disorder sexual 'deviations' (variations) are specifically excluded from the Mental Health Act 1983 (s.1.3). Some offences can only be committed by a person of a specific sex. Under English law the sexual identity or gender of a person is defined by chromosomal pattern, not by gonadal, genital or psychological factors (post-operative transsexuals legally retain their birth gender).

Some sexual variations involve inherently life threatening practices; these include autoerotic asphyxia (using strangulation, hanging, gagging, plastic bag asphyxia, inverted suspension), electrophilia and anaesthesiophilia. When accidental deaths do occur in these circumstances associated paraphernalia may be present at the scene, such as evidence of transvestism, bondage, pornographic material or mirrors. Family members or friends who discover the body in these situations may, in an attempt to preserve the reputation of the deceased, remove certain articles. In doing so they may create a scene erroneously considered a suicide or homicide. When the truth is divulged sympathetic explanations are necessary for reassurance that these deaths are usually accidental.

Homosexuality	Same gender
Transsexualism	Belief that person is of opposite sex from own bodily sex
Fetishism	Object
Transvestism	Dressing in clothing of the opposite sex
Zoophilia	Animal (bestiality)
Paedophilia	Child
Exhibitionism	Exposure of genitals to opposite sex
Voyeurism	Spying on others undressing or indulging in sexual intercourse
Sexual masochism	Sexual pleasure from receiving pain
Sexual sadism	Sexual pleasure from causing pain
Coprophila	Faeces
Frotteurism	Rubbing
Telephone scatoglia	Lewdness
Necrophilia	Corpse
Electrophilia	Electrical impulse
Anaesthesiophilia	Using volatile substance e.g. chloroform, ether, butane

Table 6 – Definitions of sexual variations

References

Burgess AW, Holstrom LL 1974 Rape Trauma Syndrome. *American Journal of Psychiatry* **131:** 981-986.

Emans FJ, Woods ER, Allred EN, Grace E 1994 Hymenal Findings in Adolescent Women: Impact of Tampon Use and Consensual Sexual Activity. *The Journal of Pediatrics* **125:** 153-160.

Estreich S, Forster GE, Robinson A 1990 Sexually Transmitted Diseases in Rape Victims. *Genitourinary Medicine* **66:** 443-438.

Faulk M 1988 *Basic Forensic Psychiatry* Blackwell Scientific Publications, Oxford.

Home Office Statistical Bulletin, Notifiable Offences. 1995 Research and Statistics Department, Home Office, Croydon.

Keating SM, Allard JE 1994 What's in a Name? Medical Samples and Scientific Evidence in Sexual Assaults. *Medicine Science and the Law* **34:** 187-201.

Murphy SM 1990 Rape, Sexually Transmitted Diseases and Human Immunodeficiency Virus Infection. *International Journal of STD & AIDS* **1:** 79-82.

Rothbraum BO, Foa EB, Riggs DS, Murdoch T, Walsh W A 1992 Prospective Examination of Post Traumatic Stress Disorder in Rape Victims. *Journal of Traumatic Stress* **5:** 455-475.

Smith JC, Hogan B 1988 *Criminal Law,* 6th Edition Butterworths, London.

Smith NC, Van Coeverden de Groot HA, 1983 Gunston KD Coital Injuries of the Vagina in Non-virginal Patients. *South African Medical Journal* **64:** 746-747.

Willott GM, Allard JE 1982 Spermatozoa - their Persistence after Sexual Intercourse. *Forensic Science International* **19:** 135-154.

Wilson EM 1982 A Comparison of the Persistence of Seminal Constituents in the Human Vagina and Cervix. *Police Surgeon* **22:** 44-45.

12

ACCIDENTAL INJURY AND TRAFFIC MEDICINE

A Marsden

INTRODUCTION

Case studies

Study A

The police give chase to four joy riding youths who have stolen a high perfor-mance car and driven it at speed through their local town. The police find the vehicle crashed into a wall and written off. The youths have "legged it". Later some youths are arrested on suspicion of taking a motor vehicle without the owner's consent - all vehemently deny being the driver! Only a close examination by the police surgeon reveals the tell tale imprinting sign of a lap and diagonal seat belt across the main suspect's right shoulder, left chest and right hip!

Study B

A man is apprehended by the police for driving the wrong way up a one way street. The police officer asks the police surgeon to attend believing the culprit to be driving under the influence of drink or drugs. The driver, mildly confused, protests his innocence. A clinical examination by the doctor raises the possibility of new onset diabetes with hypoglycaemia – a suspicion confirmed by laboratory testing.

Study C

The ambulance is asked to convey a motor cyclist to hospital for a check up after a fatal accident where the motor cyclist has killed an elderly pedestrian who stepped in his path. The motor cyclist is thrown some distance from his bike, striking a wall. The paramedic arrives at the scene to find the motor cyclist blowing into a screening breath analyser while leaning up against the police patrol car. In answer to direct questions the biker complains of pain and stiffness in his shoulder and neck. Later in hospital a cross-table radiograph reveals an unstable fracture dislocation of the 5th and 6th cervical vertebrae.

Study D

The drunken driver of a fast car insists on signing himself out of A&E after a high velocity head on crash in which the other driver is killed. Apart from his intoxication he seems to have come off remarkably well with no injuries apparent to the hospital doctors. He is taken to the police custody suite and the police surgeon is called to confirm that he is fit for interview. He dies one hour later while awaiting the doctor's arrival – from a rupture of the thoracic aorta.

Such case studies emphasise the necessity for clinical forensic examiners to be aware of the mechanisms of violent injury – particularly in relation to traffic accidents – and to appreciate the factors affecting a person's ability – or inability – to control a motor vehicle. Forensic physicians are likely to put such knowledge to use at the scene of a crime or accident or when attending to a suspect, prisoner or witness after a violent episode either at hospital, in the police station medical examination suite or in their own surgery.

ACCIDENTS ON THE ROAD

Despite changes in car and road design and improvements in transport safety, road accidents still account for approximately 4,000 deaths in the United Kingdom each year, the greatest single cause of death in adults up to the age of 50 years. Most deaths occur in the 15-24 age group. Car and pedestrian accidents each account for approximately 40% of the death toll; powered two wheeler accidents for about 10%.

In traffic medicine a knowledge of the mechanism of injury and the way this influences pattern and severity of injury are singularly important. Factors influencing the type and severity of injury include:

a) The kinetics of the impact

   i the speed of travel and force of impact

   ii the position of the injured person in the vehicle

   iii the direction of the impact

b) The vehicular design and the presence and use of restraint systems

c) The effect of secondary injury from ejection, overturning or other hazard such as fire

The kinetics of the impact

The way that violent injuries occur in vehicular (and other) accidents are explained by an understanding of Newton's laws of motion. A body at rest will remain at rest and a body in motion remain in motion unless acted upon by some external force (Newton's first law of motion). For example, though a car may be brought to an abrupt stop by collision with a stationary object such as a tree or telegraph pole, the car occupants, if unrestrained, will continue in motion until stopping by coming into contact with, for example, the dashboard, windscreen or steering column. This phenomenon has been described as "the secondary accident".

Injuries are produced because the energy of motion (kinetic energy) is converted into other forms of energy, such as mechanical energy or heat. Energy can neither be created nor destroyed, only change in form. For every action there is an equal and opposite reaction (Newton's third law).

The degree of kinetic energy contained by a moving object is given by the formula

$$\text{kinetic energy} = \tfrac{1}{2} \, mv^2$$

It is the weight or mass (m) of the vehicle or impacting object and its velocity (v) which are responsible for the amount of physical damage caused by energy transfer from a moving object. Of these, the velocity is, by far, the most important factor – a principle which is of major importance in understanding the damage caused by missile ballistics (see chapter 8).

Thus, putting these factors together, an accident may be considered serious when:

a) the speed is greater than 25 mph with an unrestrained victim (over 35 mph when restrained)

b) there has been intrusion into the cabin from the engine compartment or lateral intrusion of more than 1 m or

c) there has been ejection of a victim

A number of change-of-speed injuries, especially in relation to deceleration, are common in traffic accidents. They will be described when considering, in turn, the major types of motor vehicle collisions:

- head-on or frontal impact
- lateral or side impact
- rear impact.

Head-on or frontal impact

The phases of injury from deceleration in a frontal impact follow a typical pattern (fig. 1). An unrestrained driver telescopes forward in the seat with some extension

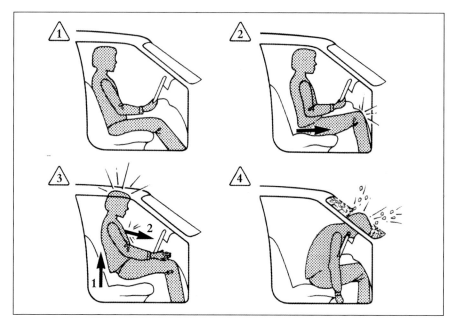

Figure 1 – Sequence of deceleration injuries

at the lumbar spine and marked knee contact with the fascia. The forces of deceleration then throw the body upwards and forwards so that the crown makes contact with the roof frame and the chest is thrown forwards against the steering wheel. Next comes a forward flexion injury of the cervical spine, before the head comes to rest in contact with or, often, through the windshield. The typical pattern of injuries sustained is shown in fig 2.

The most frequent cause of death in car accidents is head injury (70%) followed by multiple injuries and shock (8%), chest injuries (6%) and abdomino-pelvic injuries (4%).

Head injuries show various pathological features: fractures of the skull, intracranial haematoma, intracerebral laceration and contusion, brain stem and basilar damage. Flexion/extension injuries of the cervical spine are common and should not be overlooked. Chest injuries include, as would be expected, fractures of the chest wall, contusions to lung and heart from blunt injury and pleural damage including pneumothorax.

A specific vehicular injury worthy of note is rupture of the thoracic aorta: presumably as a result of deceleration, the aorta tears at its weakest point, the junction of the arch and the descending aorta. On occasions, the tear is limited to the intimal layer, the vascular leak tamponaded within the mediastinum; such patients may survive long enough to allow a vascular repair to be undertaken.

Abdominal trauma includes, in descending order of frequency, blunt injuries to the liver, spleen and kidney. Fractures of the pelvis or dislocation of the hip may be associated with injury to the knee or thigh from dashboard contact.

Lateral Impact

When a vehicle is struck from the side the energy of impact is concentrated on the side wall of the chest resulting in lateral flail chest, lung contusion or ruptured liver or spleen. Bone or joint injury to the shoulder and pelvic girdle is also common.

Rear Impact

A common entity, when a stationary or slow moving object is struck from behind. On impact, the front vehicle shoots forwards and, without properly adjusted head restraints being fitted, soft tissue sprains to the neck are common. When the front of the vehicle is forced by a shunt from behind to concertina into a stationary vehicle ahead there is a capacity for damage from a "secondary impact" of the frontal or deceleration type.

Use of restraint systems

The pattern of automotive injury has been changed by restraining systems, including seat belts and passive head restraints (see *Medical Effects of Seat Belt Legislation in the United Kingdom*, HMSO, 1984). Life threatening chest and facial injuries are extremely rare in the patient wearing a properly adjusted seat belt. However, the change in the axis of movement has resulted in an increased incidence of sprains of the neck and, by the same mechanism, there has been a

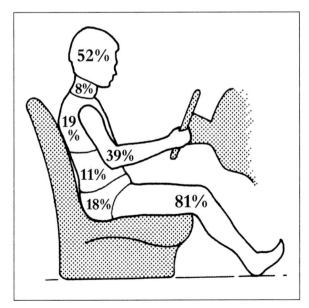

Figure 2 – The areas most frequently injured in front seat occupants (from Road Research Laboratory statistics)

relative increase in the severity of head injuries from windscreen contact in drivers. Seat belts themselves give rise to injury: strains in the lumbar area are common and abdominal visceral injuries are also described.

Air bags, designed to cushion forward motion of front seat occupants in deceleration injuries, are being increasingly fitted to modern motor vehicles. They have been shown to be of use in the 65% to 70% of collisions that occur between the headlights. Under development are air bags for passive restraint in side and rear impacts, though it will be some time before these are standardised in all motor vehicles. Despite the apparently alarming manner in which air bags are deployed (by an explosion which causes rapid inflation and deflation of the bag), air bag injuries are few with occasional abrasive injuries to the arms and chest and possibly injuries caused by the occupant's glasses. Forensic examiners should be aware, of course, of the dangers of non deployed air bags in automobile accident sites which they may be asked to attend.

Secondary injury from ejection or other hazards

The ejection of an unrestrained occupant from a vehicle increases the risk of death by a factor of six. One out of 13 ejection victims suffers a spinal fracture. Obviously, from an understanding of the laws of motion, the further that a victim has been thrown from the vehicle, the greater the potential for serious injury.

Burns seldom cause death in automobile accidents. In one series of 1292 deaths, the cause was ascribed to burning in only three cases.

ROLE OF THE FORENSIC MEDICAL EXAMINER IN TRAFFIC ACCIDENTS

A number of specific and discrete injuries have been described which relate to the mode of impact, speed of the vehicle and the disposition of the passengers within the vehicle.

Accompanying these discrete injuries may be all manner of lacerations, contusions and abrasions of the soft tissues, either from direct contact or from the impact of missiles, including flying glass and pieces of road furniture. Forensic physicians should remember the importance of securing and properly preserving trace evidence when attending to a road victim: this may take the form of embedded pieces of windscreen glass, fragments of paint or upholstery fibres.

When called to attend or examine a traffic accident victim, pay careful attention to the circumstances and the surroundings. Check for an obvious cause of the accident, though remembering that things are not always what they seem. Often the accident and the resulting lethal injuries are a consequence of sudden death from natural causes. It has been deduced, from the imprinting of the accelerator pattern on the sole of the victim's shoe, that suicide was intended. Check the seat belt position and whether head restraints were used. Retain the crash helmet in the case of the injured motorcyclist or pedal cyclist or horse rider; it may later provide valuable clues to the pattern of head injury. Search around the wreckage for other bodies (particularly a child who may be ejected some distance from the crash), dentures (which may be essential to restoring the facial skeleton of the living or to aiding the identification of the dead) or other clues to the nature and type of accident. Do not move casualties unless it is essential – extrication of the living is a specialised procedure for the accident team.

Emergency treatment and forensic assessment form only part of the total responsibility of doctors involved in the investigation of accidents. Accident prevention should be an important aspect of this work. Only after careful analysis of the causes and effects of accidents can thought be given to how such accidents may be avoided and the extent of injury further reduced. This area deserves greater effort and expenditure.

Notwithstanding advances in accident and injury prevention and in trauma surgery, the death toll from road traffic accidents remains unacceptably high. Large numbers of serious accidents are associated with recklessness, often in the young, the criminally prone or those who show no regard for speed limits, traffic regulation, drink/drive laws or safety restraints.

LEGAL ASPECTS OF TRAFFIC MEDICINE[1]

Drinking and driving

More than 1,000 people are killed in Great Britain each year as a result of drinking and driving. Almost a quarter of those killed in road accidents in 1993 had a blood alcohol concentration exceeding 80 mg/100 ml; in 10% of cases this was 200 mg/100 ml or over. The figures rise to 55% and 25% respectively when considering deaths between 10.00 pm and 4.00 am and greater still on Friday and Saturday nights.

The proportion of road accident fatalities with blood alcohol levels above 80 mg% among different age groups of road users was are shown in table 1.

---

1 Much of this section of the chapter is reproduced from the first edition, with the permission of Dr James Dunbar.

AGE	MOTOR VEHICLE DRIVER	MOTOR CYCLE DRIVER
16-19	20%	16%
20-24	24%	16%
25-29	34%	16%
30+		

Table 1

One tenth of all road accidents causing injury are due to driving with excess alcohol in the blood.

The metabolism of alcohol with respect to traffic procedures

The nature of the substance, alcohol, and its metabolism is described on pages 173-176 in chapter 9.

A unit of alcohol (for example, 25 ml of spirits) increases the blood alcohol level within the first hour by approximately 15 mg/100ml in a man (20 mg/100 ml in a woman).

Figure 3 shows the cumulative aspect of repeated drinks on the blood alcohol curve described in chapter 9.

In a healthy person 90% of the alcohol is cleared from the blood by the liver at a rate of about 15mg/100ml per hour. In convicted drink drivers this rate averages 20 mg/100 ml per hour, but ranges from 10 to over 40 mg/100 ml/hour (fig.4).

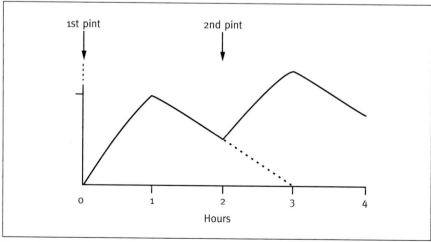

Figure 3 – Cumulative effect of alcohol ingestion

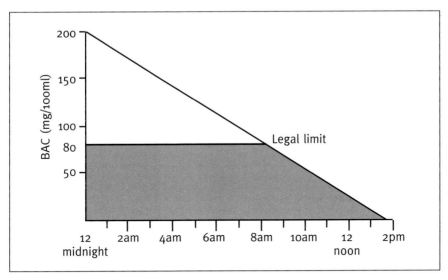

Figure 4 – Elimination of alcohol

Most of the alcohol is broken down by alcohol dehydrogenase and most of the remainder by the microsomal enzyme oxidising system (MEOS). The activity of MEOS may be increased by several drugs and by chronic alcohol abuse. This may explain the increased drug and alcohol tolerance of heavy drinkers. A third, and in normal circumstances unimportant oxidative pathway, is mediated by the enzyme catalase.

It follows from this that the breakdown of alcohol is non-linear. This has implications for calculations to work out what the alcohol level was at some time other than when the blood sample was taken.

Sometimes drivers arrested after completing their trip claim to have consumed alcohol between completion and arrest - the 'hip flask' defence. Recently, prosecutions have been successful against drivers who were below the legal limit at the time of blood sampling, but were judged, on the basis of back calculation, to have exceeded the limit at the time of an accident. Despite the opinion of the House of Lords in dismissing an appeal (*Gumley v Cunningham* [1989] Road Traffic Reports, 49) these calculations are based on assumptions of uncertain validity, for enough reliable information is seldom available. Certainly the complexity of biochemistry involved is beyond most police surgeons who should not undertake this work but refer it to forensic scientists.

The Effects of Alcohol on Performance

At blood alcohol concentrations of 30 mg% impairment occurs in cognitive function, motor co-ordination and sensory perception.

With increasing levels of intoxication beyond 50mg% the following effects occur on the central nervous system.

- Slurring of speech

- Unsteadiness

- Drowsiness

- Impaired reasoning and memory

- Reduced perception

- Decreased concentration

Paradoxically, while alcohol gives a feeling of well being it actually depresses brain function, lessening muscular control and co-ordination, lengthening reaction time. Vision is blurred and awareness decreased, especially in the dark. The ability to judge speed and distance is impaired, as is the capacity to deal with the unexpected.

Not only do all of these factors adversely affect driving performance, but alcohol impairs judgement to the extent that drivers under the influence genuinely believe that they are driving better than they are.

The risk of being involved in an accident increases sharply beyond the legal limit. The likelihood of an accident and of that accident being serious, increases disproportionately with higher alcohol levels (fig. 5). For young or inexperienced drivers, the risk increases from well below the legal limit, even after the first drink. At the legal limit the risk is twice as great; but for young and inexperienced drivers five times as great. At twice the legal limit the accident risk is twenty times as great. This relationship between alcohol level and accident risk led to the introduction of a legal limit in 1967.

This major legislative landmark made it an automatic offence to drive, or attempt to drive, or be in charge of a motor vehicle in a public place if the blood alcohol level exceeded that limit. The Act also introduced a screening breath test, which, if positive, was to be followed by an evidential blood or urine test taken at a police station.

Road traffic legislation

The Transport Acts of 1981 and 1982 and the Road Traffic Act 1988 provide for the following principal offences.

- Driving or attempting to drive a motor vehicle while unfit to drive through drink or drugs.

- Being in charge of a motor vehicle while unfit to drive through drink or drugs.

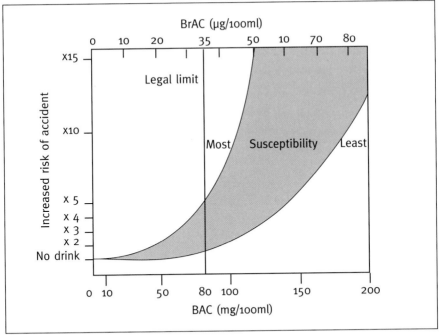

Figure 5 – Risk of road traffic accidents related to levels of alcohol in the blood (BAC) and breath (BrAC).

- Driving or attempting to drive a motor vehicle on a road or other public place after consuming so much alcohol that the proportion of it in the person's breath, blood or urine exceeds the prescribed limit.

- Being in charge of a motor vehicle on a road or public place after consuming alcohol, so that the proportion of it in the person's breath, blood or urine exceeds the prescribed limit.

- Failing to provide a specimen for analysis, when driving or attempting to drive.

Legal limits

In the United Kingdom, the current legal limits are:

Blood – 80 milligrammes per 100 ml of blood (mg%)

Breath – 35 microgrammes per 100 ml of breath (μg%)

Urine – 107 milligrammes per 100 ml of urine (mg%)

The Acts enable the police to require a driver to provide specimens for these tests while at a hospital following a road accident, unless the doctor in immediate charge of the case believes that this will be prejudicial to the proper care or treatment of the patient. Specimens may not be taken from an unconscious patient.

United States	100 mg / 100 ml	legally drunk	variable fines
	80 mg / 100 ml	driving under influence of drink	
Germany	80 mg / 100 ml	legal limit	fine of £200
	>110 mg / 100 ml	unfit to drive	1 year ban
Netherlands	>50 mg / 100 ml	police fine of approximately £150	
	>80 mg to 1300 mg/100 ml	Public prosecutor fine up to £350	
	>1300 mg/100 ml	increasing scale of fines, loss of licence and imprisonment	
France	>50 mg/100 ml	fine	
	>80 mg/100 ml	suspension	
	Spot checks and random testing		

Table 2

Conventionally, breath alcohol levels are converted to equivalent blood levels by applying a factor of 2300, but the two cannot be accurately compared. Breath alcohol levels rise faster and fall earlier than venous blood alcohol levels.

It is appropriate, at this stage, to discuss the strong arguments for the reduction of the 'legal limit' for driving of the blood alcohol level.

There is no standard 'safe limit' or legal limit and there is much variation across the world (see table 2).

Most scientific opinion favours a general legal limit of 50 mg/100ml blood. This is the level at which accident risk increases for all drivers. As young, inexperienced drivers already face an increased accident risk at the 50 mg/100 ml level, there is a case for lowering the legal limit to 20 mg/100 ml for that group, although to have two different thresholds would lead to practical complications in enforcement.

The introduction of evidential breath testing is itself a further reason for lowering the limit to compensate for the fact that breath testing takes the lower of two readings and is set to give the driver the fairest interpretation of blood:breath ratio. The overall practical effect of this has been to raise our legal limit and thus to 'underprosecute' drivers.

Random breath testing

Studies abroad show that many drivers would escape prosecution if the legal limit remained at 80mg/100ml after the introduction of random breath testing (RBT).

As a residue from the previous night's drinking a large proportion of drivers in the morning traffic have alcohol levels in the range 50–80 mg/100 ml, itself an indication of dangerousness in these drivers. The effect of RBT would be enhanced by a 50 mg/100 ml legal limit. Random breath testing is the best deterrent measure, for the greater the likelihood drinking drivers see of being caught, the greater the deterrence. A constable is already permitted under Section 163 of the Road Traffic Act 1988 to stop vehicles at random in order then to decide whether there are grounds for requiring a sample of breath for testing. These grounds exist where the constable has reasonable cause to suspect that a motorist has alcohol in his body; that he has committed a traffic offence while his vehicle was moving; or that he has been involved in an accident. RBT permits the police to set up highly visible check points on the road at any time or place and test all drivers who pass by. To implement this in Great Britain would require a change in the law. As long ago as 1976, the Blennerhasset Committee, in considering all aspects of the power to test drivers, concluded "that discretion should be unfettered. We believe this to be essential both to the simplification of the law and avoidance of loopholes, and for its better enforcement. It is central and fundamental to the reforms we propose, and accordingly we recommend that the circumstances in which a constable may require a specimen of breath from a driver for screening purposes should not be specified."

Scientific evaluation of RBT in Finland and Australia has shown the following advantages:

- RBT saves lives; perhaps between 400 and 1000 a year could be saved in this country.

- RBT deters social drinkers from drinking and driving and catches problem drinkers who form that group most likely to have road traffic accidents.

- RBT means that fewer drivers face prosecution, due to its deterrent effect.

- RBT pays for itself, the Australians reckoning that for every dollar spent on random testing 20 dollars have been saved.

- RBT is popular, three-quarters of drivers in this country favouring its introduction; its popularity would increase after it was introduced.

Effects of drugs on driving

The law concerning driving or being in charge of a vehicle while under the influence of drugs is less rigidly defined, placing greater emphasis on the opinions of both police officer and police surgeon. In numerical terms, cases involving alcohol greatly outweigh those involving drugs.

Nevertheless, it is worth bearing drugs in mind in every case and, if circumstances seem to warrant it, directing the police officer's thoughts to the possibility of drug action. Since drugs and alcohol are frequently combined, apparent drunkenness accompanied by a characteristic smell on the breath may in fact be a drug-induced condition combined with a small amount of alcohol.

The definition of impairment bedevilled road traffic legislation for many years until the introduction of legally defined limits of alcohol concentration provided an alternative procedure which could avoid the question altogether. The problem still remains in drug cases, with no foreseeable likelihood of concentration limits being set. Evidence from eye witnesses and police officers may well be important, but evidence from a doctor will obviously carry considerable weight. The laboratory analyst's role in any given case is to specify that drugs which were capable of producing impairment were present, but not to state that any particular person was impaired.

The compounds involved

Alcohol is a simple chemical present in a drinker's body fluids in comparatively massive amounts, easily detected and measured by gas chromatography (GC). The term 'drugs' embraces a host of different compounds, present in very much smaller amounts and which are very much more difficult to detect. In these days of polypharmacy, two or more quite different drugs are frequently involved. To confuse the issue further, metabolites may be present, some of which are biologically active.

Benzodiazepines account for a sizeable proportion of the drugs detected. In a number of these cases the driver has been taking medication on prescription, and some 'impaired' cases involve patients who have committed the offence unwittingly.

In drugs cases, information must be provided before analysis can begin: any drugs the driver may have in his possession (or may admit to taking or having been prescribed) or used syringes and needles. All such facts are useful to the toxicologist trying to decide the best course of analytical action and information should be passed on to the case officer for transmission to the analyst.

Unidentified preparations should be sampled and submitted to the laboratory. A single unit-dose will be sufficient and ensures that drugs are not removed from patients who may need them. In some cases drugs of misuse will be found on a driver and seized by the police officer for laboratory testing to substantiate charges under the Misuse of Drugs Act.

Diabetic patients may have become unfit as a result of dietary neglect or drug regimen. Scientific evidence of hypoglycaemia is achieved by blood-glucose determination. Forensic science laboratories do not generally undertake such testing and the police surgeon should be advised to make arrangements for analysis at a hospital biochemistry department.

The analysis

Considerable reliance is placed upon chromatographic methods, particularly thin-layer and gas-liquid chromatography (TLC and GLC). The latter in combination with mass-spectrometry and computerised data handling (GC-MS-COM) is perhaps the most sensitive, sophisticated and versatile weapon in the toxicologist's armoury.

Immunologically based methods such as radioimmuno-assay (RIA) have proved useful for morphine like substances. The laboratory has the capability of detecting cannabinoid material in blood or urine, although confirmation of the results by alternative means is not yet possible.

Road traffic act procedures

Police surgeons spend a substantial part of their time in procedures concerned with the Road Traffic Acts, and it is therefore wise to be fully cognisant of the procedural aspects of drink–drive enforcement.

Police procedure

A constable in uniform may require a person driving or attempting to drive or in charge of a motor vehicle on a road or other public place to take a breath test if he suspects the person:

a) of having been drinking; or

b) of having committed a moving traffic offence

In addition, where an accident has occurred, a constable in uniform may require any person whom he has reasonable cause to believe was drinking or attempting to drive or was in charge of the vehicle at the time of the accident, to take a screening breath test.

A person who:

a) is unfit to drive, or

b) has provided a positive breath test, or

c) has refused/failed to take a breath test

will be arrested and taken to a police station. Once at the police station, the driver will be required either to provide two evidential specimens of breath or, if the machine is not available, a specimen of blood for analysis.

The subsequent procedure depends on which offence appears to have been committed.

Driving while alcohol exceeds the prescribed limit (s5 RTA)

In these cases, the normal procedure is for the police to request the driver to provide two specimens of his breath. This does not involve the police surgeon. Only if the subject is asked for, and subsequently agrees to supply a specimen of blood, is the police surgeon called. In cases where alcohol exceeds the prescribed limit no examination is carried out to assess the driver's fitness to drive.

During the first year of evidential breath testing much controversy surrounded its accuracy. Doubts about the possibility of interference by other infra-red absorbing substances, bacterial action, gastro-oseophageal reflux and respiratory problems led to an official report on the performance of the evidential breath analysers by Sir William Paton FRS. Most of the anxieties about evidential breath testing have been overcome and the few remaining exotic defences are best left to experts. Police surgeons are unwise to become involved in these defence cases.

A driver whose breath result is between 35 and 50 micrograms alcohol per 100 ml has the option to replace the breath result with a laboratory test on blood or urine (which is chosen is at the discretion of the police officer); the driver is given part of the specimen to have analysed if he so wishes. In Scotland, drivers whose lower of the two results is in the range of 36-39 µg will not be prosecuted. Blood samples are taken by a medical practitioner; should it prove impracticable to divide such a sample, it is competent to take another, again with the driver's consent, for him to have analysed.

Driving while unfit through drink or drugs (s4 RTA)

In these cases the police surgeon normally has two tasks, both requiring the subject's consent: to assess by examination the subject's fitness to drive (see below) and to take a specimen of blood for analysis if he concludes that the motorist's fitness is impaired.

The subject will have been told of the intention to call a doctor (a police surgeon) to examine him on behalf of the police, and he will also be given the opportunity of calling a doctor on his own behalf for whose fee he would be responsible.

Driving while unfit through drink or drugs – breath test negative

When a driver either refuses to give a breath test or the result is negative at a police station but the custody officer (or the officer in charge of the station) still considers from his own observations and the testimony of witnesses that there is sufficient evidence of impairment, the subject will be examined by the police surgeon in the same way as a person who has been arrested for driving while unfit and who had been given a positive breath test (in other words, the procedure reverts to that available under s4).

The police surgeon's role

With the testing in the Courts over the past few years of proposed 'defences' to drink driving prosecutions, most police forces have tightened up their procedures and issue very rigidly enforced, legally validated, protocols to their staff. Police surgeons should avail themselves of these protocols and play their part in adhering to them - usually this is by following a precise printed algorithm completed by the officer in the case. To support these procedures, forces usually provide "Jiffy Bags" containing the necessary equipment for doctors to withdraw venous blood samples for alcohol analysis. Each kit normally contains:

Two plastic drums and caps ('securitainers')

Two rubber-topped glass injection vials each containing as preservative a mixture of citrate and fluoride

Two labels, for attaching to the glass vials

One adhesive plaster

One alcohol-free cleansing towelette

One 5 ml disposable syringe and needle

One envelope, printed with advice to the person supplying the specimen

Readers should be aware of some parts of the procedure which have given rise to problems in the past.

1. The subject should have given consent prior to the police surgeon being contacted.

2. The police surgeon should identify himself to the subject. He should satisfy himself that:
   a) the subject has consented to providing a sample of blood (consent should be sought in the presence of the police officer);
   b) there are no medical reasons why a specimen of blood cannot or should not be taken.

3. The "jiffy bag" should be opened in the presence of the police surgeon – it should be complete and in date. The details on both the labels should be identical and completed in the same hand.

4. No swabs other than the officially provided swabs should be used.

5. The blood sample must be taken in the presence of the police.

6. The Road Traffic Act requires that the specimen of blood be divided into two parts by the police surgeon in the presence of the driver, one for the Forensic Science Laboratory and one for the subject's own analysis. The doctor is NOT permitted to take two separate specimens from the subject, unless legitimate medical reasons prevent the taking of a large enough sample at the first attempt.

7. It is for the doctor to say how the blood specimen should be taken. If the doctor asks for a venous sample from the arm and the defendant only consents to a capillary specimen from his finger, that will amount to a refusal to provide a specimen (*Rushton v Higgins* [1972] *Criminal Law Review* 440). The defendant cannot insist on the blood being taken from a particular portion of his anatomy such as his big toe (*Solesury v Pugh* [1969] 2 All ER 1171). If a doctor asks to take a specimen of blood in accordance with general medical practice and is met with an offer to provide it in a different way, that is considered as a refusal. Some drivers intimate that they suffer from a pathological fear of needles; if a phobia of this kind does exist, it is associated with bradycardia which is difficult for anyone to achieve voluntarily. Many otherwise normal people feel faint during venepuncture and exhibit symptoms; recumbency is the answer.

8. When an analysis is required for alcohol only, 5 ml of blood should be taken (2 - 2½ ml per vial). The specimen should be injected in equal parts through the rubber tops of the glass vials which are then shaken vigorously to mix the blood with the preservative. The doctor should sign the two labels and ensure that these are attached to the vials. The labelled vials are placed in the 'securitainers' and the caps secured after the driver has been given the opportunity to select and retain one sample. This 'securitainer' is placed in the envelope provided, sealed and later handed to the driver with a list of qualified analysts.

9. If both the police surgeon and the prisoner's own doctor attend the police station and the prisoner insists on his own doctor taking the specimen, then he has not refused, for the Act does not specify that the specimen will be taken by the police surgeon (*Bayliss v Thames Valley Police Chief Constable* [1978] *Criminal Law Review* 363). This does not appear to be the position in Scotland; certainly the procedure should not be delayed until the arrival of the general practitioner who will act only as a witness.

10. If a medical examination is required and if the accused consents to a medical examination, this should be conducted outwith the presence of the police.

11. It is not permitted to remove evidential samples from unconscious subjects not able to consent under these procedures.

Medical examination under Section 4 RTA 1988

The aim of this examination is to determine whether there is any medical explanation to account for the driver's impairment. Clinical examination to determine drunkenness is notoriously unreliable at blood alcohol levels below 200 mg /100 ml. The common medical explanations for impairment include:-

a) Head injury
b) Cerebral tumour
c) Cardiovascular accident - epilepsy

d) Multiple sclerosis

e) Acute vertigo

f) Hypoglycaemia

g) Hyperglycaemia

h) Thyrotoxicosis

i) Uraemia

j) Hepatic failure

k) Fatigue

l) Carbon monoxide poisoning

m) Psychosis

n) Drugs

In Scotland, the clinical examination under Section 4 of the Road Traffic Act is conducted in the absence of police officers except when the blood sample is being taken, which they witness (*Reid v Nixon,* 1948 JC 68). An examination requiring the active co-operation of the driver may only be conducted with his consent.

If the driver refuses consent, observations can be made, though this is of dubious value and certainly will not exclude medical explanations. Nevertheless, evidence obtained in this way may still be led for the Crown. The blood or urine sample, or both, should be regarded as part of the examination.

Clinical examination

Scottish police forces use a nationally agreed pro forma, a practice which might profitably be followed elsewhere. The significant features are:

Medical history	Epilepsy? Diabetes? Current medical treatment?
Memory	Chronological account of events that day?
Food and drink	When was the last meal taken? What alcohol intake is admitted to?
Demeanour	This is not particularly reliable, but the state of clothing, soiling with vomit and other aspects of demeanour are worth recording.
Pulse *Blood pressure* *Respiration*	
Central nervous system	The most accurate test for alcohol is nystagmus. Penttila & Tenhu's paper (1976) is essential reading. The following test should be carried out:-

Finger to finger
>
Finger to nose
Walking a straight line
Turning rapidly
Standing on one leg
Standing on both legs with eyes closed
Picking up small objects from ground

Eyes	Suffused conjunctivae
	Inequality of size of pupils
	Reaction to light and accommodation
	Visual acuity
Breath odour	Smell of alcohol, cannabis, solvent or ketone
Urine	Separate consent should be obtained for urine testing, explaining its clinical value
Injuries	

At the end of the examination the doctor may have excluded any illness simulating alcohol intoxication, but confirmation that impairment is caused by drugs or alcohol will come when the results are obtained from the analyst.

Hospital procedure

While a person is at hospital as a patient he shall not be required to provide a specimen of breath for a breath test or to provide a specimen for a laboratory test unless the medical practitioner in immediate charge of his case has consented. To be valid, this consent must be obtained by the police surgeon from both doctor and driver.

There are very few medical circumstances which preclude sampling; police surgeons may need to remind accident and emergency staff of this. Members of the hospital staff are, however, in the best position to say whether or not the driver may be examined.

Blood specimen kits, identical to those held at police stations, are available at the hospital or are brought there for the police surgeon's use and the procedure for obtaining the sample is exactly the same as at a police station. Hospital staff are not involved in sampling for Road Traffic Act purposes.

In the case of an unconscious driver whom the police surgeon believes to have been drinking, a powerful argument is available that consent before a sample is taken is not required, on the basis that the doctor's duty to society outweighs his duty to the patient/driver. It has yet to be tested that evidence derived in this way will be accepted by the courts. In *Friel v Dickson* 1992 SLT at page 1080, the accused had a blood alcohol of 128 mg%, had had doses of narcotics to alleviate the pain of a road accident in which his legs had been trapped and was unable to provide a breath specimen. The police surgeon explained who he was and asked if the driver consented to the supply of a blood sample; the accused made no reply, simply holding out his arm rigidly, which the doctor took as tacit consent. The driver was not convicted. On appeal by the prosecutor, the judges ruled that initial consent must be obtained by the police officer in the context of an explanation by the constable of the purpose for which the specimen is required and the consequences flowing from a refusal; that does not relieve the medical practitioner from obtaining fresh consent to the taking of the specimen before he takes it. The consent which is required in the circumstances is consent by a person who is conscious of what he is doing and has heard and understood the request for it.

Medical aspects of fitness to drive

Though, operationally, guidelines on the aspects of fitness to drive are more the prerogative of the occupational physician than the forensic examiner, all doctors nevertheless should be familiar with *Medical Aspects of Fitness to Drive* published by the Medical Commission on Accident Prevention. An *At a Glance* booklet which is reproduced in summaries at the end of each chapter of the main book is also available from the Commission.

A number of drugs and diseases affect fitness to drive. Each time a diagnosis is made or a prescription given to an adult, the doctor should consider whether it affects fitness to drive.

The regulations on medical fitness differ for ordinary and for Passenger Carrying (PCV) or Large Goods (LGV) licences. An ordinary driving licence is valid up to the age of 70. Every licence states that a driver is obliged to report to DVLA any potential or actual medical disability which may affect his driving. Few are aware of this and doctors should bring it to the patient's attention where relevant.

Medical examination of elderly drivers for motor insurance purposes is common. These examinations should not take the form of an ordinary medical examination, but include an evaluation of how age has affected the patient as a driver. Much useful information is gained by watching the patient enter the consulting room and undress. They frequently have difficulty standing on one leg while undressing or unbuttoning. Reaction times can be measured by simple tests such as catching a 12 inch ruler by clapping both hands which start by being six inches (15 cm) apart. When in doubt, a doctor should have no hesitation in inviting the patient to take him for a drive.

General medical conditions

Many medical conditions affect driving. Some drivers will have had their cars modified and it is surprising the extent to which this will overcome physical disability. Again, a trial drive with the patient is frequently the best test of fitness. The main medical conditions affecting driving are:

1. Fatigue

2. Illness

    A Cardiovascular system
   - a) angina or infarction
   - b) hypertension or side-effects of treatment
   - c) arrhythmias
   - d) aortic stenosis or incompetence
   - e) heart block

    B Diabetes
   - a) diet
   - b) hypoglycaemia
   - c) impaired vision
   - d) insulin
   - e) neuropathy

    C Epilepsy

    D Nervous system
   - a) stroke – i giddiness, fainting
     - ii visual field loss
     - iii hemiparesis
   - b) Parkinson's
   - c) multiple sclerosis
   - d) vision
   - e) vertigo
   - f) limb weakness
   - g) sensory defects
   - h) cerebellar inco-ordination
   - i) deafness
   - j) migraine

    E Mental illness
   - a) psychosis
   - b) psychopathy
   - c) substance abuse

    F Vision
   - a) acuity

b) fields

c) diplopia

d) colour vision

e) dark adaptation

G Head injury and other locomotor problems

a) post traumatic epilepsy

b) loss of concentration

c) weakness

d) stiffness

e) artificial limbs

H Ageing

a) medical examination from age 70

b) senescence

Drugs

Many prescribed drugs affect driving. The effects tend to be worst at the beginning of treatment and advice should be given to stick to the dose, to try the drug when at home in the evening with the car garaged for the day and not to combine with any self medication.

Prescribed drugs:

1. analeptics/barbiturates
2. tranquillisers
3. anti-depressants
4. anti-psychotics
5. anti-histamines
6. narcotics
7. analgesics
8. anaesthetics

Illicit drugs:

1. prescribed, such as diazepam
2. opiates
3. cannabis
4. hallucinogens

LGV/PCV drivers

The conditions for heavy goods vehicle and passenger carrying vehicle drivers are more stringent. The licence requires a medical examination, but the decision on fitness is made by medical staff of the DVLA on the basis of the examining doctor's report. The main conditions affecting fitness to drive in this group are:

1. Cardiovascular system
   a) angina, myocardial infarction
   b) heart block/pacemaker
   c) arrhythmia
   d) syncope
2. Diabetes – diet and biguanides allowed
3. Epilepsy
   a) after age 3 = bar
   b) lung carcinoma = bar (cerebral secondary)
4. Progressive nervous diseases
5. Psychosis or low IQ
6. Visual defects

ACCIDENTS IN THE HOME

Some examples of home accidents are described (see box below) but it is useful to carry in one's mind a classification such as that employed by the Department of Trade in its Home Accident Surveillance Scheme.

Accidental knocks may be difficult to differentiate from deliberate blows. The single injury is usually accidental, whereas multiple blows suggest assault. Often, in non-accidental injury, the significant features are that bruises are of different ages or show different patterns. Accidental knocks most often involve the exposed surfaces of the body (back of head, nose, shoulder blades, elbows, knees, shins)

---

1. Struck by or bumped into somebody or something
2. Cut or piercing injury (includes effects of splinters)
3. Ingestions to the mouth, eye or other orifice including swallowed or inhaled substances but excluding poisoning
4. Burns and scalds
5. Explosions
6. Suspected poisoning
7. Mechanical suffocation
8. Near-drowning or submersion
9. Accidents involving electric current or radiation
10. Over-exertion
11. Fall, trip or stumble

---

whereas deliberate blows are also applied to unexposed, unprotected areas (within the orbits, the 'safe' triangle of the neck, the flanks). Knowledge of injury pattern is essential in founding a firm diagnosis of non-accidental injury in children (see chapter 7).

There are primary and secondary patterns of injury. An example is the tendency of falling objects to strike the front of the head, the shoulders and the front of the chest; the victim may then fall backwards striking the back of the head on the floor.

Fractures of the neck of the fifth metacarpal, with their associated soft tissue hump over the outer metacarpophalangeal joint on the back of the hand, are hardly ever caused by an accidental knock (unless the assailant, in failing to strike his victim, accidentally hits an unyielding surface, such as a wall).

A common domestic injury resulting often from a very slight knock is the pretibial laceration seen in the post-menopausal female. The flap of paper-thin skin is often extensive, but it is usually viable and should not be detached.

Wounds from knives, scissors or tin cans happen commonly in the home. They are usually easy to distinguish from non-accidental knife wounding (see chapter 8).

Glass is frequently involved and, with its sharp cutting edge, can cause deep stab wounds involving vessels, tendon or nerve. Splinters of glass may break off to remain in the wound as foreign bodies. Again, it is fairly easy from the pattern of injury to tell whether the incident was deliberate or accidental.

Wounds to the toes from rotary lawnmowers and to various parts of the body from other gardening tools happen commonly at the start of the gardening season.

All sorts of objects, from foodstuffs to pieces of toy, can become inhaled or ingested. They rarely involve the forensic physician unless there is alleged to be negligence in a manufacturing process; toys or other objects which break up to become swallowed should be submitted to the local trading standards department for their scrutiny.

Scalds at home are common, usually due to an inquisitive toddler pulling over a pan of hot or boiling water. This produces a circumscribed area of thermal injury over the shoulders, upper arms and trunk. Beware the multiple splash scalds to the trunk and face sustained when hot liquid is thrown at the victim. Beware, also, scalding in the glove and stocking distribution of arms or legs or of the buttocks, the dunking injury of child abuse (chapter 7, fig. 10).

Domestic explosions are uncommon but may result from the striking of a match in the presence of leaking gas. An unusual cause of explosion is that following the accidental mixture of toilet cleanser with strong household bleach: chlorine may be liberated from the lavatory pan in large quantities and sometimes with explosive force. The occasional case of explosive injury to the hands and fingers from home-made firework manufacture is seen every year.

In the context of home accidents, carbon monoxide poisoning is worth a reminder. This is still rife despite the change to domestic natural gas supply. It follows incomplete combustion of any carbonaceous fuel. At the scene of a suspicious death in the home, especially when the subject is lying close to a gas fire, consider carbon monoxide high on the list of causes. In a warm environment the classic cherry-red hue of the skin is unusual; it is certainly not seen in the living. It will be found in areas of hypostasis, especially when the body is examined in the cold atmosphere of the mortuary. If signs suggesting combustion problems — a blocked flue, soot on the ceiling, excessive condensation — are present, further investigations of this probable cause may well avert a full-blown murder enquiry. (A useful videotape on carbon monoxide poisoning has been produced for the medical profession and is available on free loan from British Gas.)

The fall in the home: 'Did he fall or was he pushed?' Investigators at the scene will be looking for accidental causes such as a loose stair rod, a cracked floor board, a carelessly left obstruction or a slippery surface. It is frequently very difficult to distinguish an accidental from a natural or deliberate fall and, of course, it is here that the detailed autopsy comes into its own.

ACCIDENTS AT WORK

Works accidents may result from the special problems of the working environment or from the particular equipment used in industrial processes.

The effects of inclement working environments are seen particularly in mining accidents, at sea and in off-shore installations. To the problems of remoteness and difficulty of access may be added the effects of extreme temperatures and changes in pressure (dysbarism).

Industrial equipment is, by its nature, liable to produce major injury. The equipment is often heavy and the large forces generated will cause crushing or avulsive damage, including mechanical suffocation or strangulation, traumatic amputation and tissue dehiscence. Rotating rollers or wheels produce tangential, degloving wounds. Fingertip amputations from circular cutting blades remain common. Steam and heat may be used in pressing or sealing machines and mechanical wounding may be compounded by thermal injury.

The use of machine guards, automatic cut-outs and safety equipment, the vigilance of factory inspectors and the influence of health and safety at work legislation have all dramatically cut the number and serious effects of accidents occurring in the workplace.

Further Reading

British Medical Association June 1989 *Guide to Alcohol and Accidents* BMA London.

British Medical Association 1988 *The Drinking Driver*, London, BMJ publishing group.

British Medical Journal, leading article, 1996 Alcohol – Pushing the Limits **312**: 7–10.

Committee on Safety of Medicines: Current Problems in Pharmaco-vigilance. 1995, 21 (page 10-10) Drugs and Driving.

Denny R.C. 1986 *Alcohol and Accidents*, Cheshire, Sigmund Press.

Department of Health and Social Security, Research Report No 13 1985 *Medical Effects of Seat Belt Legislation in the United Kingdom* HMSO, London.

Gogler E. 1965 *Road Accidents* in *Documenta Geigy* CIBA-Geigy, Macclesfield, UK.

Institute of Alcohol Studies 1987: *None for the Road*, IAS, London, 1987.

Institute of Alcohol Studies 1987: *Drinking and Driving – Controlling the Massacre*, IAS, London, 1987.

Mason JK (Ed) 1993 *The Pathology of Trauma*, 2nd edition, Edward Arnold, London.

Medical Commission on Accident Prevention 1995 *Medical Aspects of Fitness to Drive*, 5th edition MCAP London.

National Association of Emergency Medical Technicians 1994 *Pre-Hospital Trauma Life Support Manual,* 3rd Edition, Mosby - Year Book, Inc, Missouri.

Penttila A & Tenhu M. 1976 Clinical examination as medico-legal proof of alcohol intoxication. *Medicine, Science and the Law* **16**:95-102.

Royal College of Physicians Report, 1987 *The Medical Consequences of Alcohol Abuse: A Great and Growing Evil*, London.

Blood Alcohol Levels in Road Accident Fatalities in Great Britain – 1993. 1995, LF 2072 Transport Research Laboratory. Crowthorne

13

THE SCENE OF CRIME
AND TRACE EVIDENCE

I Shaw, I Hogg, B Rankin

The solution of many crimes, and certainly all major ones, depends to a large extent on scientific support for the investigation team. This can cover a wide spectrum of specialisms both inside and outside the police service, and includes the police surgeon. Initial crime scene examination is mainly carried out by police or civilian Scenes of Crime Officers (SOCOs) supplemented by other experts where their specific knowledge and expertise is required. The formation of Scientific Support Departments within police forces has varied greatly from force to force but the majority incorporate personnel responsible for photography, fingerprint, marks/impressions and some forensic examination either as individual or multi-functional disciplines. In Scotland, ballistic and suspect document examination often falls within the scientific support department's remit.

Detailed analysis of trace elements left at a scene by the perpetrator and subsequent comparison with samples taken from a suspect will frequently solve a case, therefore it must be ensured that a complete and comprehensive examination of the scene is carried out and that all material seized is properly packaged and preserved for future analysis. The potential value of the information gained from such a careful examination is so important that those who have access to the scene for whatever purpose must appreciate the severe consequences of displaying a careless or haphazard attitude. In order that all the disciplines present at a scene accomplish their full potential a recognised order of examination is followed or, where conflict occurs, proper discussion is held with the senior investigating officer (SIO).

PRESERVATION OF THE SCENE

Scientific support in some form has always been an integral part of crime scene investigation, but with advances in latent fingerprint development techniques, photography and forensic science the importance of evidence gleaned from a scene by scenes of crime officers and forensic scientists has become in some cases the lead investigative tool rather than taking a 'support' role. In order that all available evidence can be taken from a scene, the integrity of the location concerned is of paramount importance.

In this regard, the initial steps taken by the first officer attending can greatly assist an enquiry. Careful thought has to be given to the circumstances which present themselves to the officer. External locations present the greatest challenge. Control and preservation of evidence can require fast and decisive action because of the weather. Where death has occurred, the immediate area surrounding a deceased may have to be protected from the elements, with particular attention being paid to preserving any access or egress route. Internal locations generally present the officer with a more controlled environment, but still place vital importance on the immediate area surrounding the deceased and the entrance and egress routes of the perpetrator. These include paths, common entrances, back courts/gardens, pavements and even roadways. The officer has to be aware of the damage he can do or allow others to do while the locus is under his control and to this end he has to form a protected/controlled area as quickly as possible and identify a common route or path to be used by all personnel approaching and leaving the scene. Thereafter, access to this area must be restricted to essential personnel until the arrival of the photographer, SOCO and, where relevant, the forensic scientist. Those who have no specific task to perform, no matter what their rank or position, must be excluded from the scene. At times, overriding considerations such as the need to save life or prevent further injury, to ascertain that life is extinct, to search the premises for further victims or perpetrators, justify contravening this principle, but this should be strictly controlled.

Experience over the years has identified a number of areas where actions at a scene have destroyed potential evidence or introduced cross contamination. Examples are shown in table 1.

Where any action has been taken which disturbs the scene, even inadvertently, it should be brought to the attention of the senior investigating officer. Close control must be maintained of all persons entering a scene. At major incident scenes large numbers of personnel from a variety of disciplines can be expected to require access. These can include police, fire service, ambulance, utility services, local authority employees, service personnel. Detailed logs are kept, noting arrival and departure times of all persons and are generally situated at the access to the controlled area. The activities of all these people must be co-ordinated in order that the actions of one do not prejudice the actions of another, and it is for the senior investigating officer, having considered the requirements of the case, to programme operations in such a way as to maximise the benefits he can gain from the disciplines present.

Use of telephone	—	Addition/obliteration of fingerprints
Use of washing facilities	—	Obliteration of blood-stained fingerprints on and around basins; flushing of possible evidential material from sink trap
Use of toilet facilities	—	Flushing of possible evidential material from toilet; addition/obliteration of fingerprints.
Use of towels	—	Cross-contamination
Smoking at scene	—	Addition of cigarette stub and ash
Unnecessary handling of weapons	—	Addition/obliteration of fingerprints; possible injury.
Use of bare hands to open door	—	Addition/obliteration of fingerprints
Careless use of gloved hands	—	Obliteration of fingerprints
Standing on footwear/tyre impressions	—	Obliteration
Standing on wet blood	—	Additional footwear impressions
Moving the body or clothing of deceased	—	Photographs should be taken first
Covering body with blanket	—	Introduction of extraneous fibres
Entering crime scene without protective clothing/footwear	—	Cross-contamination

Table 1

TECHNIQUES USED AT THE SCENE

Photography

Photographs taken at a crime scene are used as evidence in subsequent court proceedings to give a visual impression of the location concerned and to detail particular aspects of the scene which yield specific information required by the senior investigating officer. It is important, therefore, that the scene is not disturbed before the arrival of a photographer, enabling him to capture a true record of the scene as left by the perpetrator. The photographs also assist witnesses (including the police surgeon) to recall the scene and their actions. On arrival at a scene the photographer would consult the SIO to determine which views must be taken. The senior investigating officer is ultimately responsible for deciding which photographs are taken, but the photographer, using his professional knowledge and experience, will offer advice and ensure that sufficient photographs are taken. Normal practice is to record progressively as the photographer enters, in order to capture the scene undisturbed and to maintain continuity. Crime scene photographs fall into three main categories:

1. Long views: showing general location and conditions.

2. Intermediate views: showing more detail of general areas and high-lighting specific sections to relate close-up photographs to the general scene.

3. Close-up views: detailed perspective of potential evidential material.

Long and intermediate views should always be taken using a standard 50mm lens to guarantee that no distortion is present in the photographs; where possible, they are taken from eye level, ensuring that witnesses can relate to any views they would have witnessed at the scene. Close-up views can be taken with a variety of lenses or close-up attachments.

Long views illustrate the general situation and several shots may be required to cover a large area. In difficult locations, aerial photography is frequently used to complement the ground shots. Where the crime takes place indoors, it is common practice to photograph the exterior of the building and the surrounding area.

Medium views cover the general area surrounding the deceased, showing conditions in general and relating the overall scene to specific items and places. If located indoors, all the rooms within the premises would be photographed with views taken from each of the four corners. Views of the deceased from a variety of angles are taken using a standard 50mm lens and must be recorded before any disturbance has been caused. Where possible, a photograph of the deceased's face is taken for use in identification.

Close-up views are used to record particular items of evidence at the locus, or visible wounds, bruises, discolouration and abrasions on the deceased; if, during an examination, the doctor notices any of these features he should draw them to the attention of the photographer. More specific detailed photographs of all wounds and so on are taken at the post-mortem on the directions of the pathologist.

Injury photographs are taken at right angles to the subject using a scale, ensuring that prints can be reproduced to actual size. In certain circumstances ultraviolet photography can be used to photograph injuries months after the visible signs have disappeared.

Most police forces now video major crime scenes; although these are occasionally produced in court, their main function is to provide a comprehensive record of the scene for briefing and de-briefing purposes.

Where the offence is one of assault, cruelty or rape, the doctor should consider requesting photographs to be taken, although he should remember that to the police, the purpose of photography is to compile a book of photographs for production in court; because of this the views requested, particularly in cases of a sexual nature, should be suited to the court, rather than to a medical lecture.

Fingerprinting

The examination of a crime scene for visible and latent finger and palm print impressions by scenes of crime officers can lead to an expeditious identification of the person responsible. Numerous major crimes are solved exclusively by the identification of fingerprint marks from the locus being attributable to one specific person, placing them at or near the scene of the crime.

Techniques available to the SOCO are developing continually, although aluminium and other powders are still widely utilised at the locus in the examination of dry, smooth surfaces. These powders are brushed over the surface with any resultant impression either photographed or lifted by means of a low impact adhesive tape which is then placed on to a clear acetate mount and retained for comparison and subsequent court proceedings.

Many other surfaces can be examined for latent impressions using a variety of individual or sequential chemical treatments to give results which a few years ago would have been impossible.

Some of the surfaces and related treatments are listed below:

Paper/cardboard	–	Ninhydrin
Wet paper	–	Physical developer
Hard plastics	–	Superglue
Polythene bags	–	Metal deposition
Adhesive tape	–	Gentian violet
Vinyl/rubber/leather	–	Superglue
Raw wood	–	Ninhydrin
Bloody surfaces	–	Amido black
Fabric	–	Radioactive sulphur dioxide

In addition to the above treatments, surfaces can be examined by the use of fluorescence. This involves examination of an article with a high intensity light source to produce a fluorescent effect from either naturally occurring chemicals in a fingerprint or ones which have been introduced during treatment.

It can be seen that the contamination of any surface within a crime scene, even with gloved hands, must be avoided to ensure the best possible conditions for the SOCOs to carry out their examinations.

Articles most likely to come to the attention of the doctor include weapons and medicine bottles which should not be handled without consultation with a qualified SOCO. If a doctor has handled any item by necessity or accident, he should notify the SOCO or, in his absence, a police officer at the locus.

Ballistics

Examination of the scene of a shooting incident will reveal a great deal of information about the type of weapon used, the distance over which it was fired, the position of the firer and, often, whether what happened was accidental, suicidal or homicidal.

When a shot is fired from close range, the clothing and the skin of the victim can disclose various features which, by subsequent ballistic testing of the weapon concerned, are used to estimate the range and direction of shot. Accordingly, it is important that any such marks or injuries be photographed (with a scale, as in fig. 1) for future analysis, and that extra care be taken with the victim's clothing to preserve any residue, particles of propellant or projectiles for similar reasons.

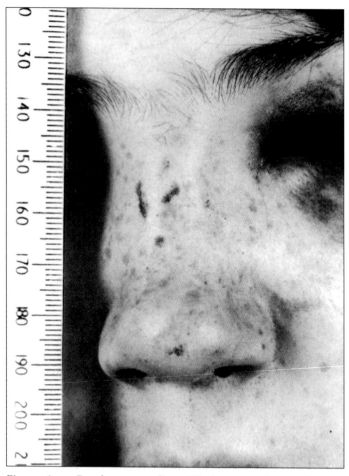

Figure 1 – Gunshot wounding. Black eye and tattooing on nose. Note centimetre scale. *This photograph and figure 2 are reproduced by courtesy of the Chief Constable of Strathclyde.*

Projectiles come in an enormous variety of shapes and sizes. What conforms to the normal idea of a bullet shape is seldom found. Bullets and other projectiles deform very readily on impact, often shattering into many pieces of such diverse shape that they are recognisable as projectiles only to the informed eye. For example, the copper/nickel jacket of a pistol or rifle bullet can separate from the lead core; unless care is taken to recover all parts, the ability to match the bullet to a specific weapon could be lost. Photographs of bullets, projectiles and cartridge components are shown in fig. 2.

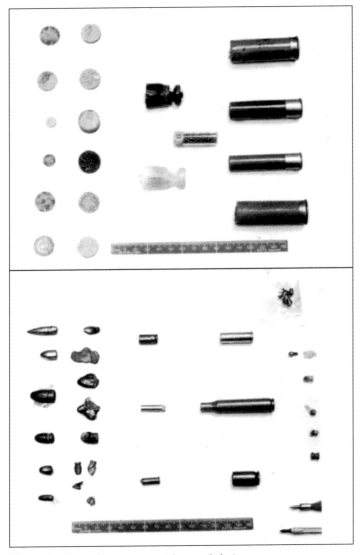

Figure 2 – (top) Shotgun cartridges and their components.
(bottom) Cartridge cases and projectiles, many grossly deformed.

DOCUMENTS

Document examination and handwriting do not normally come within the scope of a scene of crime examination, but police surgeons should be aware that injudicious handling of paper material could cause difficulties.

One of the examinations carried out on paper uses the ESDA (electrostatic detection apparatus) which will visualise very fresh fingerprint impressions, footprints and indented writing on the paper. This evidence is easily destroyed. Paper is also subjected to chemical treatments to raise latent fingerprints; careless handling with bare hands may impart further impressions, wholly or partially obliterating the writing on the document, so preventing handwriting comparison. Even to fold or smooth paper may interfere with analysis.

THE DOCTOR AT THE SCENE

The primary reason for the attendance of the police surgeon is usually to pronounce life extinct, which should be done as soon as the doctor arrives. Where death is obviously due to foul play this may be the doctor's only function, but where the circumstances surrounding the death are not clear a preliminary examination may be required at the scene.

Before gaining access to the immediate area surrounding the deceased the doctor should confirm with the SIO present if a designated route into the scene has been established and whether the scene has been photographed. Care must be taken in approaching the deceased, even along the pre-determined route, in order that footprints, fingerprint and other forensic trace evidence is not destroyed. Should signs of life be found, subsequent actions to revive the patients take priority, but the doctor should bear in mind the preservation of evidence whenever possible.

If the deceased has not been photographed, movement of the body, clothing or surrounding items should be delayed, but where circumstances dictate and any disturbance of the scene has been caused, the photographer and officer in charge of the enquiry must be informed: it is then recorded that the photographs do not represent the scene as found. No attempt should be made to return the scene to its original state for photography. When, during an examination, a doctor declares a death suspicious he should stop and have the scene photographed.

Even where initial evidence points to a sudden death, subsequent post-mortem examination may reveal foul play and a murder inquiry be initiated. The doctor should therefore ensure that in all circumstances a satisfactory examination has been carried out and attention paid to evidence preservation. Professional litter such as discarded gloves and instrument wrappings must be removed from the locus for disposal.

THE ROLE OF THE FORENSIC SCIENTIST

The role of the forensic scientist is to carry out appropriate scientific examinations in support of the investigation of crime. The purpose of these examinations may be:

- to determine if a crime has been committed. Examples here would be determining the level of alcohol in a driver's blood sample or identifying a substance as a controlled drug.

- to provide corroborative evidence. For example, linking a suspect to the victim by demonstrating that semen on a vaginal swab could have come from the suspect.

- to provide intelligence. Identifying a suspect from blood left at the scene of a crime through the DNA Database would be an example here.

While most of the work is carried out at the laboratory, the forensic scientist will often undertake examinations at the scene of crime. Examinations at the scene may be of vital importance in helping to establish exactly what went on. The interpretation of bloodstains can help to identify the location and nature of an attack. The identification of several seats of burning may establish the cause of a fire as arson. Attending the scene also allows the forensic scientist to select the most appropriate material for detailed examination back at the laboratory.

Most laboratory examinations are, however, carried out on material selected and recovered by others such as SOCOs, police officers, the pathologist or the police surgeon. In many instances the forensic scientist may have little knowledge of the circumstances of the case beyond those provided on the case submission form and associated documents such as medical examination forms.

The importance of a relevant and complete picture of the alleged circumstances, together with a clear requirement in terms of what the investigator is seeking to establish, cannot be over emphasised. Using this information, the forensic scientist will identify how best to approach the examination, which scientific methods to employ and how to interpret the findings and reach conclusions that address all the relevant points of the case.

The type of scientific evidence employed in the investigation of crime covers a wide range of scientific expertise from molecular biology to metallurgy. In the past, laboratories have tended to be organised by scientific discipline. However, recent changes in the ways in which the police investigate crime, together with new developments in forensic science, have resulted in cases benefiting from a new approach to the way in which they are investigated in the laboratory.

Instead of being organised into divisions such as 'Biology' or 'Chemistry' the modern forensic science laboratory is now more likely to consist of units based around crime types such as volume crime (burglary, theft, criminal damage), serious crime (homicide, robbery, sexual offences) and drug offences. Each unit will consist of scientists who, together, embrace all the knowledge and skills necessary to investigate the types of cases allocated to their unit. Supporting these crime based units will be service units providing specialist analytical support, such as chemical analysis or DNA profiling.

The types of scientific examinations that are undertaken in the laboratory may be broadly categorised into physical, drugs and toxicological, and biological.

Biological examinations

In the past, biological examinations have been associated primarily with providing corroborative evidence in cases of violent crime. Changes in the way that crimes are now investigated, coupled with new scientific developments, have resulted in the evidence from biological examinations being applied to a wider range of crime and to all stages of the investigative process. However, of greatest importance to the police surgeon will be the types of evidence associated with violent crime.

By its very nature, violent crime may often result in close, prolonged physical contact between the suspect and the victim, the scene of crime, and weapons or implements that may be associated with the crime. The inter-relationship between all these elements is shown in fig. 3.

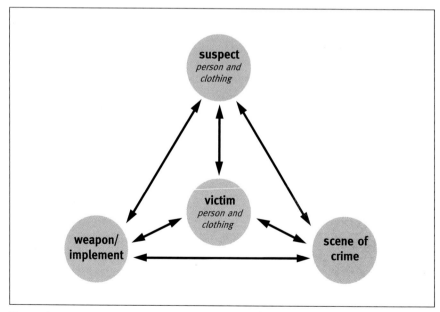

Figure 3

Depending on the type of the crime, the degree of contact, and the nature of the scene, there are opportunities for the transfer of a wide variety of evidence types. In addition, other aspects of evidence such as blood stain distribution or damage to clothing may be present. The type of trace evidence which is of greatest significance to the police surgeon is that derived from body fluids.

Body fluids

The forensic scientist is able to identify and analyse a number of body fluids. Some fluids such as blood and semen can be identified with certainty, whereas the forensic scientist may only be able to provide an opinion as to the likelihood of certain other materials such as saliva or vaginal secretions. While most of the body fluids encountered in casework are human, the forensic scientist is also able to provide an opinion as to the species of origin of animal material.

The identification of blood and semen involves the initial use of presumptive tests which locate likely stains. Semen is confirmed by identifying spermatozoa on slides which have been stained with haematoxylin and eosin. In the absence of spermatozoa, perhaps as a result of vasectomy, the presence of other components such as choline and seminal acid phosphatase can be used to confirm semen.

The identification of spermatozoa on internal vaginal swabs is of particular importance as it can confirm recent sexual intercourse. However, care must be taken in using the findings from vaginal swabs to indicate time since intercourse. Spermatozoa may persist in the vagina for up to 72 hours, and on rare occasions even up to a week. The presence of bleeding does not prevent the taking of swabs or the identification and subsequent analysis of semen; it can however affect the survival of spermatozoa in the vagina. It is important for the police surgeon to obtain a recent sexual history from the subject, as such information may be vital in helping to interpret the scientific findings.

In cases of oral sex, semen may be recovered from face and mouth swabs and saliva samples. Similarly, semen can be recovered from skin swabs or clippings of matted pubic hair. In cases of buggery, semen may be recovered from anal swabs.

The examination of vaginal or anal swabs for lubricants may be of importance where the attacker has used a condom or has used a lubricant to aid penetration. Penile swabs can also be examined for traces of lubricants as well as vaginal material, faeces, saliva and blood. As well as being the source of lubricants, a discarded condom can link the attacker to the crime through the analysis of the semen contents and vaginal material and/or blood from the outer surface. Swabbings from bite marks may yield traces of saliva.

Several methods are available to the forensic scientist for establishing the likely donor of body fluids. Tests for blood groups such as ABO, and polymorphic enzymes and serum proteins such as Phospho-Gluco-Mutase (PGM) and Haptoglobin (Hp), while still used on occasions, have largely been replaced by DNA profiling.

DNA PROFILING

The origins of DNA profiling – multi locus probes

DNA profiling has revolutionised forensic science since its introduction in 1986. Based on the discovery of Professor Sir Alec Jeffries at Leicester University in 1984, the original Multi Locus Probe technique (MLP) offered a significant advance on the conventional blood grouping techniques that were then the order of the day. The profiles produced by the MLP method were a complex pattern of up to 16 or more bands. With a chance of 1 in 4 people sharing any one band, the likelihood of 2 unrelated people having the same profile of 16 bands has been calculated at one in many millions. However, the very complexity of the MLP profiles could cause difficulties in interpretation, particularly in those cases where there was DNA from more than one person.

While the MLP method proved to be highly discriminating it was not very sensitive. The technique worked best on those materials, such as semen, that were able to yield relatively large amounts of chromosomal DNA. This was complemented by the ability to separate the DNA from semen from other sources such as vaginal material or blood. However, to get a result from bloodstains, where the only sources of suitable DNA are the nucleated white cells, required a stain the size of a postage stamp and obtaining results from saliva was rarely possible.

The introduction of single locus probes

Many of the problems associated with the MLP technique were reduced by the introduction of the Single Locus Probe method (SLP). This method resulted in far simpler profiles of just two bands or sometimes even only one. This simplification of the profile was accompanied by a large reduction in discrimination such that it was necessary to combine the results from 4 or more independent SLPs to get back to the discriminating power of the MLP method. This apart, the improved sensitivity of the SLP method meant that results could now be obtained from smaller amount of material which resulted in DNA profiling being applied to a much wider range of crimes.

The simplification of the profiles meant that results could now be interpreted more easily from mixtures of more than one individual. In addition, the simpler profiles enabled machine reading of DNA results, which permitted the storage and retrieval of SLP profiles on a computer, opening the way for the creation of a limited DNA database.

The way forward – polymerase chain reaction

The quest for increased sensitivity also led forensic scientists to look at the novel Polymerase Chain Reaction technique (PCR). Through carefully controlled cycles of heating and cooling a targeted area of the DNA molecule can be induced to make several hundred thousand exact copies of itself. Tiny amounts of starting DNA can be amplified until there is sufficient to analyse.

The early application of PCR targeted a region of the DNA molecule that coded for the Human Leucocyte Antigen (HLA) - DQa. This permitted limited HLA typing of a sample using DNA analysis. The increase in sensitivity meant that forensic scientists could now get results from bloodstains smaller than a match head and also from material such as saliva and even aspermic semen. The increased sensitivity also meant that results could be obtained from samples where the DNA had degraded, leaving only minute amounts of intact DNA.

With only one HLA type being targeted, the discriminating power of this early PCR based method was very low with chances of a random match being 1 in 100 at the very best. The low discriminating power of HLA - DQa restricted the use of PCR to cases where other methods of DNA profiling or blood grouping had failed or there was insufficient material to attempt any other test.

The limitations of HLA - DQa led quickly to the development of alternative PCR based methods. In 1994 the Forensic Science Service (FSS) launched a new PCR based method of DNA profiling which analysed areas of DNA known as Short Tandem Repeats (STR). The first implementation of STR improved the level of discrimination to a 1 in 10,000 chance of a random match. This was soon followed by the introduction of a second generation STR method which saw the level of discrimination restored to that of MLP and SLP with a chance of a random match now back up to 1 in several millions.

STR results can be obtained from any material that yields chromosomal DNA. Small bloodstains, traces of semen, saliva from cigarette ends and envelope flaps, a single hair root, can all give results. A measure of the sensitivity of the technique can be gauged by the fact that results have even been obtained from spermatozoa recovered from microscope slides that had been prepared 10 years earlier from material in a rape case. Even though the material on the slide had been fixed, stained in haematoxylin and eosin and mounted in a xylene based mountant, STR profiles were still obtained. Profiles have also been obtained from histological preparations, including cervical smears.

The use of semi-automated equipment coupled with computer aided analysis and interpretation of results means that DNA profiles can now be obtained within 48 hours compared to the 14 days for the early MLP method. Semi-automation, which also helped to reduce the cost of analysis, combined with computerisation, enabled the FSS to introduce the world's first national DNA database.

The DNA database

A DNA database has been the goal of forensic scientists and the police since the introduction of DNA profiling in 1986. The improvements in technology, combined with the recommendations of the 1993 Royal Commission on Criminal Justice, led to the establishment of the national DNA Database in April 1995. The introduction of the database was supported by changes to the Police and Criminal Evidence Act codes which included the reclassification of mouth swabs as non-intimate samples and confirmation that plucked hairs (excluding pubic) are also non-intimate samples. Such samples could now be taken by a police officer, without consent, where the subject has been charged or reported for, or convicted of, a recordable offence.

Samples from suspects are submitted to the Birmingham laboratory of the FSS for analysis and inclusion on the DNA database. Material found at the scene of a crime which is suitable for DNA profiling is submitted to the local forensic science laboratory for analysis and the results of these analyses are also put on to the database. Comparison of profiles from suspects and crime stains is a continuous process. As the result from each new suspect is added, that person is searched against all the outstanding crime on the database. Similarly, as the result from each new crime stain is added, that sample is searched against all suspects. As well as linking a suspect to a crime, the database also links crimes. It does this by matching the results from different crimes that have been committed by the same person, even if that individual is not on the database.

The results from the database may not be used as evidence directly but only as intelligence. Having established a link between a suspect and a crime the police are informed. Should the police wish to pursue the case using DNA evidence they are then required to take a further sample from the suspect. It is the result from this further sample that will be put before the court as evidence to connect the suspect with the crime.

The application of DNA profiling

The use of DNA profiling is not restricted to demonstrating the link between an individual and material arising from the commission of a crime. A DNA profile is a combination of components of the profiles of one's parents, so DNA profiling can be used to investigate paternity. Whilst most paternity investigations will be in support of civil cases involving disputed paternity, issues of probate or immigration, they may also be used in criminal cases to establish incest or to support the identification of the remains of a victim where more conventional means have failed.

The area of casualty identification in mass disasters is one in which DNA profiling is being used increasingly. The benefits of STR, which can often yield results from poor quality DNA, come into their own when applied to badly burnt or decomposed human remains. If no soft tissue remains, results may even be obtained from bone.

The future of DNA

Improvements in DNA profiling are resulting in a major reappraisal of the position of some other types of biological evidence, particularly of blood grouping. Methods that were the mainstay of forensic biology only 10 years ago are now being phased out with only a restricted capability being retained to deal with the exceptional case.

Our experience to date suggests that DNA technology is likely to change again. The analysis of mitochondrial DNA has already been used in a restricted number of cases, the most notable being the identification by the FSS of bones from the family of the last Czar of Russia. The greater use of mitochondrial DNA will enable DNA profiles to be obtained from an even wider range of material, including the shafts of hair.

The forensic scientist can already identify sex from DNA and research is continuing into the identification of inherited characteristics such as hair colour, eye colour and racial type. From a small spot of blood left at the scene of a crime, the forensic scientist of the future may be able to provide the investigators with a limited physical description of the person that they are looking for.

PHYSICAL EXAMINATIONS

The ubiquitous evidence type at virtually every scene you attend will be footwear impressions. In reality, there are no "Peter Pans" flying about; these impressions will be there, and any comparison of the scene footwear impressions with suspect items of footwear will have the potential to produce conclusive evidence. In other words, one can say that a particular shoe made a particular impression at the scene - an unequivocal link between the two. So, one of the first rules at an scene is "don't put your foot in it". Always use the pathways provided and work with the SIO and crime scene manager to ensure your correct route.

What other evidence types may be present? Any list of evidence types will not be exhaustive and they can all provide a vital link in the investigation depending on the circumstances. Evidence types are not case specific. This means that, when you are attending a serious assault, a specific number of evidence types are not to be considered to the exclusion of others. A scene initially appearing to be a suicide may change into a murder investigation; many other evidence types may then be pertinent.

Below is a list, with the accompanying strength of evidence of various evidential materials, to be used as a general reference. But beware, it is worth emphasising again that evidence types are not case specific, they are circumstance led. This means that evidence types traditionally considered of limited value or of limited significance may well turn out to have greater significance. Equally, the presence of a conclusive link between a person and a scene can become valueless, if, for example, the person later fully admits to being at the scene.

The presence of glass on the floor or ground at the point of entry may suggest the possibility of glass on the clothing of the perpetrator. However, the surface of the glass at the scene can be extremely useful for contact traces such as fingerprints and footwear impressions.

Some evidence types are normally perceived as conclusive, such as fingerprints, a physical fit between two parts of one object, multiple paint layers, shoe and toolmarks. Other evidence may be considered as providing strong support, such as body fluids and plucked root hairs for DNA, multiple fibre mixtures from several sources, rare glass or a mixture of glass types. There can also be what is regarded as moderate evidence, such as ordinary window glass, container glass, a single fibre type, semen and saliva grouping, single paint layer. Finally, but not least, there can be limited evidence such as soil (unless it contains rare materials), sand, brick dust, plaster, mortar – general building material – and faeces. As said previously, the list is not exhaustive and the evidence types are circumstance led.

Other materials such as liquids thrown into a person's face, for example, ammonia or sulphuric acid, or materials used to inactivate a burglar alarm, for example, spray foam or other spray materials can also be encountered.

Only by knowing the circumstances of the case, applying common sense to a sequence of events, and working within the investigation team can relevant evidence types be gathered by members of the investigation team. One of the most difficult aspects of scene investigation is that the contact trace materials cannot always be seen with the naked eye. It is true that some contact trace materials can be easily seen, whereas others can be seen only with the additional help of various light sources. Many of the physical evidence types such as glass and paint will be minute and will not be seen by the naked eye. With so wide a range of evidence types, there may be only one opportunity to collect the evidence, and it needs to be collected in an uncontaminated state. It does not need anyone to put a foot in it!

Other types of physical evidence often encountered are tyre impressions, tool/instrument impressions and physical fits. As with footwear impressions, individual tyre marks are identified using a combination of size, pattern, wear and distinguishing damage marks. If visible, these marks or impressions are photographed before any treatment is carried out, then, depending on the surface, the marks either lifted or cast. Where marks are faint or latent they can be enhanced using a variety of treatments.

Tool/instrument impressions can be produced by various means but, in practice, tend to be chisel or cutting type tools. Marks are identified to individual tools by microscopic comparison of the striations caused by the cutting surface. Impressions are photographed before being cast, using a suitable material.

Any damaged or separated items found at a locus, which could have an elemental part missing, are preserved. Subsequent enquiries may recover items, attributable to the perpetrator, which constitute an exact physical fit. These items are photographed separately and then fitted together to show the fit.

DRUGS AND TOXICOLOGICAL EXAMINATIONS

By far the greatest number of drug examinations are in connection with the Misuse of Drugs Act 1971. The Act covers more than 100 controlled substances, including cannabis, diamorphine (heroin) and morphine, cocaine and 'crack' cocaine, LSD, amphetamine and MDMA (Ecstasy).

In addition to basic identification, detailed examinations may be carried out to establish the concentration of the drug and the presence of adulterants or impurities. Such detailed examinations may be important in helping to substantiate charges of supply or possession with intent to supply. A range of other forensic examinations may also be carried out to establish links between seizures, including the comparison of material, such as cling-film or polythene bags, used to package the individual 'wraps'. Forensic scientists are often called to the scene of illicit laboratories. Their involvement in such cases is crucial, not only to confirm what is being manufactured, but also to establish the method and scale of production. A scientific presence at such scenes is also vital in ensuring that the manufacturing process is shut down safely.

The 1990s has seen a significant increase in the illegal cultivation of cannabis. Using modern hydroponic growing methods combined with specially selected varieties of the plant, it is possible to produce cannabis in the UK which more than rivals that smuggled in from abroad in terms of both yield and strength. These 'home-grown' varieties are often referred to as 'skunk' owing to their pungent smell.

Toxicology investigations generally involve the analysis of body fluids for alcohol, drugs and poisons and may be associated with sudden deaths, poisonings or the effect on behaviour arising from the use of these substances. Sudden death may be suicidally, accidentally or deliberately induced. In the case of the living, toxicology examinations are commonly associated with offences against the Road

Traffic Act and involve driving under the influence of alcohol and/or drugs. Examination for alcohol and drugs is frequently requested for the suspects and victims in other serious offences such as assault, rape and homicide.

THE MEDICAL EXAMINATION – THE REQUIREMENTS OF THE FORENSIC SCIENTIST

Contamination

We have already seen how important it is that the police surgeon takes all possible care to avoid contaminating evidence at the scene of crime. The same care needs to be taken when examining patients and taking samples. Ideally, any doctor who visits the scene of the crime or who examines the victim should not examine any suspects in the same investigation. If a separate doctor is not available the examiner must be able to show that different outer clothing was worn for the examinations of the different parties. Similarly, it is important to use different examination rooms. Any instruments used to collect samples or assist in the taking of samples, such as proctoscopes, must be new, disposable ones. All these necessary precautions are mirrored in the laboratory, where different scientists will conduct the initial examinations of the items from the victims and the suspects.

At every scene attended, the forensic medical examiner must consider a core group of evidential materials, such as blood, semen and saliva. Beyond these, what other evidence types and evidential materials could there be? What influences will these have on the investigation? These questions are at the heart of good practice during an investigation and should be at the forefront of the forensic medical examiner's mind.

Information

The importance of information to the forensic scientist has been referred to earlier. In sexual offences, the vehicle for this information is the Sexual Offences Form. This form will accompany the laboratory submission and should provide the scientist with the necessary background information. Of particular importance are relevant dates and times, such as the date and time that samples were taken and the date and time of the last previous act of intercourse. In cases where a sexual offences form is not required, the police surgeon should ensure that the investigating officer is aware of any information that may be relevant to the forensic scientist.

Samples

The samples to be taken will depend on the type and nature of the crime. Table 2 provides a check list of the more usual samples. The police surgeon should discuss beforehand with the investigating officer, or with the officer present at the medical examination, exactly what is known about the case and what samples are required. If there is any uncertainty about the need for a particular sample it may be better to take it as there is unlikely to be a second opportunity. If a sample considered necessary cannot be taken for a medical reason, that reason should be recorded.

In using the table, police surgeons in Scotland must remember that the provisions of the Police and Criminal Evidence Act do not apply. The Prisoners and Criminal Proceedings (Scotland) Act 1993 gives a constable authority to take from prisoners and detained persons fingerprints, palm prints and impressions of an external part of the body as he thinks it reasonably appropriate. Under the Act, a constable may, with the authority of an officer of a rank no lower than inspector, take hair by cutting or combing; samples from under nails; any external swab of the body. Reasonable force is authorised in carrying out these provisions. Warrants must be obtained if samples requiring invasive techniques are sought.

Swabs

Only plain, sterile untreated swabs should be used. Charcoal or albumen coated swabs must never be used, nor should swabs be placed in transport medium. Make sure that the swab stick is returned to the same tube that it was taken from. The recommendation of the FSS is that all swabs should be frozen as soon as possible following the examination to help counter any allegation of contamination. In some areas outside England and Wales, drying may still be preferred.

Vaginal, anal and mouth swabs

To maximise the recovery of material, 2 swabs should be taken from each chosen area, for example, 2 external vaginal swabs, 2 internal anal swabs.

Penile swabs and swabs from bite marks

Unless the site is already moist the swab should be pre-moistened with sterile distilled water or freshly drawn tap water, not saline.

Control blood samples for DNA profiling

Control blood samples are needed to establish the DNA profiles of the various parties in an enquiry. Only one blood sample of a minimum of 5ml is required. The blood should be taken into the anticoagulant EDTA; the sample is stored frozen and frozen as soon as possible following the examination. Sampling systems such as the Monovette® system are suitable for taking and storing blood samples but care must be taken when freezing blood in glass containers lest the cap be damaged or become detached.

Blood for alcohol

Blood for alcohol should be stored in vials containing fluoride/oxalate at the

Table 2

EXAMINATION TYPE	SAMPLES REQUIRED		GBH AFFRAYS	MURDER SUSPECTS	DRUG / DRINK DRIVING	ARMED ROBBERY	BURGLARY	SUSPECT POISONING DRUGGING	RAPE Female Victim	RAPE Male Suspect	BUGGERY Female Victim	BUGGERY Male Victim	BUGGERY Male Suspect	P.A.C.E. NOTES
CLOTHING/ PAPER	Clothing and sheet of paper		✓	✓	❖	❖	❖	❖	✓	✓	✓	✓	✓	Authority of the Custody Officer needed to remove clothing
INTIMATE	Urine (preserved)		❖	❖	❖	❖	❖	❖	❖	❖	❖	❖	❖	WRITTEN CONSENT NEEDED can be taken by Doctor, SOCO, police officer
	Blood (EDTA)	For DNA analysis	✓	✓		❖	❖		✓	✓	✓	✓	✓	WRITTEN CONSENT NEEDED **To be taken by a Doctor ONLY**
		For grouping	❖	❖		❖	❖		❖	❖	❖	❖	❖	
	Blood (preserved)	For alcohol/ drug/ solvents	❖	❖	✓			✓	❖	❖	❖	❖	❖	DETAINED / CHARGED PERSON Authority of Superintendent or higher rank needed for **ALL** intimate samples
	Penile swab			❖						✓			✓	
	Anal swab	External		❖ ❖							✓✓	✓✓	✓✓	
		Internal									✓✓	✓✓	✓✓	
	Vaginal swab	External		✓ ✓ ✓					↘ ❖ ↘		↘ ❖ ↘			
		Low internal												
		High internal												
		- and -												
	Cervical swab	If 2+ days after offence		❖					❖		❖			
	Pubic hair	Combings (comb to be submitted with combings)		❖					✓	✓		✓	✓	
		Pulled / cut		❖					❖	✓	❖	❖	✓	
	Fragments	Paint, glass etc. from wounds	❖	❖		❖	❖		❖	✓	❖	❖	✓	
	Nose samples	For firearms residues		❖		❖			❖	❖	❖	❖		

EXAMINATION TYPE	SAMPLES REQUIRED		GBH AFFRAYS	MURDER SUSPECTS	DRUG / DRINK DRIVING	ARMED ROBBERY	BURGLARY	SUSPECT POISONING DRUGGING	RAPE Female Victim	RAPE Male Suspect	BUGGERY Female Victim	BUGGERY Male Victim	BUGGERY Male Suspect	P.A.C.E. NOTES
NON-INTIMATE	Saliva			❖		❖	❖		❖	❖	❖	❖	❖	A) WHERE WRITTEN CONSENT NEEDED
	Mouth swab	Not for DNA database		❖					❖		❖	❖	❖	*Samples to be taken from:* VICTIMS – by Doctor ONLY
	Skin / Hair samples	For firearms Residues		❖		❖				❖				DETAINED PERSON – by Doctor, SOCO, Police Officer.
	Head hairs combings	For alien hairs (Comb to be submitted with the combings)		❖					❖		❖	❖	❖	
		For paint, glass etc.	❖	❖		❖	❖			❖	❖	❖	❖	B) NO WRITTEN CONSENT NEEDED WHERE – PERSON CHARGED / REPORTED / CONVICTED /
		For fibres	❖	❖		❖	❖		❖	❖	❖	❖	❖	DETAINED FOR A RECORDABLE OFFENCE
	Head hair	Pulled / cut	❖	❖		❖	❖		❖	❖	❖	❖	❖	Police Officer ONLY to take samples. Authority of
	Fingernail samples							❖				❖		Superintendent or higher rank needed where the suspect has
	Skin samples	From various parts of the body eg. for blood, semen, saliva; From bite marks	❖	❖			❖		❖		❖	❖	❖	not been charged, reported or convicted of a recordable offence.
	Cosmetic traces on skin			❖						❖			❖	
	Medical examination form			❖					✓	✓	✓	✓	✓	

Key ✓ – Essential samples – always take.   ❖ – These samples may be required - consider taking

Table 2 *continued*

concentration specified for blood alcohol analysis. Vials supplied for specimens of blood taken under the Road Traffic Act are suitable for this purpose.

Blood for drugs

If there is no requirement for alcohol, a minimum of 5ml, taken into a vial containing an anticoagulant should be sufficient for most purposes. Where there may be a requirement for alcohol as well as drugs, RTA vials should be used. No more than 4ml of blood should be added to the standard RTA vial and if a larger blood sample is obtained it should be divided between two or more vials.

Urine for alcohol & drugs

Urine should be placed in vials containing preservatives at the concentration specified for urine alcohol analysis. Containers as supplied for specimens of urine taken under the Road Traffic Act are suitable for this purpose.

Saliva

Saliva samples should be taken from the victims of oral sex into plain sterile 'universal' tubes. The sample should be frozen as soon as practicable following the examination. Unless there is a specific request, there is no longer a requirement to take control samples of saliva for blood grouping purposes.

Control head hair

The characteristics of a person's hair may vary along the length. For this reason complete hairs are required. The sample should consist of a minimum of 10 plucked hairs plus a further sample of at least 15 hairs which should be cut next to the scalp. The hairs should be representative of the subject and may need to be taken from more than one point on the head.

Control pubic hair

A minimum of 25 hairs is required. Ideally 10 of these hairs should be plucked with the remainder cut next to the skin. Failing this 25 hairs cut next to the skin may be acceptable.

Fingernail samples

When the intended laboratory examination is to seek traces of blood, nail clippings should be taken in preference to nail scrapings. This is because the patient's own DNA from material sloughed off by scraping may swamp any DNA from a foreign source.

Clothing

Dry clothing should be packaged in paper bags or sacks. Paper sacks with polythene inserts may be available and these offer the dual benefit of a container from which any residual moisture can escape, combined with a means of viewing the article without opening the bag. If clothing is wet it should be packaged temporarily in polythene bags until it can be dried. Items which are to be examined for solvents or accelerants should be sealed in nylon bags.

Other items

Sharp items such as knives, pieces of glass or syringes should be packaged in rigid containers to prevent injury to anyone handling the package. Special tamper-proof evidence bags may be available for packaging controlled drugs.

Labelling

All samples taken by the doctor must be labelled and sealed in a particular and precise way, otherwise difficulties arise at court about the origins of samples produced. With items such as containers, tubes and swabs, it is good practice to use an adhesive label in addition to the police Criminal Justice Act (CJA) exhibit label as this label may become detached from the container. Do not use fountain pens or other types of pen where the ink may run should the label become damp.

Each label should bear the following:

- Name of patient
- Date, time and place taken
- Type of sample
- Person taking sample
- Other details required on the CJA label

CJA exhibit labels should also bear a reference number which is usually formed from the initials of the person taking the sample, followed by a serial number. For example, the first sample taken by Dr ABC would be ABC/1, the second ABC/2, and so on. If more than one person is examined in a particular enquiry, item numbers should continue in series. No two samples in an enquiry should bear the same number, even if taken from different people on different days.

Exhibits are described as productions in Scotland. The police officer who corroborates the evidence of the doctor who takes the samples is responsible for completing labels and assigning numbers to them. The doctor must sign the label in the appropriate space. Containers with their own labels should be initialled by the doctor who should add the date and time.

Sealing

Sealing packages and containers safeguards the integrity of evidence by preventing any material from escaping or entering. The presence of a seal also serves to indicate if there has been any attempt to open the container.

When sealing bags, turn over the top 3cm or so, then turn the flap created over again, securing it with adhesive tape which is long enough to fasten the ends on the reverse of the bag and seal any gaps at the edges.

Swabs and blood samples should be placed in polythene bags which should be sealed in the fashion described above. Where samples are to be stored frozen or refrigerated, the use of special freezer tape is advised. Specimens of blood and urine taken under the Road Traffic Act have special arrangements covering the security of the samples which must be complied with fully.

FORENSIC SCIENCE IN THE UK

England and Wales

The provision of forensic science in England and Wales has undergone considerable change in the 1990s. Prior to 1991 the Forensic Science Service (FSS) was funded centrally as part of the Home Office. In 1991 the FSS was established as an executive agency of the Home Office and required to recover its full economic costs through direct charging.

The introduction of direct charging led to the creation of a market place for forensic science where the police as customers were free to choose how to make the most cost effective use of forensic science. At the same time, the FSS gained the freedom to offer its services to a wider customer base, including lawyers acting for the defence. An expanded FSS was formed in April 1996 following the merger of the Metropolitan Police Laboratory with the original FSS laboratories, creating a national service covering the whole of England and Wales.

The creation of the market place has seen the entry of other general providers, such as the Laboratory of the Government Chemist, British Rail Scientifics and the British Textile Technology Group and specialist providers such as Cellmark UK and University Diagnostics Ltd in the field of DNA and Document Evidence Ltd which specialises in document and handwriting analysis. There are several other companies which concentrate on providing expertise to the defence.

Northern Ireland and Scotland

The arrangements for Northern Ireland are similar to those in England and Wales in that the Northern Ireland Forensic Science Laboratory operates as an executive agency which is funded through direct charging, its principal customer being the Royal Ulster Constabulary.

Scotland is somewhat different in that the provision of forensic science remains the direct responsibility of the police. There are four laboratories, the largest being that operated by Strathclyde Police in Glasgow. Lothian & Borders, Grampian and Tayside Police operate laboratories in Edinburgh, Aberdeen and Dundee respectively. Those forces without their own facilities pay for examinations to be carried out at one of these four laboratories. Defence work is undertaken mainly by the universities.

14

DEATH AND ITS INVESTIGATION

P Dean

It is clearly to the benefit of the community as a whole that any sudden, unnatural or unexplained death is investigated thoroughly. A range of medical and legal factors and their implications must be considered. The first step in the process of investigation is to determine that a death has actually occurred; this may often be very obvious indeed, but declaration of death merits further discussion.

CONFIRMATION OF DEATH

The United Kingdom, unlike some countries, does not have a legal definition of death, and the diagnosis of death is therefore entirely a matter of clinical medical judgment. Colloquially, reference is often wrongly made to 'certifying death' in these circumstances, whereas the doctor is actually confirming the fact that death has occurred. The separate process of issuing a medical certificate of cause of death will be described later.

The point at which death can be said to have occurred may not always be immediately apparent. Numerous medical consequences flow from this, such as the implications for organ donation and transplantation, but there may also be significant legal consequences, both civil and criminal. In a multiple fatality such as an aeroplane or a car crash, the sequence in which deaths have been determined to occur in a family group may have profound effects on inheritance. There has recently been debate and proposed legal reform concerning the unavailability in England and Wales of a murder charge for an assailant whose victim survives on a ventilator for more than a year and a day.

Knight (1991) notes that there is wide variation in the rate at which different tissues and organs die, resulting from their range of vulnerability to oxygen deficiency. He observes that skin, bone and muscle may survive hypoxia for a long time, whereas nervous tissue is very vulnerable to it, and that the motility of white blood cells for at least six hours after cardiac arrest makes the concept of 'vital reaction' less certain.

Clinically, the fact of death is usually confirmed after determining the absence of carotid pulse and heart and breath sounds, with additional possible signs such as segmentation changes in the retinal vessels. Care must be taken to listen to the chest for an adequate period of time, minutes rather than seconds, and to be aware of and to avoid the particular pitfalls presented by hypothermia, overdoses of drugs such as barbiturates, apparent drowning, cachexia and coma, and electrocution. Attempts at resuscitation should, of course, commence if there is any doubt, and in some circumstances ECG or EEG confirmation may be necessary.

Where organ donation is an option, cardio-pulmonary function is maintained artificially, and the concept of brain death becomes important. Brain death should be diagnosed by a consultant, preferably the one in charge of the patient's clinical care, and by another doctor of consultant or senior registrar level who is clinically independent of the first. This is discussed further in the relevant Code of Practice (Cadaveric Organs for Transplantation, A Code of Practice including the Diagnosis of Brain Death; Health Departments of Great Britain and Northern Ireland Working Party, 1983). In these circumstances, the time of death is recorded as the time at which death was conclusively established, and not earlier at the time of the original injury or insult, or later at the time at which artificial support is withdrawn or the heartbeat finally ceases.

EXAMINATION OF THE BODY
AND ESTIMATION OF TIME OF DEATH

In circumstances where the doctor is called to the scene of a death that has occurred some time previously, questions arise as to whether it was natural or unnatural, if unnatural whether accidental or intentional, and if intentional whether suicidal or homicidal. The question of time of death also commonly arises in this context. Estimation of time of death is the source of a great deal of debate both in and out of court and, in common with much in the medico-legal field, it is an area where extreme care must be taken not to over interpret what one sees, and not to make dogmatic, unsupportable and potentially inaccurate statements which may either inadvertently mislead a murder investigation, or may, alternatively, lead to a miscarriage of justice. It will be considered in the overall context of the examination of the body, but further and more detailed reference material on changes in the early post mortem period is recommended in the reading list at the end of this chapter.

Any available history should be taken first, in keeping with basic medical principles, and then any useful evidence that can be derived from initial examination of the scene should be considered. The subject of detailed scene examination has already been dealt with in chapter 13, but clearly the doctor must be mindful of any local physical or environmental factors, such as the presence of fires and domestic heating, open windows or recent ambient temperatures, that might affect the rate of change in the early post mortem period. To avoid losing or disturbing evidence, any detailed examination of the body at the scene in a death that might be suspicious, including the route by which the body is approached, should only be undertaken after discussion with the officer in charge of the investigation, and after appropriate photographic recording of the scene (see page 254).

The initial flaccidity of the body that occurs after death is replaced after a very variable period of time by rigor mortis. This may commence in the first two to four hours, more noticeably in the smaller muscles such as those around the jaws and fingers, become established by nine to twelve hours, and start to wear off after twenty-four to thirty-six hours as the protein in the muscle starts to break down. Its onset is due to the failure to resynthesise adenosine triphosphate from adenosine diphosphate as the muscle's store of glycogen reduces after death, which leads to the overlapping actin and myosin fusing and resultant muscle stiffness and loss of elasticity.

The onset is delayed while residual glycogen stores allow for the resynthesis of ATP, and it follows that this latent period will be influenced by the amount of glycogen present initially. The onset of rigor will be influenced, therefore, by the nutritional state and the amount of activity in the period preceding death, and it may develop sooner, for example, in a death following a struggle or convulsions. Its duration and subsequent reduction as muscle decomposition proceeds is dependent on temperature and will, therefore, also be very variable. The marked variability of onset and duration of rigor mortis reduce its usefulness in estimating time of death considerably. Cadaveric spasm, an extreme variant where rigor appears instantaneously after death, is much less common and less well understood. Consideration should also be given to other effects of temperature on the tissues, such as extreme cold freezing the joints and muscles, and extreme heat causing contractures as in the pugilistic attitude sometimes seen in fire victims.

Post mortem hypostasis or lividity results from the gravitational pooling of blood, particularly of erythrocytes, in vessels. Its onset is also very variable, and it may start to appear in the first hour after death, become more fully established over the following six to nine hours, and remain until putrefaction supervenes. It is seen in dependent areas, although there may be paler areas of sparing if pressure of the body on a firm underlying surface empties the vessels in those compressed areas. If seen in non–dependent, and therefore inappropriate, parts of the body it indicates that the body was moved after death. This effect, however, may not be long lasting and the old concept of hypostasis fixing in one position is no longer felt to be correct. The onset of hypostasis is too variable to be of any great use in estimating time of death, and it may be difficult to see if the person has a lot of fat or has lost a lot of blood, but note should be taken of its colour, which may be cherry red due to carboxyhaemoglobin in carbon monoxide poisoning, pink due to undissociated oxyhaemoglobin in hypothermia, a deep red due to blood remaining fully oxygenated in cyanide poisoning, and grey brown in methaemo-globinaemia.

Temperature loss from the body after death has long formed the basis for much discussion, opinion and research when considering the time elapsed since death. The traditional concept of an estimate of time based on the body temperature declining at 1.5 degree Fahrenheit (0.9 degree Centigrade) an hour after death is fraught with inaccuracy. Bodies cool at different rates if clothed or naked, thin or obese, indoor or outdoors (dependent on factors such as the presence or absence of wind, rain, ambient temperature or immersion). Moreover, body cooling progresses in a sigmoid rather than a linear manner. The picture is further complicated by lack of knowledge of what the body temperature was at the time of death, for example raised through illness or physical activity or reduced through hypothermia, and the presence of a plateau of a few minutes to a few hours before body cooling starts which, because of its variability, is of unknown duration in any individual case.

Should the temperature be taken at the scene or in the mortuary, by whom, and from what orifice or location? The temperature of exposed skin will clearly be more susceptible to environmental factors than the rectal temperature, but if a rectal temperature is taken, photographs and relevant swabs and samples should be taken prior to this to avoid interference with potentially vital evidence. This may therefore be more appropriately conducted in the mortuary, but even with considerable care in controlled circumstances, recording errors may still arise, for example from the thermometer or probe being inadvertently sited in a bolus of faecal material. Much experimental work has been conducted using sequential measurements in different sites, and results have been the subject of complex analyses in order to try to improve the level of accuracy.

Other research methods have looked at biochemical changes in blood, cerebro-spinal fluid, and ocular fluid, in particular at an approximately linear post mortem increase in potassium in the vitreous humour, and other tissue changes, such as post mortem muscle excitability, have been examined.

Other physical findings that have traditionally been looked for include the early colour changes in the right iliac fossa due to putrefaction, which may be present after the second day depending on temperature, and eye changes such as corneal opacity due to desiccation after approximately twelve hours, and dark marks on the sclera known as 'taches noires sclerotiques'. The various forms of insect life to be found on the body after death may, if the opinion of an expert in forensic entomology is sought, give much useful information about time and season of death and whether the body has been inside or outside and, in cases of suspected poisoning, toxicological examination of maggots found on a decomposing body has proved revealing.

Injury has been dealt with in a previous chapter but clearly, subject to the constraints imposed by access to the body at the scene and consultation with the senior officer as to the extent to which the body may be touched or disturbed, examination should include assessment and recording of any injuries present, noting any features of particular forensic significance such as the presence of tentative cuts on the neck or wrists, or the presence of defence injuries. The position of clothing may be of significance, and the relationship of the body to any relevant objects in the vicinity, such as weapons, furniture if inside, and any particular items such as medication containers that may be of relevance should also be documented.

After a consideration of the body at the scene, one must then consider the legal framework in which sudden, unexplained, violent or unnatural deaths are investigated, the responsibilities that these impose on the medical practitioner, the procedures for disposal of bodies, and how these systems developed. In England, Wales and Northern Ireland, the coroner has the statutory duty to inquire into these deaths, and in Scotland, as will be discussed later, they are investigated by the procurator fiscal.

HISTORICAL ASPECTS

The history and development of medical jurisprudence in general and death investigation in particular are closely linked, and the office of coroner has evolved over the eight centuries since the office was formally established in 1194, from being a medieval official concerned with protecting royal revenues to an independent judicial officer charged with the investigation of sudden, violent or unnatural death for the benefit of the community as a whole.

The early coroners performed a variety of functions and investigated any aspect of medieval life that had the potential benefit of revenue for the Crown. Suicides were investigated, as the possessions of those found guilty of the crime of 'felo de se' or 'self murder' would be seized by the Crown. Suicide continued to be classed as a crime until as recently as the Suicide Act of 1961 (in common parlance people still refer to 'committing' suicide) but aiding and abetting remains one. It is significant that the standard of proof required by a coroner to record a verdict of suicide remains the criminal standard of 'beyond reasonable doubt' rather than the civil standard of 'a balance of probabilities' required for most other verdicts.

The early coroners also investigated a wide variety of other features of medieval life, ranging from shipwrecks and fires to the discovery of buried treasure in the community which, as 'treasure trove', remains a statutory duty of the coroner today, although in modern times this has more to do with preserving antiquities than protecting royal revenues.

From the earliest days of their office, coroners were involved with the investigation of sudden death, although for very different reasons from those of today. In the years after the Norman Conquest, to deter the murder of Normans by the local population, a heavy fine was levied on any village where a dead body was discovered on the assumption that it was presumed to be Norman, unless it could be proved to be English. The fine was known as the 'Murdrum', from which the word 'murder' is derived, and the coroner's long association with sudden death began as many of the early coroners' inquests dealt with this 'Presumption of Normanry' which could only be rebutted by the local community, and a large fine thus avoided, by the 'Presentment of Englishry'.

In response to legal, administrative and social changes, the coroner system continued to adapt over the centuries, but in the nineteenth century major changes took place in relation to the investigation of death in the community.

Despite the fact that autopsy had been performed in Italy as early as 1286 and continued to develop there for both public health and forensic purposes, prior to 1836 no attempts had been made in this country to certify any medical cause of death. The method of recording the number of deaths also left much to be desired, and consisted of two women 'searchers' who were appointed in each parish, and who would view the dead bodies and record the numbers of deaths.

Not only was this system very inaccurate, and often caused panic in the population during times of epidemic when higher numbers of deaths were recorded than were actually occurring, but corruption also presented problems as searchers were bribed not to inspect some bodies too closely. Following a Commons Select Committee on Parochial Registration in 1833, registration of births and deaths was introduced in the first Births and Deaths Registration Act in 1836, which also imposed duties on the coroners concerning, among other things, the issue of burial orders.

In addition, concern that uncontrolled access to numerous poisons and inadequate medical investigation of the actual cause of death was leading to many undetected homicides resulted in further changes: the Coroners Act of 1887 diminished coroners' fiscal responsibility, leaving them to become more concerned with determining the circumstances and the actual medical causes of sudden, violent and unnatural deaths.

DEATH CERTIFICATION

The statutory basis for this is contained in Section 22 of the Births and Deaths Registration Act 1953 which provides that 'In the case of the death of any person who has been attended during his last illness by a registered medical practitioner, that practitioner shall sign a certificate in the prescribed form stating to the best of his knowledge and belief the cause of death and shall forthwith deliver that certificate to the registrar'.

It is essential that care is taken to ensure that the Medical Certificate of Cause of Death is completed properly and will not be rejected by the Registrar of Births and Deaths. This avoids both unnecessary distress to grieving relatives waiting in a register office trying to register a death, and subsequent anger directed at the individual doctor by those bereaved whose grief has been added to in this manner.

This involves a knowledge and recognition of those deaths that must be reported to the coroner, which are defined below, and in such a case the coroner's office should be contacted by telephone at the earliest possible opportunity for further guidance and advice.

The Registrar of Births and Deaths scrutinises all Medical Certificates of Cause of Death, and has a statutory duty under section 41(1) of the Registration of Births and Deaths Regulations 1987 to report the death to the coroner if it is one

a) in respect of which the deceased was not attended during his last illness by a registered medical practitioner; or

b) in respect of which the registrar

   i has been unable to obtain a duly completed certificate of the cause of death; or

   ii has received such a certificate with respect to which it appears to him, from the particulars contained in the certificate or otherwise, that the deceased was not seen by the certifying medical practitioner either after death or within 14 days before death; or

c) the cause of which appears to be unknown; or

d) which the registrar has reason to believe to have been unnatural or to have been caused by violence or neglect or by abortion, or to have been attended by suspicious circumstances; or

e) which appears to the registrar to have occurred during an operation or before recovery from the effect of an anaesthetic; or

f) which appears to the registrar from the contents of any medical certificate of cause of death to have been due to industrial disease or industrial poisoning.

Arrangements usually exist for notifying deaths that occur within 24 hours of admission to hospital at a local level. This is not a statutory requirement, but it avoids the registrar otherwise questioning a certificate where it appears that the patient may not have been in hospital long enough to enable the cause of death to be fully established, or where it appears that the patient was not attended during the last illness by a registered medical practitioner other than treatment given in extremis by hospital staff.

Section 41 (1) of the Registration of Births and Deaths Regulations defines most, but not all, of the instances when a death must be reported to the coroner. One exception that must be considered by any forensic or prison doctor is a death in custody which, rather than being notified through the registrar, will be reported directly to the coroner by the appropriate prison or police authority. Any medical practitioner must be aware, however, that since a recent judicial review of a coronial decision in such a case, a prisoner who dies while a patient in hospital is still considered in legal terms to be in custody whether under guard or not. Such deaths must, therefore, be reported to the coroner whether natural or not, rather than being registered in the normal manner.

Where the death is entirely natural and does not fall into any of the above categories, care must be taken to ensure that the certificate is completed correctly, and the correct format employed, to ensure that the Medical Certificate of Cause of Death is acceptable to the Registrar of Births and Deaths. Advice on this was given in a letter to doctors from the Office of Population Censuses and Surveys in 1990, which reminded doctors that the certificates served both a legal and a statistical purpose, and indicated some of the common certification errors that occur.

The letter pointed out that there is no need to record the mode of dying, as this does not give any assistance in deriving mortality statistics, and stressed that it is even more important not to complete a certificate where the mode of dying, for example shock, uraemia or asphyxia, was the only entry. The need to avoid the use of abbreviations was emphasised, as these may mean different things to different doctors and can lead to inaccuracy and ambiguity, for example 'M.I.' which might mean mitral incompetence or myocardial infarction, or 'M.S.' which might mean mitral stenosis or multiple sclerosis.

If the cause of death is one that is often recognised to be employment-related but is known not to be in the case in question, then the addition of the words 'non-industrial' on the certificate after the cause of death can avoid subsequent rejection by the registrar.

An immediately available and useful set of notes and directions is contained in books of blank Medical Certificates of Cause of Death, and compliance with these will avoid many of the common problems that arise. This will assist with the correct inclusion and positioning of any relevant antecedent diseases or conditions, and will help to ensure that part I, and where appropriate part II, are filled in correctly and in a sequence which is logical.

A survey (Start et al 1993) revealed significant and similar numbers of failures to recognise which deaths are reportable in all grades of doctor from junior to senior, and any doctor, regardless of seniority, who is uncertain about an aspect of death certification or referral would be best advised to seek the guidance of the local coroner's office at the earliest opportunity to resolve the matter and to avoid subsequent problems and the distress to relatives (and doctors) that these can cause.

Problems can also arise from a doctor's well intentioned desire to keep certain sensitive diagnoses off the Medical Certificate of Cause of Death. To withhold such information would not seem to be lawful (Schutte 1991) as the doctor's statutory duty is to state 'to the best of his knowledge and belief the cause of death' on the certificate.

At the present time, about a third of all deaths in England and Wales are reported to coroners. In 1994, out of a total of 551,600 deaths, 185,000 were reported, and the sequence of events that ensues is as follows.

NATURAL DEATHS

If further enquiry reveals that the cause was natural a post mortem examination is not required, the coroner will issue a Form 100A, which notifies the registrar that the death was due to natural causes, and the attending doctor will then be advised to complete a Medical Certificate of Cause of Death in the usual manner.

In the majority of cases reported to coroners, however, a post mortem examination is still required to ascertain the cause of death, and if this reveals that the cause of death is natural, the coroner will issues a Form 100B, which notifies the registrar of the cause of death, and that the coroner will be taking no further action.

The registrar, having received either the Medical Certificate of Cause of Death from the attending doctor, or Form 100B from the coroner, is then able to register the death and issue a disposal certificate to allow for arrangements to be made to dispose of the body.

In 1994, post mortem examinations were ordered on 125,200 of the 185,000 reported deaths. This proportion has declined steadily as the number of deaths requiring neither post mortem nor inquest has increased.

UNNATURAL DEATHS AND INQUESTS

If the cause of death is found not to be natural, either from the history of the circumstances of the death or from the post mortem examination, the coroner has a statutory duty to conduct an inquest under Section 8 (1) of the Coroners Act 1988, which provides that:

Where a coroner is informed that a body of a person ("the deceased") is lying within his district and there is reasonable cause to suspect that the deceased –

a) has died a violent or unnatural death;

b) has died a sudden death of which the cause is unknown; or

c) has died in prison, or in such a place or in such circumstances as to require an inquest under any other Act, then, whether the cause of death arose within his district or not, the coroner shall as soon as practicable hold an inquest into the death of the deceased either with or, subject to subsection (3), without a jury.

Prior to the Coroners (Amendment) Act 1926, every inquest had to be held with a jury, but in most inquests now, the coroner sits alone. Section 8(3) of the Coroners Act 1988, however, provides that:

If it appears to a coroner, either before he proceeds to hold an inquest or in the course of an inquest begun without a jury, that there is reason to suspect –

a) that the death occurred in prison or in such a place or in such circumstances as to require an inquest under any other Act;

b) that the death occurred while the deceased was in police custody, or resulted from an injury caused by a police officer in the purported execution of his duty;

c) that the death was caused by an accident, poisoning or disease notice of which is required to be given under any Act to a government department, to any inspector or other officer of a government department or to an inspector appointed under section 19 of the Health and Safety at Work etc. Act 1974; or

d) that the death occurred in circumstances the continuance or possible recurrence of which is prejudicial to the health or safety of the public or any section of the public, he shall proceed to summon a jury in the manner required by subsection (2).

The conduct of an inquest is governed by The Coroners Rules 1984, and the function and range of an inquest, as well as the controversial subject of what used to be referred to as 'lack of care' but is now more properly considered as 'neglect', was usefully examined and re-affirmed by the Court of Appeal in *R v North Humberside Coroner*, ex parte Jamieson [1994] 3 WLR 82.

Rule 36 of the Coroners Rules 1984 (Matters to be Ascertained at Inquest) provides that:

1. The proceedings and evidence at inquest shall be directed solely to ascertaining the following matters, namely –

   a) who the deceased was;

   b) how, when and where the deceased came by his death;

   c) the particulars for the time being required by the Registration Acts to be registered concerning the death.

2. Neither the coroner nor the jury shall express any opinion on any other matters.

and Rule 42 (Verdict) provides that:

No verdict shall be framed in such a way as to appear to determine any question of –

a) criminal liability on the part of a named person, or

b) civil liability.

An inquest is a fact finding enquiry rather than a fault finding trial, and the proceedings are inquisitorial rather than adversarial in nature. The Master of the Rolls, giving the judgement of the court in *R v North Humberside Coroner*, cited above, stated that it is the duty of the coroner to 'ensure that the relevant facts were fully, fairly and fearlessly investigated'.

The coroner initially examines a witness on oath, after which relevant questions may be put to the witness by any of those with a proper interest in the proceedings, either in person or by counsel or solicitor. Those who have this entitlement to examine witnesses are defined by Rule 20 of the Coroners Rules, although the coroner has discretion to include other people, who do not appear to have a 'proper interest'.

Evidence given on oath before a coroner may subsequently be used in proceedings in other courts, and Rule 22 provides that:

1. no witness at an inquest shall be obliged to answer any question tending to incriminate himself, and

2. where it appears to the coroner that a witness has been asked such a question, the coroner shall inform the witness that he may refuse to answer.

This protection against self-incrimination applies only to criminal offences, and not to possible civil or disciplinary proceedings, and it does not allow a witness to refuse to enter the witness box itself.

Of deaths reported to coroners in 1994, inquests were held on 20,800, or about 11%. The commonest verdicts were death by accident or misadventure, recorded in 18%. It is interesting to note that the Home Office 'Statistics of Deaths

Reported to Coroners' in 1994 also revealed that the verdicts of death from industrial diseases have almost doubled in the last ten years (from 5% in 1984 to 9%) and that verdicts of death from drug abuse have also increased.

In addition to those duties relating to unnatural death that are provided for by s8 (1) of the Coroners Act 1988, section 30 provides that a coroner shall continue to have jurisdiction to inquire into any treasure which is found in his district. This last vestige of the coroner's medieval duties remains on the statute book, although in modern times it is for the purpose of preserving antiquities rather than for any financial benefit to the Crown.

DISPOSAL ARRANGEMENTS

The Births and Deaths Registration Act 1926 prohibits disposal of a body except where there is a registrar's certificate or on the coroner's order and, as stated above, the registrar, having received either the Medical Certificate of the Cause of Death from the attending doctor, or Form 100B from the coroner, is able to register the death and issue a disposal certificate to allow for arrangements to be made to dispose of the body. This disposal certificate is then delivered to the undertaker, who must notify the registrar after the burial takes place. In cases where an inquest is to be conducted, a Burial Order must be issued by the coroner to enable the burial to take place. In Scotland, the registrar's acknowledgement of registration (Form 14) is required by the cemetery or crematorium superintendent before disposal may take place.

Strict controls exist where a cremation is requested, to prevent evidence of crime being lost, and the Cremation Regulations prescribe the use of particular forms, dependent upon the situation:

Form B is signed by the registered medical practitioner who issued the Medical Certificate of Cause of Death and who must, for this purpose, have viewed the body after death.

Form C is a confirmatory certificate signed by a doctor who has been registered for at least five years, and who was not involved in the care of the patient, and who must have examined the body after death, and seen and questioned the doctor who signed Form B. The doctors should not be professional partners, or related to each other or to the deceased. Form C can now be dispensed with in hospital deaths where a post mortem has been conducted.

Form D is issued after a post mortem examination conducted where the medical referee of the crematorium requires further information to confirm the cause of death.

Form E is a cremation certificate issued by a coroner, and replaces Forms B and C. It can be issued whether or not the coroner has decided to hold an inquest. The

Scottish equivalent issued by the procurator fiscal (Form E (1)) includes the medical cause of death. Cremation of persons dying abroad requires authority from the Secretary of State.

Form F is the authority to cremate the body from the medical referee of the crematorium.

Form G is the completion certificate from the cremation superintendent, once the cremation has taken place.

Form H is used where a body has undergone anatomical examination according to the Anatomy Act 1984.

Where a request is made to take a body out of the country for disposal abroad, whether it was originally a coroner's case or not, this can only be done with a coroner's Out of England Order. This is to ensure that a body is not lost from the jurisdiction until it is certain that there has been no foul play. The same also applies to requests for a burial at sea, where additional notification must be given to the District Inspector of Fisheries.

DEATH CERTIFICATION IN NORTHERN IRELAND

The coroner system in Northern Ireland is similar to that operating in England and Wales, although there are certain differences. Coroners in Northern Ireland are appointed by the Lord Chancellor, unlike those in England and Wales who are appointed by the local authority, the appointment then being subject to the approval of the Home Secretary before it can take effect. In Northern Ireland, only barristers and solicitors are eligible to become coroners, whereas in England and Wales doctors of no less than five years standing are also eligible. The Medical Certificate of Cause of Death in Northern Ireland, unlike the certificate in England and Wales, does not have a Notice to Informant; the medical practitioner in Northern Ireland is required to issue a Medical Certificate of Cause of Death if he or she has attended and treated the deceased within twenty-eight days, rather than fourteen days as in England and Wales, and is satisfied that the cause of death was natural.

The medical practitioner in Northern Ireland has a statutory duty to refer reportable deaths to the coroner, in addition to the registrar, and a statutory obligation not to issue a certificate in those cases, whereas in England and Wales the doctor who has attended the deceased in the final illness has the statutory duty to report deaths to the coroner. It is, of course, a standard and appropriate practice for doctors in England and Wales to report relevant deaths to the coroner themselves at the earliest opportunity, despite the absence of a statutory obligation to do so.

Where a death is reported in England and Wales the coroner 'shall (that is, must) hold an inquest if the death falls within s8 (1) of the Coroners Act 1988, as discussed earlier. In Northern Ireland the relevant statute, the Coroners Act (Northern Ireland) 1959 (as amended) states that the coroner 'may' hold an inquest, thus introducing an element of discretion.

The jurisdiction of the coroner in England and Wales arises from the presence of a body within his or her district, irrespective of where the death occurred, and therefore also covers deaths that occur abroad when the body is returned to the district. In Northern Ireland, however, the coroner only has jurisdiction if the death takes place, or the body is found, within the district.

As in England and Wales, there are rules in operation, the Coroners (Practice and Procedure) Rules (Northern Ireland) 1963 (as amended). In jury cases, coroners in England and Wales can accept a majority verdict as long as no more than two jurors disagree, whereas in Northern Ireland, only a unanimous verdict can be accepted from a jury.

DEATH CERTIFICATION IN SCOTLAND

Section 24 of the Registration of Births, Deaths and Marriages (Scotland) Act 1965 places a duty on a registered medical practitioner who has attended the deceased during the last illness to complete a Medical Certificate of Cause of Death. This certificate, like the Northern Ireland one, has no Notice to Informant. If no doctor has attended the deceased during the final illness, any other doctor who knows the cause may complete the certificate.

There is no coroner system in Scotland, where the law officer responsible for inquiring into all sudden and unexpected or unnatural deaths is the procurator fiscal, who has a statutory duty to investigate the following categories of death:

– deaths where the cause is uncertain

– deaths from accidents caused by any vehicle, aeroplane or train

– deaths from employment, whether from accident, industrial disease or industrial poisoning

– deaths due to poisoning

– deaths where suicide is a possibility

– deaths occurring under anaesthetic

– deaths resulting from an accident

– deaths following an abortion or attempted abortion

– deaths appearing to arise from neglect

– deaths in prison or police custody

- death of a newborn child whose body is found
- deaths occurring not in a house, and where the deceased's residence is unknown
- deaths caused by drowning
- death of a child from suffocation, including overlaying
- deaths from food poisoning or infectious disease
- deaths from burning or scalding, fire or explosion
- deaths of foster children
- deaths possibly arising from defects in medicinal products
- any other violent, suspicious, sudden or unexplained deaths

The medical practitioner in Scotland has a duty to report deaths in these categories to the procurator fiscal, as does any citizen under a general duty, and the Registrar of Births, Deaths and Marriages has a specific statutory duty to inform the procurator fiscal of these deaths under the 1965 Act.

The jurisdiction of the procurator fiscal is coterminous with that of the civil jurisdiction of the sheriff in whose court he appears, although where the death is criminal and the body has been moved from one jurisdiction to another, the area where the crime was originally committed will determine which fiscal supervises the investigation.

The procurator fiscal's enquiries are made in private, regardless of how the death was caused, although a public enquiry may be held if the relatives persuade the fiscal of the need for this. In practice, much of the investigation will be conducted by the police. Opinion may also be sought from medical practitioners involved in the care of the deceased and from pathologists, and independent experts in technical matters, if relevant. As in criminal investigations, the fiscal prepares a precognition including any witness statements, reports and conclusions.

The fiscal has a common law power to order a post mortem examination but, if difficulties are anticipated, may apply for a warrant in suspicious cases granting authority to two named pathologists to conduct the examination.

In non-suspicious cases, the procurator fiscal will only instruct a post mortem examination if the circumstances justify it, and the post mortem rate for natural deaths is significantly lower than in England and Wales. If a death is thought to be natural and the deceased's general practitioner cannot issue a certificate, a police surgeon may be asked to undertake an external examination and report the results of this to the fiscal, who may then decide to accept a certificate from the police surgeon.

If a death occurred in custody or was caused by an accident in the course of employment, the Fatal Accidents and Sudden Deaths Inquiry (Scotland) Act 1976 obliges the fiscal to hold a Fatal Accident Inquiry in public before a sheriff. Such an inquiry may also be held in some discretionary circumstances where it appears to the Lord Advocate to be in the public interest to do so; this will include some sudden, suspicious or unexplained deaths or where there was significant public concern. The procurator fiscal, or occasionally Crown counsel, will lead the evidence, and parties may be legally represented.

Further reading and references

Knight B 1991 *Simpson's Forensic Medicine* 10th edition Edward Arnold, London.

Henssge C, Knight B, Krompecher T, Madea B, Nokes L 1991 *The Estimation of the Time of Death in the Early Post Mortem Period* Edward Arnold, London

Hunnisett RF 1961 *The Medieval Coroner (Cambridge Studies in English Legal History)* Cambridge University Press, Cambridge.

Office of Population Censuses and Surveys – Completion of Medical Certificates of Cause of Death, 1990. OCPS, London

Jervis on Coroners 11th edition Foreman J, Matthews P 1993 Sweet and Maxwell, London.

Start RD, Delargy-Aziz Y, Dorries CP, Silocks PB, Cotton DWK 1993 Clinicians and the coronial system; ability of clinicians to recognise reportable deaths. *British Medical Journal* **306**:1038-41.

Schutte PK 1991 Problems in death certification *The Police Surgeon* **39**: 31-32

Statistics of Deaths Reported to Coroners: England and Wales 1994; Home Office *Statistical Bulletin* 6/95, April 1995.

The Coroners Rules 1984 HMSO, London.

The notes and directions accompanying books of Medical Certificates of Cause of Death.

15

FORENSIC ODONTOLOGY

D Clark

The forensic odontologist's role in assisting the forensic physician may be either the interpretation of marks on the body surface which may have been caused by a dentition, or identification of an individual by dental examination, either in the dead or the living. Dental examination may also include age assessment.

MARKS WHICH SHOULD RAISE THE POLICE SURGEON'S SUSPICIONS THAT AN ODONTOLOGIST IS REQUIRED

In recent years there has been a rapid increase in the number of suspected bite mark cases examined by forensic odontologists. This is believed to be due to the increasing awareness, through education, of those most likely to examine such cases rather than an increase in the incidence of this particular type of assault. In some criminal trials bite mark evidence has been the only evidence on which a conviction or acquittal has been achieved.

It is thus important that the police surgeon should consider the possibility of human bites when examining surface trauma in certain cases, particularly alleged rape and child abuse. Any circular or semicircular or short linear mark with indentations should be considered as a possible bite mark (see fig. 1). However, marks caused by various implements (for instance saw teeth, shoe heels) may mimic a bite mark. The author once examined what appeared, at first glance, to be a perfect bite mark on an elderly lady which turned out to be an injury caused by her falling against a patterned circular metal door knob.

The interpretation and presentation of bite mark evidence produces many problems even for the most experienced forensic odontologist: in brief, these

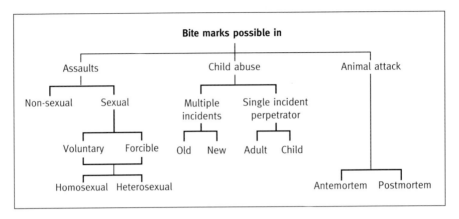

Figure 1

are the resistance and elasticity of the tissues, the degree of curvature of the body surfaces and the lapse of time. In clinical forensic medicine bite marks are usually thought of as being marks made on the skin of a human victim by the bite of a human assailant (see fig. 2). Although this is far the most common situation it must not be overlooked that the victim in a case of assault may bite the assailant in defence or may have a self inflicted bite caused by the assailant forcing the victim's arm into the mouth in an attempt to procure silence during the assault. Moreover, at scenes of crime bite marks may be found in discarded food and other materials ranging from bottle tops to woodwork. Although such marks are not within the province of the police surgeon, he will be an early visitor to the scene during an investigation of death, and his trained eye may allow him to call attention to possible bite marks on articles at the scene.

Bite marks may be made in a variety of ways: direct tooth pressure, skin pressed against the teeth by the tongue which may produce an outline of the palatal surfaces of the upper incisors and canines, or by scraping teeth over the skin as may occur when the victim is struggling violently – this produces a series of parallel marks or wounds and is often associated with bites on the nipple.

There is often limited detail and it is infrequent to observe a complete set of marks made by all the anterior teeth in both upper and lower arches: marks rarely extend beyond the second premolars. Individual tooth marks may be seen, producing a double horseshoe appearance. In other cases there may only be marks made by one dental arch or the number of teeth marks may vary from several to only one.

Animal bites

Bites are also produced by non-human vertebrates possessing teeth, most mammals, reptiles (crocodiles and alligators) and some fish (sharks and rays).

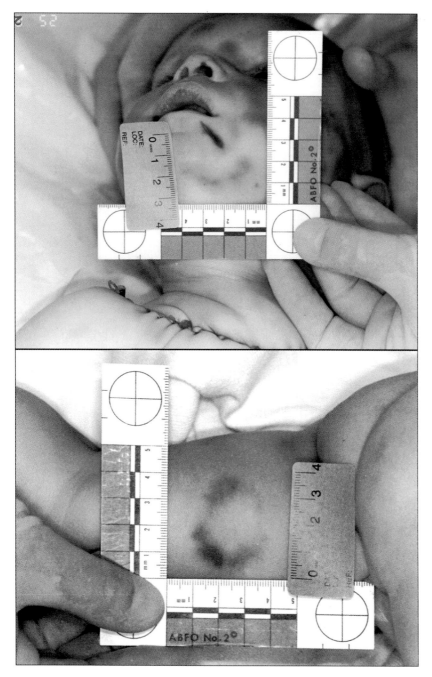

Figure 2 – Bite marks on a child on two different curved surfaces. Also demonstrated is the American Board of Forensic Odontology photographic scale, used by most forensic odontologists in the UK.
Reproduced by permission of West Sussex Constabulary

Corpses lying undiscovered may be attacked by carnivorous animals. The scientific literature lists many animals responsible for biting humans, the most common being cats, dogs and rodents; only in exceptional circumstances, such as an incident on a farm, in a pet shop or a zoo, need we concern ourselves with the rest of the animal kingdom. It is necessary, therefore, to recognise the basic differences in bite patterns.

DIFFERENTIAL DIAGNOSIS OF BITE MARK INJURIES

Animal teeth tend to puncture deeply and tear the tissue, whereas human bites are blunt and more superficial and cause abrasion rather than tearing.

Human

Ovoid or elliptical pattern. Canine areas are not unduly pronounced, with indentations broader and more blunt in appearance than those of the under mentioned animals. Petechiae caused by sucking is only seen in human bite marks.

Dog

Narrow squarish arch anteriorly; prominent pointed marks produced by canines.

Cat

Small rounded arch with puncture marks made by canines. The bite is often associated with scratch marks from claws.

Rodent

Small bites with long grooves caused by the central incisors.

Human bites may be predominantly sexual or predominantly aggressive (nonsexual) although there is often a mixed picture. In the aggressive type the teeth areused as a weapon: there is no suck mark and the bite is said to be forceful and rapid. Such bites have been observed on police officers' arms, chest or face when attacked during the course of arresting a suspect. In sexual bites the teeth are used to grip during sucking: the resulting central or peripheral suck marks are visible as petechiae, producing the characteristic reddening; this bite is said to be forceful and slow. In many such marks there maybe no visible imprint left by the teeth.

As they bite, the teeth may puncture the epidermis, causing a number of small wounds. Larger wounds, associated with a violent struggle, are produced by the incisors or canines scraping across the tissue; such wounds have been mostly noted on the areola of the female breast where the nipple has been severely traumatised or bitten off completely. Most bites do not perforate the epidermis but initially make deep impressions followed by underlying areas of bruising. In some cases

NON-SEXUAL	SEXUAL	
	Hetero-	Homo-
Arm	Breast	Breast
Leg	Neck	Upper back
Fingers	Cheek	Axilla
Hands	Arm	Arm
Chest	Thigh	Genitalia
Ears	Abdomen	Nose
	Genitalia	Buttocks

Table 1 – Common sites

a second bite may be superimposed on the first, increasing the difficulties of interpretation. Sites vary according to the types of case (table 1), but any area of the body may be bitten.

If a human bite is suspected or, in the living, is alleged, the value of this evidence must be assessed by physical examination. Immediate action will be necessary due to the rate of fading of such marks. In the living, these marks are seen most easily from one to twenty-four hours after infliction. In the dead, they may take twelve to twenty-four hours to develop, depending on the severity and on the environmental temperature.

ACTION TAKEN BY THE FORENSIC PHYSICIAN

Stop any attempt to clean up the area before it is swabbed for saliva. Swabs should be taken immediately after, not before, photographic recording, thus avoiding any subsequent suggestion in court that the evidence had been tampered with prior to photography. The only reason to vary this is when there might be a considerable delay in getting the photography undertaken.

A minimum of four swabs should be sent to the laboratory; the first three swabs must be moistened with sterile water before use.

1. Swab of bite mark area.
2. Swab of control area adjacent to the mark.
3. Swab of victim's saliva.
4. Unopened unused dry swab from same batch.
5. A sample of the victim's saliva in a sterile container where the victim is alive.

If there is likely to be a delay in delivering the swabs and sample to the laboratory they should be placed in the freezer compartment of a fridge. The swabs should not be air dried.

Request the services of a forensic odontologist, but do not delay photography until his or her arrival. The suspected bite mark must be accurately photographed by a police photographer at the earliest possible opportunity. Correct photography is vital as the forensic odontologist bases his evidence on measurements and comparisons of one-to-one photographs with dental models of suspects; unsupervised photography may result in useless prints for court presentation. Because accurate and correctly exposed photography is so important for evidence the reader is strongly advised to refer to more detailed literature on this subject (Summers & Lewin 1992).

Although police photographers are experienced in recording scenes of crime, advice is often necessary on the views required for bite marks. Essential views are:

1. At right angles to the centre of the bite.
2. The lens is aimed at an angle of 85° from the outside of the upper arch at a point in the central part of the curve.
3. The lower arch is photographed likewise.

These views should be taken first without a scale and then with a scale, both in colour and monochrome. The scale must be close to, but not obscuring any part of the bitten area, and should be attached in two planes at right angles. The self adhesive centimetre tape to be found in SOCO kits may be used and the actual tape used in the photographs should be retained for production in court. Ideally, a specially designed rigid scale for bite marks should be used (see fig. 2). A total of twelve photographs will thus be produced and those with a scale must be printed up one-to-one.

Live victims should be encouraged to present the bitten area to the photographer as it was at the time of the bite. In the same way, a dead body should be positioned as at the time of the assault, if this can be ascertained, and the photography repeated.

Ultraviolet photography will often demonstrate the mark more clearly. In 'battered babies' ultraviolet photography is particularly useful as it will demonstrate otherwise invisible marks up to six months after infliction. Therefore, the whole infant should be examined under ultraviolet radiation and appropriate areas photographed. This is of particular value when there is a history of multiple incidents.

If haemorrhage or debris has obscured part of the bite mark, the area should be cleansed after the initial photography and re-photographed. It is important to preserve the negatives carefully as these will form the exhibits when the photographs are produced as evidence.

ACTION TAKEN BY THE FORENSIC ODONTOLOGIST

He should examine the bite mark at the earliest opportunity. Daily repeat photography will usually be requested for at least the three following days. Changes in colour and bruising patterns sometimes produce results which demonstrate the bite more clearly; this applies both to the living and the dead.

An impression of the injury may be made, to reproduce its indentations and curvatures. Dental stone models will be constructed from this impression for measurements and court presentation. If the injury could have been self-inflicted, impressions of the alleged victim's own teeth will be required.

If suspects are available, alginate impressions and wax bites will be taken for the construction and articulation of stone models; these will be used in measurement procedures in conjunction with the one-to-one photographs. Before impressions are taken, witnessed written consent must be obtained. Impression taking is considered to be an intimate sample under the Police and Criminal Evidence Act 1984, so requires correct police authorisation. In Scotland, a warrant to authorise the procedure may be obtained by the procurator fiscal from a sheriff.

In child abuse cases impressions will be required from each member of the household and this may have to be extended to others who have frequent contact with the youngster.

Finally, having obtained models and photographs, the forensic odontologist will undertake a number of measurement and comparison techniques and produce a report on his findings for the court. Unlike fingerprint evidence, there are no recognised minimum 'points of correspondence'.

ODONTOLOGY'S PLACE IN IDENTIFICATION

Most of the population have, at some time, received dental treatment. Dental surgeons are required to record treatment and retain dental records for up to five years, but many retain these for longer periods. At the present time identification by the comparison of dental records with a post mortem dental examination record is the most successful method. This may change in the future as the incidence of dental disease continues to decrease coupled with the decrease in attendance at dental surgeries due to the increasing costs of treatment. As DNA techniques become less expensive and results are obtained faster it is possible that this technique may eventually depose odontology as the most successful identification method.

The police attempt to obtain dental records of persons reported missing, to compare these with the dental chartings of victims. In many instances clues to identity result in police enquiries to local dental surgeons, either close to the missing person's residence or place of employment, who make antemortem records available for comparison during or after the dental postmortem. This has been a consistently successful method, particularly in mass disasters.

At dental postmortem examination notes are made of the number, position, rotation, diastemas and anomalies of the teeth and the types, material, shape and surfaces of the restorations. Resection of the jaws may be undertaken for radiographic examination and age assessment. Radiographs will indicate the presence of unerupted or buried teeth, root treatments and metal pins and posts used in restorative treatment. Age assessment is also undertaken (see below).

Smiling photographs have a part to play in dental identification, as they demonstrate the angles and positions of the anterior teeth and assist where dental records are not available or of poor quality. Such photographs have also been used where skulls have been recovered and the technique of video or photographic superimposition used to match the shape and position of the teeth in the photograph with those in the skull (*R v West* (unreported) Winchester Crown Court 1995). For superimposition it is preferable to use a photograph straight on as in a passport photograph. It is also important to be able to ascertain the focal length of the lens used – such information is readily available in the passport kiosks used in shops.

Dental records do vary in quality, most dental surgeons only recording the work undertaken by themselves. At present there are no regulations in the UK requiring a dental surgeon to note all existing dental restorations at the patient's first attendance, nor are there requirements for a patient's records to be forwarded to a new dentist when a patient makes a change. In some areas of the world it is mandatory to mark dentures with the patient's name; few dental surgeons in the UK did so until recent years. Dental identification, arguably the most consistently successful method, particularly in mass disasters, would be much easier if these simple requirements were met.

AGE DETERMINATION FROM THE TEETH

Dental age is estimated by comparing the dental development status of a person of unknown age, using lateral oblique and/or orthopantomograph radiography, with published dental development surveys. A likely chronological age for that individual can then be deduced. This method is of value up to around the age of twenty-one years and is particularly accurate, but once the adult dentition is fully formed accurate age assessment by dental means becomes difficult without the removal of a tooth for microscopical analysis. The forensic physician is more likely to require a reference table for those under twenty-one (table 2).

Emergence and exfoliation times of deciduous teeth

TOOTH	EMERGENCE		EXFOLIATION	
Central incisors	6-8	months	6-7	years
Lateral incisors	7-8	months	7-8	years
Canines	16-20	months	9-12	years
First molar	12-16	months	9-11	years
Second molar	20-30	months	10-12	years

Emergence times for permanent teeth

MAXILLARY TEETH	EMERGENCE		MANDIBULAR TEETH	EMERGENCE	
Central incisor	7-8	years	Central incisor	6-7	years
Lateral incisor	8-9	years	Lateral incisor	7-8	years
Canine	11-12	years	Canine	9-10	years
First premolar	10-11	years	First premolar	10-12	years
Second premolar	10-12	years	Second premolar	11-12	years
First molar	6 -7	years	First molar	6-7	years
Second molar	12-13	years	Second molar	11-13	years
Third molar	17-21	years	Third molar	17-21	years

Table 2

Reference

Summers R, Lewin D 1992 *Forensic dental photography* in *Practical Forensic Odontology* Butterworth-Heinemann, Oxford, 188 -205.

Further reading

Two useful books for the forensic physician to have on the shelf:

Whittaker DK, MacDonald DG. 1989 *Colour Atlas of Forensic Dentistry*. Wolfe Publishing, London

Clark DH. (Ed) 1992 *Practical Forensic Odontology*. Butterworth-Heinemann, Oxford

16

DEALING WITH A MAJOR DISASTER

A Busuttil

A major disaster (etymologically, an abnormal star) or an emergency may be defined as:

> *any event that occurs with or without warning, and causes or threatens to cause death or injury, damage to property or to the environment and disruption of the community, and whose effects are of such a scale that they cannot be dealt with by the emergency services, the National Health Service and the local authorities as part of their everyday activities, and therefore require the mobilisation and organisation of special and extra services.*

From the point of view of the police, a major incident does not require them to carry out activities which they would not deal with in their everyday work, but such tasks appear to be more complicated because of the large scale of events, the heightened interests of the community and the public media, and the necessity to bring the incident to a swift conclusion, so enabling the particular community to return to normality.

POLICE OBJECTIVES IN THE AFTERMATH OF A MAJOR INCIDENT

The clinical forensic examiner will be working closely with the police in such emergencies, so there should be a complete understanding of the primary objectives of police activity:

1. In conjunction with the other emergency services (mainly the ambulance and fire services) the first priority is the saving of life. The task of the police is to facilitate the recovery and removal of casualties from wreckage, then their treatment and transport to hospital by those who are appropriately trained and equipped to carry out such duties, not to put themselves and others at risk by attempting this themselves.

2. In the disruption and disorder amounting to chaos which may be experienced by those actively involved in or affected by the incident, and inevitably also by those responding to it, the police co-ordinate the responses and activities of the emergency services and other organisations and restore order as promptly and effectively as possible.

3. Whatever the nature of a major incident, some form of inquiry must look at causation of the incident. In addition to an inquiry, a criminal trial and almost certainly civil litigation must ensue.

In the light of this, the police regard any major incident site as a scene of crime requiring a thorough investigation. It has to be preserved as much as practicable, and to be managed in as structured a manner as incidents of a smaller scale. Thus, the fewer the people at the scene, particularly those who are not essential to the rescue efforts and to the investigation, the better. The police, together with forensic scientists and photographers, will proceed with preserving the evidence; they will also keep out those who have no business to be there.

One of the cardinal aspects of crime scene investigation is to photograph the body in the original position in which it was found. This also holds true in a major incident; bodies should be moved only if they hamper the activities of the rescuers and their access to the living, if they would be lost or further damaged if not moved, or if they are too exposed to the public gaze and the attention of the media where they are. If they must be moved, statements will be obtained in due course from those carrying out this displacement, to ensure full documentation and continuity of evidence-gathering.

4. Although the police have to carry out an investigation in all instances, others have a legitimate, and sometimes a statutory, right to proceed with their own specialised investigations. As appropriate to the incident, these include the Air Accident Investigation Branch, the Maritime Accident Investigation Branch, Railway Inspectorate, the Board of Trade, the Department of Transport, and the Health and Safety Executive, or a combination of these. The investigation initiated by any of these bodies is independent of that carried out by the police, but the police have a duty to facilitate such additional investigations, and to co-ordinate their efforts and collaborate with them. Companies and other establishments whose premises, personnel and equipment (for example, an aircraft company) have been involved in a disaster may wish to carry out their own private investigation which would also be assisted by the police.

5. In the British Isles, the police traditionally accept the role of collating and disseminating information about causalities involved in the disaster. The casualties of a major incident are various:

a) The injured, who require treatment on site and, when necessary, transport for further treatment in hospital.

b) The deceased, who require to be identified accurately and promptly and their remains returned to their relatives accompanied by the appropriate documentation for disposal according to their wishes. Life may be pronounced extinct on site either immediately or after triage and resuscitation; there will often be other deaths en route to hospital or in hospital after treatment. All the fatalities related to a particular incident should be dealt with by the same mortuary team.

Although it has generally been customary for a doctor to diagnose death, there are no statutory obligations requiring this; indeed, when severe mutilation or burning has taken place, personnel who are not medically qualified may take on this role. It is prudent to have a medical practitioner subsequently confirm death, preferably with the body still in situ. This event must be documented fully with the name of the doctor and the timing. The time that life was formally pronounced extinct is often the time inserted in the death certificate, with the consequent influence on probate and other civil legal matters, not least if members of the same family have succumbed together (commorientes).

c) the uninjured survivors who do not need treatment, but urgently desire to pass on messages to their relatives.

d) evacuees who may be shocked, have no roof over their heads and have lost property, urgently require shelter and somewhere to rest and recuperate. A Survivor Reception Centre will be set up by the local authority (social work and housing departments) with the co-operation of such voluntary organisations as the Red Cross, Salvation Army, Women's Royal Volunteer Service.

e) relatives and friends, urgently seeking accurate and full information about those who may have been involved in the incident. Difficulties of communication with those dealing with the incident will result in people taking to their cars and making a visit to the scene, adding further to the chaos.

It is salutary to remember that all the survivors, injured and uninjured, in an incident are potential witnesses whose personal details must be accurately recorded, and the information that they can supply about the incident carefully documented in statements.

In conjunction with the ambulance services and the NHS, detailed, well rehearsed and updated plans are in existence to deal with the casualties on site and to transfer them to designated hospitals.

A casualty bureau established by the police receives inquiries, collects and collates information about missing persons over the telephone, by fax or as written documents (for example, general practice or hospital notes). In turn, when information becomes available, the bureau arranges for messages to be passed on through local police forces. This involves a major deployment of resources by the police and the putting into operation of sophisticated telephone call interception and diversion techniques. Doctors may sometimes be better equipped to gather detailed information about complex medical conditions and past surgical operations: this is yet another role for some of the police doctors.

6. If there are any deaths in a disaster H. M. Coroner (in Scotland, the Procurator Fiscal) must be informed at a very early stage, and instructions obtained. All police officers in such an incident have a role to play as coroner's officers or as agents of the procurator fiscal.

There is a requirement to ensure continuity of the chain of evidence and for a full investigation of each death. After being photographed and labelled on site, bodies are transferred, perhaps through an interim collection point established close to the site of the disaster, to a mortuary. The body collection point may be an open air area, a building such as a gymnasium or swimming pool, or an inflatable tent. The labelled bodies (the label is attached to a limb) are placed into sealable body bags (also labelled) at the scene; these labels have now been largely standardised on a national level. The body bags should not be opened again for any reason until the body has reached the mortuary and the post-mortem examination commences.

If the incident has involved several deaths there may be an early requirement for a temporary mortuary plan to be set into motion – usually by the police on the instructions of the coroner or fiscal, and in close collaboration with the local authority. This must be equipped, manned and fully commissioned; appropriate secure and reliable communication links are established at an early stage with the casualty bureau and the coroner or fiscal.

Formal identification of the deceased is carried out by an identification commission chaired by the coroner or procurator fiscal.

7. In any large or unusual incident there is potential for superimposed criminal activity such as looting. Commonly, members of the public with no direct involvement in the incident seek to observe the incident with their own eyes, and travel far and wide to do this; an even stranger phenomenon is the quest to collect souvenirs of such incidents. These activities hamper both the emergency services and the investigators.

The police will set up cordons to attempt to prevent such incidents and will be responsible for the security of the scene. Attempts will also be made at an early stage to ensure that the public are not exposed unduly to scenes of carnage and suffering; screens may have to be erected for this purpose. Road blocks and diversions will be put in place for similar purposes.

8. There is a legitimate quest by the public media for accurate and up-to-date information about the incident and the evolution of the emergency responses to it. All such communications are channelled through a police press office staffed by trained personnel. This office will be the only source of information, ensuring that it is strictly and carefully controlled. The press have to be given appropriate facilities and kept fully briefed; they should be able to ask questions at the regular press conferences held for them.

PLANNING FOR DISASTERS

The effectiveness of the response to a major incident is greatly enhanced by appropriate planning, by regular training, testing and exercising, and by continuous updating and modification of plans. Local authorities are obliged only by their general duty of care to formulate such plans; a failure to do so can lead in due course to successful litigation and the award of substantial damages (as in Cardiff judgement against South Glamorgan District Council in 1979 following the severe flooding in Cardiff).

The Civil Defence Act 1948 enables the Home Secretary to introduce regulations affecting both the functions of local authorities and the provision of specific grants to reimburse the costs incurred in meeting such requirements. The Civil Protection in Peacetime Act 1986 allows civil defence grants to be used for making preparations for peacetime emergencies. These Acts are reinforced by the Civil Defence (Grant) Regulations 1987 and the Civil Defence (Local Authority Functions) Regulations 1993 which spell out in detail these specific requirements. The Control of Industrial Major Accident Hazards (CIMAH) Regulations 1990 implemented the European Council Seveso Directive following on the Seveso incident in Northern Italy in 1976; this introduced the concept of off-site planning for installations handling large quantities of hazardous substances to protect the public in cases of accidents.

Planning of this nature must ensure a carefully co-ordinated team effort, involving all those who have a legitimate and essential role to play when disaster actually strikes.

THE AMBULANCE SERVICE

The ambulance service carries the principal responsibility for:-
   a)   saving lives

b) prompt dispatch of sufficient ambulances, medical, paramedical and other logistical support to the incident site

c) overall management and safety on site of NHS staff and of resources

d) setting up and management of triage and casualty clearing areas

e) alerting of receiving hospitals

f) setting up on site of effective communications systems with other medical facilities

e) a proper interface with the police and other emergency services, especially the fire brigade

f) effective and efficient evacuation in order of priority of all casualties to the appropriate hospitals.

THE CLINICAL FORENSIC EXAMINER

There is a tendency for doctors to volunteer their professional services or attempt to join in the work of the emergency services, particularly in a well publicised incident which involves numerous casualties: a doctor who has worked closely with the police will feel that his professional services and clinical skills could be required in a major incident to assist with the treatment of casualties on site. This inclination to help should be avoided at all costs, and only those doctors who have been specifically called out and to whom specific duties have been pre-assigned, should attend. When they so do, they should be briefed fully and in detail as to the very specific tasks which are allotted to them and they should stick strictly to these.

There are duties which clinical forensic medical examiners can apply themselves to on site. Where the place of doctors called out specifically by the police is written into disaster plans, and rehearsed during major incident exercises, the police doctors and all other emergency services become totally familiar with these roles.

Once the living casualties have been transported away, and the incident site made safe, clinical forensic examiners are eminently qualified to carry out the following tasks:

In liaison with the coroner or fiscal and the pathologist called out to the incident (the supervising pathologist) they may visit the scene, formally pronounce life extinct and assist with placing the bodies in bags after they have been tagged and photographed in situ, and their exact location identified accurately on a map or by some other means. Relatives and others who wish to pay their respects are often keen to visit the exact spot where specific bodies were found.

In liaison with police, any human remains have to be identified as such, and collected. If the incident involves several fatalities and extensive mutilation, as in an aircraft crash, an early decision is taken about which body parts are to be specifically labelled, and tagged similarly to the intact bodies. All body parts have to be identified (sometimes difficult in rural areas, because of admixed animal remains) and collected not only from the aesthetic and humanitarian points of view but also because these form an important adjunct to the pathological examination. A portion of skin with a tattoo, a prosthesis, a portion of a jaw, a finger or fingers might be enough to be able to state that a particular person has perished in the particular disaster. Furthermore, these fragments may contain vital information in terms of embedded foreign bodies that they have been in the vicinity of an explosive device.

Advice on kitting out with protective clothing the personnel concerned in body retrieval, and briefing them about health and safety matters, may often require an input from police doctors. This must be co-ordinated and integrated with the informed advice from the local environmental health department and consultants in communicable diseases.

A watchful eye is kept on all personnel for the development of features suggesting the onset of an acute post-traumatic stress reaction. All participants in the disaster need to feel cared for by those to whom they answer, and this caring attitude has to be maintained throughout the incident. This topic is explored further in chapter 17.

Amenities for the bereaved who visit the scene or who wish to view the bodies of the deceased should be carefully attended to. As part of the mortuary plans for major incidents, appropriate facilities for the bereaved to view the body in dignified surroundings, then to recuperate and collect their thoughts should be provided. Formal visual identification is not usually resorted to, and thus the viewing of bodies can be delayed until they are in a more presentable state, and perhaps even until they have been embalmed, if the investigations are prolonged and bodies have to be repatriated. Adequate medical support to deal with acute bereavement reactions and with the stress on relatives' physical and psychological health is no less important.

As part of the response by the police and by the local authority in providing full support and care for evacuees and for the wider local community, the professional skills of police doctors may also be called upon in dealing with emergency medical problems in this displaced community.

MORTUARY PHASE

The establishment of a temporary mortuary is likely if there is a significant number of fatalities. This will be in a building (for example, hanger, ice-rink, warehouse) separated from the local hospital or public mortuary to ensure that the activities of these two mortuaries can still proceed during the disaster investigation. This site may require to have attached to it facilities for radiological examination of the cadavers, odontological identification, fingerprinting, the storage of specimens (toxicological, histological, DNA) removed from the deceased and the refrigerated interim storage of the cadavers and other retrieved human remains. Space must also be provided for storing securely the personal effects of the deceased.

When the body bags are eventually opened in the mortuary, standard forms (such as those produced by Interpol) are used to log all relevant information derived from the external, and if indicated, the internal examination of the bodies.

In carrying out their examinations, the pathologists would value the assistance of medically qualified persons in transcribing the autopsy findings during the post-mortem examinations: it does expedite the documentation of this information and it also shields inexperienced personnel from the sights necessarily associated with the mortuary.

All the information gathered has to be written down contemporaneously; doctors are better able to cope with the swift and accurate transcription of this. It may perhaps be worth noting that tape-recording of this information is a recipe for a further disaster, given the multitude of tapes which may be erased, lost or re-used.

IDENTIFICATION

Definitive identification of an individual who has perished in a major disaster is ultimately the responsibility of the coroner or the procurator fiscal, who must be convinced that there is an adequate match on a number of pre-determined criteria. In practice, such decisions are often taken on a committee basis by the Identification Commission, chaired by the coroner or the fiscal, on which the police and other relevant agencies involved in the investigation are represented. For example, it may be decided that identification would only be accepted if two of the following three items match: personal features, fingerprints and odontological details.

Identification is often a lengthy process of gradual elimination and exclusion. Computer programs such as CRISIS (Zeebrugge incident) and HOLMES (Lockerbie air disaster) have to be used to assist with such investigations. The main identification criteria are the following:

Visual – This method is rarely favoured in major incidents, and is obviously useless in the presence of mutilation, burning, or fairly advanced decomposition; this method is not only inhumane, but often one fraught with potential for error.

In their state of emotion and shock, bereaved relatives may find themselves coming to the wrong conclusion.

When few victims are involved, this method can prove to be entirely valid and rapid. It may be supplemented by taking photographs of the faces of the deceased, and using these as a preliminary screening method to avoid having to show too many bodies. This method was used in the Hillsborough stadium disaster.

Photographs – The use of photographs from family albums, from passport and visa applications for matching purposes is to be treated with great caution, but may be helpful for screening and supplementary identification.

Personal and stomatic details –

a) *General information:* approximate age, ethnic features, height, weight, build, colour of hair and eyes, length of hair, balding, patterns of the facies, pierced ear lobes, body hirsutism, and so on.

b) *Specific information:* for example scars, tattoos, birth marks, amputations, circumcision, old injuries.

c) *Occupational data:* carbon pigmentation of the facial skin in miners, callosities on hands and feet in manual workers.

d) *Medical complaints:* psoriasis, eczema.

Clothing – This is described in layers, photographed and subsequently (particularly if intact) laundered or dry cleaned to enable its demonstration to the relatives. Patterns of suits and dresses, labels, sites of previous repair, may all be useful.

Personal effects –

a) *Contents of pockets:* – all items in the pockets are removed, catalogued and described. Note that any documents carried by the deceased may be useful particularly if a series of them are present bearing the same name and address.

b) *Jewellery* – if firmly attached to the body (rings, earrings) may be particularly useful. These items may have to be cleaned before they are shown to the bereaved. If the body is mutilated, these items may be displaced internally into other parts of the body e.g. necklaces into the thorax.

All items retrieved are eventually returned to the bereaved.

Fingerprints (and palm prints) – in the United Kingdom they can only be matched with prints retained on criminal records and perhaps on the files of the armed forces. If these become of major importance in identification, prints may be taken from personal items in the office, workplace or home for comparison purposes (this had to be done in the Piper Alpha disaster).

Fingers which have become dehydrated after death or are partially decomposed may still yield good prints if they are appropriately treated in the laboratory - this may necessitate the removal of the fingers or the hands (as done in the Marchioness disaster).

Details of the feet – Foot-prints are kept on record by some armed forces. Chiropodists also retain a vast amount of detail about feet and their records may assist in identification.

Teeth – The characteristics of the teeth are retained to a large extent even in the presence of severe mutilation and decomposition, and also after burning (at least the back teeth). Details are covered in chapter 15. Research has shown that it is always preferable that dentists work in pairs, double-checking each other's work (in terms of corroboration of evidence, this is mandatory in Scotland).

Radiological – features may assist in ageing the individual, particularly in children. In addition, anatomical abnormalities such as a cervical rib, and metallic foreign bodies (prostheses, metal sutures) may be demonstrated. The three-dimensional configuration of the frontal sinuses are unique to individuals.

If the disaster involves the possibility of an explosive device or gun-shot injuries, extensive radiography is used in the attempt to identify such a device from shrapnel and other foreign material embedded in the bodies of the deceased. Personnel in the mortuary require proper protection during radiological examinations.

Serological tests – unless an ante-mortem specimen of blood is available it is unusual to have access to more than the A B O and Rh blood groups. If blood is available other blood groups and polymorphic proteins (for instance, phospho-glucomutase – PGM) may be looked for.

DNA – A sample of spleen or muscle (iliopsoas is satisfactory) may serve as a source of DNA provided this is retained at minus 20°C. This must be compared with a tissue specimen (blood, semen, bone marrow) or with a profile obtained by elimination using blood or buccal scrapes from siblings, children and other relations (this was done in the Air France disaster near Strasbourg).

Heavy contamination with aviation fuel (kerosene) and other chemicals may render such laboratory testing difficult, if not impossible.

Facial reconstruction – computerised or soft tissue building-up techniques may have to be resorted to.

As an example, the methods of identification used successfully in the Lockerbie air disaster are presented in table 1.

NUMBERS OF DECEASED IDENTIFIED	METHOD USED
18	Odontology alone
78	Odontology & fingerprints
118	Odontology & methods other than fingerprinting mainly personal effects
13	Fingerprints alone
78	Fingerprints and odontology
17	Fingerprints with methods other than odontology
14	Methods other than odontology and fingerprinting
253	TOTAL

Table 1 – Identification methods used in the Lockerbie investigation

SPECIAL INSTANCES

Some disasters will involve the spillage of chemical agents and corrisives, or irrespirable gases, or even the leakage of radioactivity. Before the retrieval of any fatalities commences expert advice must be obtained to ensure that none of the personnel involved in their recovery is exposed to dangerous situations which can be catered for and avoided. Chapter 9 of 'Emergency Plannng in the NHS' deals specifically with chemical contamination incidents.

OPERATIONAL DEBRIEFING

After the investigation of the incident has been completed, it is essential that all the relevant documents are made available for any eventual court or inquiry purposes.

Similarly the lessons learnt from each individual incident are unique and it is essential that in any final debrief after the incident, the doctors called by the police should be fully involved.

Further reading

ACPO Emergency Procedures Manual 1995 HMSO, London.

Adshead G, Canterbury R, Rose S 1994 Current provision and recommendations for the management of psycho-social morbidity following disaster in England. *Criminal Behaviour & Mental Health* **4**:181–208.

Alexander D, Wells A 1991 Reactions of police officers to body-handling after a major disaster. A before and after comparison. *British Journal of Psychiatry* **159**; 547–555.

Allen AJ, 1991 *The Disasters Working Party - Planning for a caring response*. Department of Health, HMSO, London.

Welsh Office, Health and Social Work Department 1993 *Arrangements to deal with health aspects of chemical contamination incidents*. Health Services Guidelines - HSG (93)38, 1991 – Chapter 9 - Emergency Planning in the NHS. HMSO, London.

Busuttil A, Jones JSP 1990 *Deaths in Major Disasters - the Pathologist's Role*. Royal College of Pathologists, London.

Clark DH 1991 Dental identification in the Piper Alpha Oil Rig Disaster. *J Forensic Odonto-Stomatology* **9**(2); 37–46.

Home Office, 1994 *Dealing with fatalities during disasters* – Report of the National Working Party, Emergency Planning College, HMSO, London.

Gersons B, Carlier L, 1992 Post -Traumatic Stress Disorder: The history of a recent concept. *British Journal of Psychiatry* **161**; 742–749.

Moody GH, Busuttil A, 1994 Identification in the Lockerbie Air Disaster. *American Journal of Forensic Medicine and Pathology* **15**(1); 63–69.

Scanlon TJ 1992 *Disaster Preparedness - Some myths and misconceptions* Emergency Planning College, Easingwold.

17

OCCUPATIONAL HEALTH OF POLICE OFFICERS

WDS McLay

Until now, police officers have been excluded from the provisions of the Health and Safety at Work etc. Act 1974, but that position is about to change, under the terms of the European Framework Directive for Health and Safety. A daughter directive requires an employer to undertake assessment of the risks to which employees are put in the course of their work. At the time of writing, the legislative framework to implement the directive is not yet clear, but police forces are engaged in a process of compiling risk assessments – a process inevitably complicated, for the work performed by operational officers is so diverse and so unpredictable. Another factor is the increasing use of civilian employees on what are essentially operational tasks formerly done by police officers. The Act put duties on both employers and employees, but the responsibilities under any new statute will lie much more heavily upon employers. This puts yet another nail in the coffin of the constitutional position of the constable as an independent holder of an office under the Crown, rather than as an employee. Forces have introduced occupational health units with a varying ambit; the largest are in charge of full time occupational physicians. Despite this development, many police surgeons will continue to advise chief officers, as they have done in the past. In practical terms, too, the police surgeon is often on hand to give immediate advice or reassurance.

Fitness for the tasks set by society entails a basic level of physical health and stamina in recruits; injury and ill-health will reduce the effectiveness of serving officers, and there may come a time when capacity for continued service must be assessed. Four simple considerations have been suggested (Trottier & Brown 1994a) in assessing the officer with disease or disability: ability to do the job; safety of the public; safety of a co-worker; safety of the individual police officer. The occupational health physician's concern is to look far beyond ill-health and management concepts of reducing the number and duration of sickness absences.

The heightened awareness of the hazards of police work referred to above must be accompanied by greater understanding of officers' reaction to these. The stress occasioned by involvement in violent incidents – whether as direct victim of assault, or in policing public disorder or as a rescuer in a major incident – is not difficult to appreciate. What is often viewed less sympathetically is the distress caused by minor tragedies such as attendance at a cot death or the delivery of news about an unexpected bereavement. That procedural and organizational factors arouse so much unexpressed anger in lower ranks is scarcely credited by those further up the tree. It is not enough to have in place a mechanism to treat post-traumatic stress in the individual officer: it is necessary to mitigate needless anxiety by paying careful attention to relationships between senior officers and their subordinates, by ensuring that operational demands are well thought out and reasonable, by improving communication between the ranks.

CONDITIONS OF SERVICE
OF POLICE OFFICERS

On appointment as police officers, candidates expect to serve what is described in the regulations as an ordinary working life of 30 years. This is much shorter than the span of most other careers. They may also opt to retire after 25 years, but with entitlement to a reduced pension, on reaching the age of 50. The recruitment of older men and women will result in still shorter service, an outcome encouraged by a lengthy, controversial and only partly implemented report (Sheehy 1994).

Constables and sergeants reach their age limit at 55 but, subject to the chief constable's approval and the applicant's medical fitness, late entrants may continue to serve beyond this age to qualify for a full pension. Chief officers (chief constables, assistant chief constables and Metropolitan commanders – the post of deputy chief constable as a substantive rank has been abolished) may also retire at age 55, although they are entitled to serve for another 10 years.

Despite the positive encouragement of female recruitment, the proportion of policewomen in Great Britain is just over 13%, for they have a greater tendency to leave at an earlier age, and far fewer sit police (promotion) examinations. A recruit may be as young as 18½, the age at which cadets transfer to the regular force, but there is a financial incentive for those of 22 to join, for they are credited with age related salary increments. Selection is based on standardised examinations, interviews and medical fitness.

During the first two years, service is probationary and may be terminated if the chief constable considers the individual unlikely to become an efficient officer. Such a decision is properly taken in the light of inefficiency in a professional sense, concerns about integrity and attitude or because, within that time, some medical condition debarring further service has come to light.

CONDITIONS OF WORK

The conventional picture of the British 'bobby' is of an officer pounding the beat, but (despite strenuous and much publicised efforts to "get officers back on the streets") today's policeman spends much of his time in a car or behind a desk, where little expenditure of energy is required. When activity is called for, it is usually in sudden bursts as, for example, in a chase. It is important to encourage police officers to play games or be involved in sports from an early stage in service, and to reinforce this when they marry, a time when other interests seem more pressing: stamina and agility are assets to the operational officer.

Life style can be influenced for the better. Local health education units will provide posters and other printed material for display and distribution. Commercial organisations in the food industry will help to mount exhibitions, and advise on improved canteen catering. 'Sponsored slims' for a good cause are surprisingly popular (the British Heart Foundation is a suitable source of publicity material). Encourage the enforcement of no smoking policies.

Unpleasant conditions cannot be separated from police work! Officers are deployed to cover both sociable and unsociable hours, so must work shifts, in all weathers, learning from their first hours on the beat to cope with the wicked, the pathetic, the dying and the bereaved, the frightened victim of rape, the indignant householder who knows his stolen property is unlikely to be recovered. Accidents occur when roads are wet and busy; crime is not confined to daylight hours. The police officer is at the beck and call of society, yet his or her work is ever more minutely scrutinised. Each is personally answerable for the decisions taken in trying circumstances; this responsibility adds a great deal of stress to the officer's working day.

Shifts by themselves disrupt the normal pattern of anyone's life, and the need to ensure proper coverage by rotating the shifts exacerbates the disruption. No system has been devised which does not to some extent impair effective working, but different forces use different patterns and methods; any rotation not based on a forward change – early/late/night – is working against the physiological clock.

RECRUITS

British police forces are in turmoil at the moment, for the concept of physical fitness to be a police officer is questioned in terms of equal opportunities policies, and the analysis of work related activities with the skills necessary to perform these. Test circuits have been devised, and are in use for the Royal Canadian

Mounted Police (Trottier & Brown 1994b) as well as in some forces in the United Kingdom. It is clear that no scheme can set the same target standard for males and females (Henderson J & Gamble R 1996, personal communication). Even height standards have been largely abandoned. It is essential to discuss with the recruiting staff what policies are followed in the particular force, and to seek to influence these in the event of disagreement. Most forces now accept the advice of a working party set out in Home Department circulars. The doctor examining a recruit should have in mind an individual whose service will stretch for the following 30 years; much of the officer's career may be spent on the beat, or on a variety of tasks requiring a reasonable degree of physical fitness. Only a small proportion of officers are essentially administrators, and the number of protected posts to which unfit officers can be assigned has diminished. Some recruits have the unrealistic expectation that it is feasible to opt for a particular type of police work (popular ones are the mounted or traffic branches) in which they will spend their whole service.

Accidents cannot be foreseen, nor can illnesses be predicted, but these may well reduce the candidate's potential. Be reluctant to accept the overweight candidate (especially someone with an adverse family history), the even mildly hypertensive or the young man with a tachycardia who assures you he is normally very calm. Rejected candidates often appeal to consultant physicians; these practitioners are not good at taking stress or any other occupational factor into account, so tend to give an opinion that such an individual is fit for appointment. If a medical examination induces overreaction, what will a confrontation on the street do? Routine urinalysis and haemoglobin estimation are worthwhile, but chest X-ray is not a cost effective procedure, for disqualifying lesions are seldom found.

The national advice referred to above is summarised in table 1 (reproduced from Home Office circular 9/1995 and Scottish Office Police Circular 16/1995). These standards are likely to be modified over the course of years as experience suggests. It is unwise to take too prescriptive an attitude to these matters: approval for fitness for appointment is the force medical officer's prerogative, and he should err on the side of safety; subsequent invaliding from the force is expensive. In all of these cases, it is important not to be pushed into hasty decisions if correspondence with the applicant's general practitioner, or even referral for further investigation, will help you reach a proper conclusion.

Even less easy to quantify than physical illness are attitudinal problems or other psychological difficulties. These are more likely to be spotted by recruiting staff during extended interviews than by a doctor. Nevertheless, the line of questioning you choose may well reveal concerns which you want to discuss with police staff. In this respect, the candidate is not a patient, and must know that the history he gives will have a bearing on the outcome of the selection process. If it is your decision to reject, the details driving you to this conclusion are no concern of lay staff, but you may have a duty to urge the examinee to consult his or her general practitioner, and then to communicate with the doctor yourself.

CADETS, SPECIAL CONSTABLES AND CIVILIAN EMPLOYEES

Standards for the first of these should be very high, because it is wrong to allow them to waste time as cadets, and wrong for the resources of the service to be wasted on training if they are doubtful candidates for the force.

Special constables have a mainly auxiliary role, but they may be faced with the same hazards as their regular colleagues. Although there is no need to consider pensioning implications for them, you must remember that physical or psychological incapacity on their part could easily put the regular partner at risk. The Police Federation is made responsible by the Police Act 1919 for the welfare of special constables, but the police authority is responsible for insuring them against injury.

Most civilian employees (often now called 'Support Staff') are office bound, and no unusual features are of importance in considering their fitness. Nevertheless, police forces are large, complex organisations employing, for example, spray painters and garage mechanics whose sensitivity to allergenic materials could cause problems; risk assessments for these posts are also required. Scenes of crime officers and photographers, too, must be able to work in circumstances trying from both physical and psychological points of view. As a deliberate policy, very many civilians have been recruited to perform work formerly done by police officers; some of this work must be considered operational, carrying with it the stresses implicit in such tasks.

Traffic wardens form a group of civilians who must be capable of both patrol and points duty in inclement weather as well as having the stability to cope with discourtesy and worse from the outraged motorist. They must be able to read road vehicle registration numbers at a distance, identify the colour of a car, and read the small print on driving licences and insurance certificates.

SPECIALISTS

Members of an underwater search unit are subject to the Diving Regulations (which are under review) and must be examined at intervals by doctors approved under these regulations or by an Employment Medical Adviser (Health and Safety Executive).

For Large Goods or Passenger Carrying Vehicle drivers – complete the official form supplied by the Driving Vehicle Licence Agency.

SYSTEM	REJECT	CONSIDER CAREFULLY	COMMENTS
EYES	Squint History of detached retina History of glaucoma Radial keratotomy Photorefractive keratoplasty	Latent squint Lens implant Corneal graft with good uncorrected visual acuity	Photorefractive keratoplasty under review
Visual acuity (unaided)	Worse than 8/18 in either eye (binocular worse than 6/6 requires correction) Worse than 6/12 in either eye binocuilar worse than 6/6	Following the changes in age restrictions, consider the effects of age on acuity	Some current force standards are more strict than this where there may be special circumstances e.g. firearms in RUC. (aided) An independent with specialist eye opinion may be helpful on occasions
Colour vision	Failure on City University Test	Failure on Ishihara Test	Current City University Test rationale states 7 out of 10 correct responses is within normal limits.
EARS	Need for hearing aid Active chronic suppurative otitis media Current perforation	Any chronic ENT condition	
Hearing	More than average of 30db loss over range 500-4000Hz More than average of 20db loss over range 500-4000Hz when audiogram is taken using a sound proof booth Unilateral hearing loss of a similar magnitude	Following the change in age restrictions, consider the effects of age on hearing	Routine audiometry required at pre-employment assessment
CARDIO-VASCULAR	Hypertension requiring treatment Severe varicose veins Uncorrected congenital heart disease History of coronary heart disease Cardiac surgery - adult	Hypertension greater than 140/90 at pre-employment medical Minor varicose veins Haemorrhoids Cardiac surgery - paediatric	Defer until treated Defer until treated Routine ECG not required
NEUROLOGICAL	Any proven epileptic seizure after five years of age Degenerative neurological disease	Any episode of altered consciousness after five years of age History of migraine History of brain surgery Any significant head injury	

Table 1

SYSTEM	REJECT	CONSIDER CAREFULLY	COMMENTS
METABOLIC	Diabetes mellitus	History of thyroid disorder History of any other metabolic disorder	
Weight	BMI above 30	BMI between 25 and 30 BMI below 19	
Body fat		Percentage of body fat greater than Male 21% Female 30%	
GASTRO-INTESTINAL	Peptic ulcer Hiatus hernia Crohn's disease Ulceratice colitis Irritable bowel syndrome	Occasional dyspepsia Hernia	Defer until treated
RESPIRATORY	Non-asthmatic chronic respiratory disorders Asthma currently on treatment including inhalers Spontaneous pneumothorax on two or more occasions FEV$_1$ or FVC more than two standard deviations below predicted norm	Sinusitis, chronic URTI, hay fever Past history of asthma Spontaneous pneumothorax on one occasion FEV$_1$ less than 75%	Routine chest X-ray not required Routine spirometry required
MUSCULO-SKELETAL	History of back disorder requiring hospital treatment History of laminectomy History of major knee surgery including meniscectomy Recurrent dislocation of major joint Major foot deformities Muscle wasting - effects of cerebral palsy Chronic orthopaedic problem	History of minor back disorder History of arthroscopy including partial meniscetomy Isolated dislocation of any joint History of knee injuries not requiring surgery Significant fracture Major soft tissue injury Chondromalacia patellae	
PSYCHIATRIC	Psychotic illness Most neurotic or stress related psychiatric disorder History of drug abuse History of alcoholism History of eating disorder History of socio-pathic behaviour	History of isolated reactive depression	
GENITO-URINARY	Chronic genito-urinary disorders	Any significant disorder of reproductive system	
SKIN		Severe eczema, psoriasis, pustular acne Other chronic skin disorders	
RETICULO-ENDOTHELIAL	All RE disorders		
MOUTH		Evidence of poor dental hygiene	

Table 1– *Continued*

Authorised Firearms Officers (AFO) are required to work long and uncomfortable hours in difficult environments, but they also carry a heavy psychological burden. These officers undergo intensive physical training as well as shooting practice. In an industrial medicine context, it is as well to remember the need to ensure that firing ranges are adequately ventilated; permanent staff should have a periodic check on blood lead and porphyrin levels. Ear protectors must be worn by instructors and trainees in the range; nevertheless, their freedom from noise induced hearing loss should be checked regularly by audiometry.

Traffic officers require excellent eyesight when handling cars driven at high speed, so must use suitable lenses. As with AFOs, traffic officers commonly encounter unpleasant sights, and need a high degree of psychological stability. Motor cyclists are at risk from both road noise and the necessarily loud communication equipment in their helmets. Some forces now use helicopters with civilian pilots: their crews do not operate at heights posing great barometric hazards, but they must have good Eustachian function and hearing (again, regular screening is mandatory).

All these specialists are regularly exposed to incidents from which traumatic stress may arise. Further reference is made to traumatic stress on page 318 below.

PHYSICAL AND CHEMICAL HAZARDS

Police officers encounter many physical and chemical substances, including toxins spilled as a result of traffic or industrial accident, carbon monoxide and other fumes produced in fires, asbestos fibres released during vandalism or demolition.

During patrol in derelict premises, or in poor lighting conditions, they meet unguarded electric cables, unsafe stairways, unexpected obstacles. They are at risk of assault in all its forms, of injury in road accidents on duty or while assisting at the scene of one. There is intermittent pressure for the arming of the police; even before any official issue, many officers equipped themselves with body armour – it has proved difficult to manufacture any material proof against both bullets and knives. Incapacitating sprays (CS aerosol) are under test.

A welcome development is the institution of 'officer safety training' which is designed to give officers a greater understanding of the techniques of maintaining a safe space around them by demeanour and dominance, rather than simply by threats and the use of a baton. This is backed up by improved equipment in the form of extending batons and rigid handcuffs (and the expertise in their use). Such equipment has brought problems in its train, for the increased weight is uncomfortable and may exacerbate back pain; it is a serious hindrance to those in ordinary motor vehicles. From the point of view of the forensic medical examiner, the equipment has introduced new patterns of injury.

BIOLOGICAL HAZARDS

Operational police officers come into close contact with a wide variety of infectious disease, whether acting in a humanitarian capacity, in the process of arrest or as a result of the random effects of meeting many people in the course of the day. All officers should be immunised against tetanus. In the United Kingdom, there is a resurgence of tuberculosis, likely to be most prevalent in those living rough or those with impaired immune systems.

Far and away the greatest fear is reserved for AIDS, although hepatitis B is more common and more readily acquired by contact with infected material. A family of hepatitis strains has been identified, all with the potential for causing serious disease. There is effective immunisation for hepatitis B, but not for the others. Treatment with specific immunoglobulin is available, but must be given within eight hours. The cost of hepatitis B prophylaxis is high, but development of the disease after occupational exposure could well lead to expensive litigation, for it is a prescribed disease under the Health & Safety at Work Act. Antibody titres should be checked to assess the effectiveness of immunisation.

Of much greater importance is education in the need to treat all body fluids as hazardous, yet at the same time affirm that simple precautions are adequate, if conscientiously followed. Biting and spitting (habits which are commonly practised by drug abusers in the course of arrest, or as a means of intimidating officers and others) are, at most, an unlikely prelude to the transfer of HIV, but inoculation of a very much smaller quantity of infected material through the skin or mucous membranes could cause hepatitis.

STRESS AND ALCOHOL

Pursuit of the efficient use of expensive police manpower has led to the replacement of many officers by civilians, when the duties of the post do not require the holder to exercise police powers. As a consequence few such posts are available for the unfit officer, unless on a very short term basis. Changes in the style of policing, in public attitudes, in the investigation of complaints against the police all contribute to a rise in stress. So, too, do unexpected changes in duty hours. Careful management in this, as in other supervisory aspects, will ameliorate working conditions, reducing the resentment officers feel when they consider themselves to be treated in a cavalier manner.

Attendance at mass disasters and the use of firearms are examples already mentioned of events causing great stress to those involved. A better account of an incident by the participants is likely after an interval during which they have had time to collect their thoughts: there are sound reasons, therefore, to keep over officious investigators at bay. The actions taken by police officers will be of interest to journalists. There is a need to protect them – and relatives – from intrusive questioning; relatives certainly must be kept well informed about the wellbeing of the officers. Where an officer is involved in the death of a civilian, some form of public inquest will surely follow; adequate support must be provided by those not required to judge the wisdom of the officer's conduct.

Few are unscathed by major or life threatening incidents; emotions become engaged. Immediate supervisors need training in recognition of signs of exhaustion, physical or emotional, in those on duty; they must take active steps, as far as practicable, to protect their staff. The very normality of a measure of distress is difficult for many police officers to accept, or to admit to. The concept of post incident (some would call it psychological) debriefing is that the recognition by participants of how angry, or guilty, or scared or sad they felt will help to prevent the later onset of common stress symptoms: moodiness, irritability, poor quality of sleep, loss of affect, impaired concentration, intrusive thoughts, flashbacks. An understanding that any or all of these symptoms may occur puts them into a context allowing the officer to deal with them. There is an argument for arranging the automatic attendance of all officers involved in the incident, to prevent the obvious singling out of individuals, who may worry that they are considered weaker than their peers. The value of the technique – which essentially gives participants an opportunity to tell what happened in a supportive group led by (usually two) trained facilitators, then to speak of how they felt – has been questioned (Raphael *et al* 1995) but seems, at least on an anecdotal plane, to confer benefit. Debriefing of this type, usually held 24 to 72 hours after the incident, must be clearly distinguished from counselling, which is a form of psychotherapy designed to deal with individuals or groups suffering from persistence of symptoms. Persistence of the symptom complex for at least a month, accompanied by an enhanced startle reflex, is designated as post traumatic stress disorder (PTSD) and accepted as a basis for both litigation and criminal injuries compensation.

Stress at work, in turn, leads to conflict at home. Domestic pressures are themselves a prime source of stress, although it is more usual to lay emphasis on that arising at work. Quite apart from the more dramatic incidents referred to above, maladroit supervision, frustration, lengthy investigation of sexual abuse cases, the delivery of death messages are all part of the relentless pressure felt by many officers.

Alcohol abuse is a widespread problem in the working population, and it seems unlikely that police officers are differently affected than others. The consequences to their own careers and to the standing of the police when drunken officers become involved with members of the public are dire. It is to be hoped that most chief officers treat alcohol abuse in their force as demanding appropriate counselling rather than as a purely disciplinary matter. Good management includes the acceptance of an alcohol policy which also has the support of the representative organisations. Few officers with an established, severe alcohol problem return to productive work. So often initial improvement (perhaps under the threat of disciplinary action) is not maintained.

SICK LEAVE

Police officers are subject to the Statutory Sick Pay Scheme, as if they were normal employees (strictly speaking, for the purpose of carrying out their duties, they are not employed). Under new regulations (Regulation 46, Police Regulations 1995 and 27A of the Police (Scotland) Regulations 1976 as amended) police officers have six months fully paid sick leave, then six months on half pay; after twelve months, no payment is made. The chief constable has personal discretion to modify the strict application of the rules, discretion likely to be exercised if the absence results from injury on duty. Various conditions of service have been altered, including loss for recruits presently joining of housing allowance, and a buy out of inspectors' right to payment for overtime.

Forces should have routines for monitoring sickness absence, both to minimise it and for welfare purposes. Officers on sick leave, or with a pattern causing concern, may be referred for an opinion. To assist you in reaching a fair conclusion you should be ready to seek advice from the officer's own doctor (the response from general practitioners to requests of this kind is patchy) or from a consultant if he attends hospital. The provisions of the Access to Medical Reports Act 1988 must be considered when information is requested for employment purposes. The Act requires consent to be given by the subject of any enquiry to a doctor who has had clinical care of him as a patient; the consent may be hedged by a declaration that the patient see the report before it is sent to the enquirer. The occupational physician may be in a quandary here, for the General Medical Council (1995) requires doctors to "respect requests by patients that information should not be disclosed to third parties, save in exceptional circumstances". The legal force of this is not in dispute (*Hunter v Mann* [1974] QB 767) yet there may still be doubt as to the definition of a patient. How much 'care' may you extend to an employee before a doctor/patient relationship exists? Your own opinion will be valueless if you do not make yourself familiar with the officer's circumstances at home and at work. Very occasionally, a difference of opinion arises between an officer's own doctor who considers that sick leave is justified, and the force medical officer who takes a contrary view. Regulations require a police authority, within 28 days of becoming aware of such a dispute, to appoint (preferably with the agreement of the first two) a third medical practitioner to arbitrate; this opinion is binding on the authority.

MATERNITY LEAVE

Running in parallel with the statutory maternity provisions, policewomen are entitled to a year on maternity leave (three months being paid at the ordinary rate, but nine months without pay or housing allowance where this remains applicable). Proper arrangements must be made to protect pregnant officers when they have notified their condition. A European directive now lays a duty on employers to protect new and nursing mothers (in effect, they may not work in an operational role, even if they wish to).

PENSIONS

Service pensions are available at 25 years although, to qualify for payment, the officer must have attained 50 years of age. After serving for 30 years, the full pension is payable even to those under 50. These pensions become index-linked at the age of 55. Any officer retiring with less than 25 years service may be entitled to a deferred pension. Rather than take the full amount of the pension, most officers opt to commute part in favour of a lump sum; the calculation makes it financially attractive to serve for 30 years.

Officers may themselves request pensioning because of ill-health, or this may be proposed by the chief constable on the force medical officer's recommendation. Each case must be looked at individually. It has already been emphasised that the scope for 'tucking away' an unfit officer has been much reduced and there may be little option but the unpalatable one of premature discharge. A great benefit to pensioners who are retired prematurely on grounds of ill-health is that they may become eligible for index-linked increments immediately. The terms of an ill-health pension vary with length of service and age, and will be enhanced if unfitness is caused by an injury on duty. The size of an injury award increases in bands in proportion to what the regulations describe as greater loss of earning capacity. How a doctor is to determine this is not at all clear. He may also have some difficulty in being sure that a particular injury did result in disability sufficient to justify pensioning ('permanent disablement'). It is open to a police authority to reassess its pensioners after discharge and, if appropriate, invite the former officer to take up duty again. Police officers who are retired against their wishes may appeal to the secretary of state, on the grounds that discharge is unwarranted, or that a percentage award for injury purposes is wrong. The secretary of state appoints a medical referee to examine the appellant, and to hear representations made by him and by the chief constable.

You must resist pensioning proposals simply designed to get rid of awkward customers. Conversely, there is also potential for abuse by officers who realise that a medical discharge at 26½ years service earns the full pension, immediately index linked.

References

General Medical Council. 1995 Duties of a doctor. GMC, London

Raphael B, Meldrum L, McFarlane AC 1995 Does debriefing after psychological trauma work? *British Medical Journal* 1995; **310**:1479.

Sheehy 1994 *Inquiry into Police Responsibilities and Rewards.*

Trottier A and Brown J 1994a Occupational health in police work: a Canadian perspective. *Journal of Clinical Forensic Medicine* 1994; **1**:39–42.

Trottier A, Brown J, 1994b *Police Health. A Physician's Guide to the Assessment of Police Officers.* 1994. Canada Communication Group, Ottawa.

Further reading

The Police Pensions Regulations are set out in Statutory Instrument 1987/257, but a simpler guide prepared in the Home Office for those who need to apply the regulations and advise prospective pensioners has been written.

TABLE OF CASES

AG v Guardian Newspapers Ltd (2)
(1988) 52

Bayliss v Thames Valley Police
Chief Constable (1978) 236

Evans v Ewels (1972) 194

Friel v Dickson (1992) 238

Gillick v West Norfolk and Wisbech Area
Health Authority and ano. (1986) 121

Gumley v Cunningham (1989) 227

H v Schering Chemicals Ltd (1983) 21

HMA v Khaliq (1984) 25

Hornal v Neuberger Productions (1957) 11

Hunter v Mann (1974) 319

Lines (1844) 193

Miranda v Arizona (1966) 19

Moorov (1930) 25

Oscar Slater (1928) 27

R v Abadom (1983) 22

R v Aves (1950) 17

R v Bradshaw (1985) 21

R v Central Criminal Court, ex
Parte Francis & Francis (1988) 23

R v Cook (1987) 18

R v Crampton (1990) 20

R v Goldenberg (1988) 20

R v Hayes (1977) 13

R v Keane (1994) 56

R v Li Shu-Ling (1989) 19

R v Mallinson (1977) 21

R v North Humberside Coroner, ex parte
Jamieson (1994) 280

R v Prentice and anor; R v Adomako
(1993) 3

R v Sat-Bhambra (1988) 20

R v Scarrot (1977) 22

R v Turner (1975) 21

R v Ward (1993) 2, 21, 56

Re T (1992) 43

Reid v Nixon (1948) 237

Rushton v Higgins (1972) 236

Solesury v Pugh (1969) 236

Woolmington v DPP (1935) 11

X v Sweeney (1982) 26

TABLE OF STATUTES

Abortion Act 1967 215

Access to Health Records Act
1990 .... 43, 55

Access to Medical Reports Act
1988 .... 43, 54, 319

Age of Legal Capacity (Scotland) Act
1991 139

Anatomy Act
1984 283

Births and Deaths Registration Act
1926 282

Births and Deaths Registration Act
1953 277

Children Act
1989 .... 120, 135

Children (Scotland) Act
1995 .... 137, 139

Civil Defence Act
1948 301

Civil Evidence (Scotland) Act
1988 25

Civil Protection in Peacetime Act
1986 301

Concealment of Pregnancy Act
1809 216

Coroners (Amendment) Act
1926 280

Coroners Act (Northern Ireland)
1959 284

Coroners Act
1988 .... 280, 282, 284

Criminal Appeal Act
1968 8

Criminal Justice Act
1967 .... 18, 76, 80

Criminal Justice Act
1988 .... 12-13, 18, 46

Criminal Justice Act
1991 12-13

Criminal Justice Act
1994 46

Criminal Justice and Public
Order Act 1994 .... 13, 16, 193

Criminal Procedure (Scotland) Act
1995 .... 36, 190

Customs and Excise Management Act
1979 48

Data Protection Act
1984 .... 43, 54-55, 92

Fatal Accidents and Sudden Deaths
Inquiry (Scotland) Act 1976 286

Health and Safety at Work etc Act
1974 .... 280, 309

Homicide Act
1957 11

Human Fertilisation and Embryology
Act 1990 215

Infant Life (Preservation) Act
1929 215

Infanticide Act
1938 216

Magistrates Court Act
1980 .... 18, 76, 80

Medicines Act
1968 163-164

Mental Health Act
1983 .... 10, 171, 186, 189, 217

Mental Health (Scotland) Act
1984 190

Misuse of Drugs Act
1971 .... 48, 164, 263

Offences Against the Person Act
1861 .... 144, 215

Police Act
1919 313

Police (Scotland) Act
1967 34

Police Act (Northern Ireland)
1970 35

Police and Criminal Evidence
Act 1984 .... 2, 10, 12, 18-19, 22-23,
36, 42, 46, 49, 53, 62, 79, 103, 172, 214,
260, 265, 293

Police and Magistrates' Courts Act
1994 34

Prisoners and Criminal Proceedings
(Scotland) Act 1993 265

Registration of Births, Deaths
and Marriages (Scotland) Act
1965 284

Road Traffic Act
1988 .... 228, 231

Road Traffic Regulation Act
1984 22

Sexual Offences (Amendment) Act
1976 15

Sexual Offences Act
1956 .... 44, 193-194

Sexual Offences Act
1967.. 194

Social Work (Scotland) Act
1968 .... 31, 137

Stillbirth (Definition) Act
1992 215

Suicide Act
1961.. 275

Transport Act
1981 228

Transport Act
1982 228

Vagrancy Act
1824 194

INDEX

A

Abrasion, 113, 144-146, 149-150, 157-159, 290

Abstinence syndrome (opiate), 168-169

Actus reus, 10, 191

Administration of Justice Department, 75, 83

Adhesions
    labial, 130, 134-135

AIDS, 200, 317

Alcohol,
    absorption of, 173-175
    abuse, 227, 318
    blood concentration, 106, 174-175, 225-226
   and crime, 176
   and driving performance, 228
    'hip flask' defence, 227
    hypoglycaemia and, 97, 175
    in breath, 228-230, 233
    intoxication, 100, 106, 175, 238,
    legal limits, 9, 22
    safe limit, 230
    susceptibility of drinkers, 175
    unit of, 173, 175, 226
    withdrawal symptoms, 177-178

Alcoholism, 106, 178

Alginate impressions, 293

Amnesia
    post-traumatic, 100

Amphetamines, 166, 172

Amyl nitrite, 167

Anabolic steroids, 167

Anal
    folds, 126, 133, 209-210
    fissures, 209
      healed, 126
      in Crohn's disease, 209
    skin texture, 210
    sphincter tone, 126, 133, 210
    tags, 209

Anti-convulsant medication, 96

Anus, 126, 203, 206
    in child sexual abuse (CSA), 133
    digital examination of, 206
    injury of, 210

Appeal
    grounds of, 8

Appropriate adult, 42, 50-51, 53-54, 64, 93, 105, 108, 172, 185, 189

Approved doctor (Section 12), 64, 186

Approved social worker (ASW), 64, 93, 105, 186-188, 190

Aspirin, 104

Association of Chief Police Officers (ACPO), 33, 36

Association of Chief Police Officers Scotland (ACPOS), 36

Association of Police Surgeons, 4, 52, 57 92, 143

Asthma, 97-99

'At risk' register, 140

Authorised Firearms Officers, 316

Automatism, 96, 191

B

Baby
    shaking of, 117

Bacterial vaginosis, 134

Balance of probability, 79

Barbiturates, 168, 241, 272

Barotrauma, 68, 161

Behavioural problems, 123

Beyond reasonable doubt, 11, 19, 38, 79, 139, 276

Bite marks, 67, 113, 123, 257, 265, 287-290, 292

Blennerhasset Committee, 231

Blood alcohol concentration, 174-175, 225-226

Blood sample for drugs, 268

Blood groups, 257, 306

Blood sugar, 97

Body bags, 300, 304

Body charts, 72, 121, 143, 145, 202

Body fluids, 11, 257, 262, 263, 317

Body search
  intimate, 47, 172
  orifices, 48

Body sketches, 63, 78

Bowel sounds
  in opioid misuse, 107

Brain death, 272

Breath alcohol
  levels of, 229-230
  measurement of, 106
  test, 228, 233

Bruise/Bruising 68-70, 72, 112-113,
  125-126, 129, 133-134, 146-149 207
  290, 293
  see petechiae

Buggery, 126, 193-194, 257

Bullet
  wound, 158-159

Burial Order, 282

Burns
  cigarette, 115-116, 118, 155
  deliberate infliction, 116

C

Cadaveric spasm, 273

Candida albicans, 134, 213

Cannabis, 48, 167, 172, 238, 241
  cultivation of, 263

Capacity to give consent, 39, 50

Carbamazepine, 96

Care
  compulsory measures of, 137-138

Carol X, 26

Case conference, 112, 118, 120, 140

Casualty bureau, 300

Cell visiting
  frequency of, 94

Chaperone, 53, 60, 93, 195-196,
  200-201, 210-211

Chest pain, 95

Chief Medical Officer, Department
  of Health, 215

Chief Medical Officer,
  Home Office, 172

Child
  assessment order, 136-137
  in care, 120
  protection, 136,137, 139-141
  protection register, 140
  sexual abuse, 2, 4, 119, 128, 133-134
  rights of, 135
  valid consent of, 93

Children Act 1989, 120, 135,

Children's Hearings, 31, 138

Children's Panel, 137-138

Chlamydia trachomatis, 133, 213

Civil courts, 7, 31, 82

Clinical forensic medicine
  assessment and accreditation in, 5

Clitoris, 125, 129, 134-135, 205

Clobazam, 96

Clonazepam, 96

Cocaine, 166, 172, 263

Code of Practice
  (Mental Health Act), 186

Codes of Practice (PACE), 19-20, 42, 50-51

Cognitive function, 105, 107, 227

Coitus
  vulvar, 129

College of Justice, 31

Colposcope, 124, 206

Commorientes, 299

Complainant, 15, 85, 103, 149, 154, 194-197
  200-203, 206-208, 210-211, 213-214

Complaint, 15
  details of, 78
  examination in case of, 66

Complainer, 26, 194

Compulsory admission
  (Mental Health Act), 186-188
  (Mental Health (Scotland) Act),
    190-191

Confessions, 19-21, 28, 161
  false, 21, 103, 106

Confidentiality, 39, 51-57, 60, 64, 120,
  171-172, 201
  breach of, 52
  duty of, 40-41, 54, 57
  and personal safety, 52

Conscious level, 99, 101

Consent
    capacity of child to give, 55
    capacity to give, 50, 55
    forms, 45
    implied, 44
    informed, 55, 59
    to medical examination, 136
    to medical treatment, 43, 51
    of the child, 120, 139

Constable
    constitutional position of, 309
    probationary, 37, 310

Constabulary
    Her Majesty's Inspectorate of, 34, 38

Coroner
    deaths to be reported, 278, 280
    duties at disaster, 300

Coroner's
    Form 100A, 279
    Form 100B, 279, 282

Coroner in Northern Ireland, 283

Corroboration, 22, 49, 306
    mutual, 25

Court
    appropriate dress for, 84
    contempt of, 12, 84
    doctors at, 82
    exhibit, 200-201, 269
    productions, 269
    report for in CSA, 128

Court of Appeal
    Civil Division, 8
    Criminal Division, 8

County Courts, 7

Court Listing Office, 75

Court of Criminal Appeal, 27

Court of Session, 31, 139

Cremation Regulations, 282

Crime and drug use, 163

Crime scene investigation, 247, 254, 255, 298

Criminal Injuries Compensation Board, 214

Criminal Procedure
    Royal Commission on, 19, 51

Cross-examination, 14-15, 40, 86-88, 123

Crown Counsel, 28, 286

Crown Court, 8, 13, 82, 84-85, 88

Crown Office, 26, 28

Crown Prosecution Service (CPS), 3, 9, 36, 38, 53, 55-57, 64, 66, 77, 83-85, 88

Custody
    patient in, 94, 96
    death in, 94, 280, 285

Custody officer, 42, 44, 51, 62, 64, 79, 93-94, 97, 108, 182, 185, 234

Custody record, 46-47, 53-54, 95-96

Cyanosis, 147

D

Data Protection, 54-55, 92

Death, 2, 18, 28, 94, 161-162, 216, 220, 222, 224-225, 244, 248, 254, 263, 271-286, 288, 299-300, 310, 318
    in custody, 280, 285
    legal definition of, 271
    temperature loss after, 274
    time of, 272-274

Debriefing
    critical incident (psychological), 318
    operational, 307

Declaration of Geneva, 43

Defence medical experts, 86-88

Delirium tremens, 178

Dental
    age, 294
    identification, 293
    imprints, 206
    stone models, 293

Detainees
    care of, 2, 52, 60, 91-93, 95, 97, 101, 107

Detention
    fitness for, 44, 50, 97, 163

Diabetes
    and driving, 232
    insulin dependent, 97
    non-insulin dependent, 97

Diagnosis of NAI
    errors in, 118

Diazepam, 96, 168, 177, 241

Diminished responsibility, 11, 191-192

Diploma in Medical Jurisprudence, 5

Diplopia, 99-100, 241

Director of Public Prosecutions, 9, 36, 38

Disaster
  cost of training for, 301
  identification of victims, 304
  plans, 301-302

Disclosure
  ordered by a court, 91

District Court, 26, 36

DNA database, 255, 258
  national, 30, 260

DNA profiling, 215, 256, 258-261, 265

Drinking and driving, 225, 231
  clinical examination, 236
  enforcement procedures, 233
  hospital procedure, 238
  refusal of blood test, 236
  refusal of breath test, 234

Driving
  and benzodiazepines, 232
  and diabetes, 232

Drug abuse
  stigmata of, 105

Drug
  class A, 48, 172
  criminal intent to supply, 50
  dependence, 163, 165-166, 168,
    170-171, 186
  driving under the influence of,
    231-232, 241
  search for, 48
  tolerance, 165, 168
  withdrawal, 106

Drug database centres
  regional, 105, 172

Drug misuse
  definition of, 165

Drug misuse and dependence
  (Mental Health Act), 171, 186

Drunk and incapable, 176

E

Ecstasy, 165-167, 263

Elderly drivers
  examination of, 239

Electrostatic detection apparatus, 254

Emergency hormonal contraception, 201,
  205, 211

Emergency Protection Order, 121, 136

Employment Medical Adviser, 313

Epilepsy, 44, 95-96, 100, 236-237,
  240-242

Episiotomy scars, 209

Equal opportunities policies, 311

Erythema, 134, 144, 207
  transient, 146

Ethanol, 173

European Convention, 16-19

Evidence
  admissibility of, 10, 31
  circumstantial, 10-11
  in chief, 29, 85-86
  children of, 12-13
  confessional, 20
  control and preservation of, 248
  corroborative, 22-23
  hearsay, 17-19, 21, 25, 30, 78
  law of, 9
  opinion and expert, 21, 79
  trace evidence, 65, 162, 203, 224,
    253-255, 257, 259, 263
  types of, 10

Examination
  in cases of complaint, 66
  in chief, 14
  of child by order of court, 136, 139
  consent to by child, 120, 140
  facilities, 60, 196
  genital in girls, 123
  kits, 61, 68
  records of, 53
  refusal, 41, 121
  in sexual assault, consent for, 201
  specimens taken in, 79
  suites, 196

Exhibit(s), 60, 67, 195-196, 200-201, 210,
  214, 236, 269, 292
  numbers, 201
  officer, 60

F

Fatal Accident Inquiry, 285-286

Fellatio, 200, 208

Fingerprint marks, 247, 251

Fingertip pressure, 69, 148

Fissures,
  anal, 209
  healed, 126
  in CSA, 133
  in Crohn's disease, 209

Fitness to be interviewed, 20, 102-103, 109, 163, 167, 169

Fitness to drive, 234, 239, 241

Fluoride/oxalate, 265

Fossa navicularis
lymphoid follicles in, 134

Fourchette, 125, 128, 130, 132, 134-135, 205, 209

Frenulum
torn, 113, 123, 129

Frog position, 124

Frozen awareness, 112

G

General Medical Council, 39, 49-50, 83, 120, 319

Genitalia
redness of, 129

Glaister's globe, 124-125

Gonorrhoea, 133, 213

Gooseflesh, 107, 169

Grip marks, 69, 113-114, 129, 149

H

Haematoma, 146, 222

Haemorrhage
extradural, 99
intracranial, 101
subdural, 99

Handcuff injuries, 70

Harm minimisation, 170

Head injury, 99-102, 225, 236, 241
and abnormal mental state, 182
in road traffic accident, 222

Health and safety at work legislation, 244, 309

Health records
access to, 55

Hearsay, 17-19, 21, 25, 30, 78

Heart disease, 94

Hepatitis B, 94, 154, 170, 213-214, 317
vaccination, 170, 317

Herpes, 133

High Court, 7

High Court of Justiciary, 26, 27, 29, 31, 36

Hippocratic Oath, 43, 51

Home Secretary, 34-35, 42, 301

House of Lords, 8, 25, 27, 31

Human immunodeficiency (HIV), 94, 127, 154, 167, 170-171, 213-214, 317

Human papilloma virus, 127, 213

Hymen,
appearance of, 205
crescentic, 130-131
fimbriated, 131, 205
healed tears of, 133, 210
influence of oestrogen, 132
imperforate, 131
measurement of, 131
orifice, 125, 128, 130-132, 205
posterior edge, 124
shape of, 130-131
tears of, 131-132, 209
torn, 125
transection of, 205, 209-210

Hypertension, 104, 178, 240

Hypoglycaemia, 182, 219, 232, 237, 240
and alcohol, 97, 175

I

Identification (personal), 42, 47, 150, 225, 250-251, 260-261, 293-294, 300, 304-307

Identification Commission, 300, 304

Incised wounds, 145, 151-152, 154, 208

Indecency, 194

Independent Commission for Police Complaints, 38

Indictment, 26, 28-29

Infanticide, 216

Infectious disease risks, 94

Injecting equipment
hazards of sharing, 167

Injury
absence of in sexual assault, 207
age of, 144, 207
defence, 73, 113, 149, 152, 153-154, 208
facial, 69, 223
handcuff, 70
intentional by prisoner, 154
interpretation of, 143
photographs of, 250
road traffic accident, 220-224

self-inflicted, 119, 154
in sexual assault, 203

Illiteracy
adult, 183

Inquest, 280-282, 284, 318
nature of, 281
self-incrimination at, 281

Intercourse
intercrural, 129

Interrogation, 13, 106,160-161

Interview
fitness for, 2, 50, 103-104, 106, 109,
169

Intimate searches, 41, 46-50, 163, 172

Intoxication
alcohol, 100, 106, 175, 238
clinical signs, 176
opiate, 168

Intrauterine device (IDU), 211

Introitus, 125, 131

J

Judicial decisions
binding, 8

Justice
miscarriage of, 8, 21, 31, 272

K

Khat, 166

Knee-chest position, 124, 126

L

Labelling of samples, 60, 195-196, 269

Labial
adhesions, 130, 134-135
separation, 124
traction, 124

Labia majora
wrinkling of, 130

Laceration, 41, 70, 144, 150-151, 210, 243

Large goods vehicle licence, 239, 313

Left lateral position, 126, 203

Legal Aid Fund, 88

Lichen sclerosus et atrophicus, 135

Ligature
application of, 148

Lithotomy position, 203

Lividity, 273

Lord Advocate, 26, 28, 36, 286

Love bites, 126, 129, 146, 149, 208

LSD, 167, 263

Lubricants
use of, 209

M

Malingering and mental state, 185

M'Naghten rules, 191

Magistrates court, 7-8, 13, 82-83, 85

Major incident, 37, 248, 297-298, 301-302,
310

Malpractice
police, 19

Mania, 106

Manic depressive illness, 184

Manual strangulation, 148-149, 207

Masturbation, 129, 194

Material
undisclosed, 56
unused, 56

Medical defence bodies, 57, 82, 120

Medical Certificate of Cause of Death,
277-279, 282-284

Medical jurisprudence
history of, 275

Medical reports
access to 54-55, 319

Medical treatment
consent to, 43

Medicines
custody of, 94

Mens rea, 10, 191

Mental health officer, 190

Mental illness
simulation of, 184-185

Mental state, 20, 30, 107, 163, 168,
171, 185, 202
examination, 181-183,

Mental Welfare Commission for Scotland, 190

Methadone, 107, 169-170

Mitochondrial DNA, 261

Modesty of the examinee, 202

Motor vehicles
  air bags, 224
  restraining systems, 223

Munchausen's syndrome by proxy, 118

N

Naloxone, 171

National Criminal Intelligence Service, (NCIS), 36

Negative findings
  record of, 78

Neisseria gonorrhoeae, 213

Non-accidental injury, 2, 4, 111, 242-243

Notes
  clinical, 63, 77, 92
  contemporaneous, 64, 73, 77, 92, 94, 162, 181
  disclosed to defence, 83, 122
  examination, 83, 294
  original, 63, 83-85, 195, 201
  private, 46, 53, 56

Nystagmus, 69, 167, 176, 178, 237

O

Oath, 12-13, 27, 29, 85, 139, 188, 281

Occupational health units, 309

Office of Population Censuses and Surveys, 278

Officer safety training, 316

Opening speech, 14

Opiate withdrawal, 169

Opioid analgesics, 104

Out of England Order, 283

P

PACE
  Code C, 42, 44, 53-54, 103
  Code D 42, 45-47
  Codes of Practice, 19-20, 42, 50-51

Papilloma virus, 127, 213

Paracetamol, 104, 169

Parental rights
  transfer of, 136, 139

Parental responsibility, 120, 135-136

Passenger carrying vehicle licence, 239, 241, 313

Past medical history, 78

Patient
  health and welfare of, 91

Peak expiratory flow rate (PFR), 97, 99

Penetration
  proof of, 193

Pensions, 320-321

Perceptual disorders, 183

Periurethral bands, 134

Perjury, 85

Petechiae, 66, 113, 125, 129-130, 146, 148, 207-208, 290

Phenytoin, 96

Photography, 67, 72, 249-250, 254, 291-293

Physeptone, 107

Physical fit in forensic science, 262

Physician
  safety of, 93

Place of safety, 139, 187-188

Pleading diet, 29

Police arrest techniques, 67

Police authorities, 34-35, 60
  doctors contracted to, 62
  in Scotland, 35

Police
  duties of, 33-35
  complaints against, 28, 37, 65

Police officers
  pensions
    ill-health, 320
  permanent disablement, 320
  promotion, 37, 110
  sickness absence, 319

Police Complaints Authority (PCA), 38, 66

Police Federation, 313

Police Protection Order, 136

Polymerase chain reaction (PCR), 259

Post-ictal state, 95, 191

Post-mortem hypostasis (lividity), 273

Post-traumatic stress disorder (PTSD), 318

Post-traumatic stress reaction, 303

Precognition, 27-28, 285

Prednisolone, 99

Pregnancy, 111, 125, 133, 193, 200, 210, 213, 215-216
    termination of, 215

Prescription only medicines, 164

Prescription
    NHS, 60
    private, 94

Presumptions, 12

Prisoners
    examinations of, 43

Privilege
    absolute, 52-53, 91
    professional, 23

Procedure
    solemn, 26

Proctoscope, 206

Procurator Fiscal, 27-29, 36, 38, 191, 275, 293
    and death investigation, 283, 286
    duties at disaster, 300, 304

Proof
    balance of probability, 79
    beyond reasonable doubt, 79
    civil standard, 31
    standard of, 11, 16, 31, 79, 139, 276

Proof hearings, 138

Prosecution
    private, 26
    public, 36

Protective disposable overalls, 161

Psilocybin, 167

Psychosis, 106, 166, 178, 191,
    functional, 182-183

Pupillary dilatation, 107

Purpura, 146

Q

Questions
    leading, 14, 85-86

R

Random breath testing (RTB), 230-231

Rape, 10, 15, 26, 129, 210, 212-213, 287
    definition of, 193-194,

Rape Trauma Syndrome, 213

Raphe
    midline, 126

Registrar of Births and Deaths, 277-278

Registrar's acknowledgement of registration, 282

Relationship
    doctor/patient, 40, 61

Relationship between alcohol and crime, 176

Remand to hospital, 191

Reporter to the Children's Panel, 137

Responsibility
    dual, 40

Rigor mortis, 273

Royal Ulster Constabulary (RUC), 35, 270

S

Saliva
    samples, 257, 268
    swabs, 291
    and mouth swabs, 46, 200

Samples
    corroborate taking of, 60
    internal, 30
    intimate and non-intimates, 46-47

Scalding, 116, 243, 285

Scarring, 145, 209

Scene of crime
    bite marks at, 288
    examinations by forensic scientist, 255
    filming of, 250
    major incident site, 298
    photographs of, 249
    restricted access to, 248, 254
    contamination of, 264

Scenes of Crime Officer (SOCO), 37, 47, 65, 247-248, 251, 313

Schizophrenia, 106, 183-184

Sealing packages, 269

Secretary of State for Northern Ireland, 35

Secretary of State for Scotland, 35

Section 9 statement, 76, 82

Securitainers, 235-236

Senior investigating officer, 62, 247-249

Serious bodily harm, 144

Sexual examination kit, 196

Sexual assault
  examination of suspects, 214
  psychological consequences of, 211
  and STD prophylaxis, 213

Sexual variant behaviour, 217

Sexually transmitted diseases, 125-127, 211, 213-214

Sheriff Court, 26-27, 29, 31, 36

Sheriff
  petition to, 28

Shifts, 311

Shotguns, 155

Silence
  right of, 15-16

Skeletal survey, 111, 117-118

Skin tag, 126, 133

Skull
  fracture, 100-101
  X-ray criteria for, 100

Sodomy, 194

Solemn trial, 29

Solicitor General, 28

Solicitor-advocates, 27, 31

Soul and conscience (certificate), 29

Speculum, 125, 204-205

Spermatozoa
  in CSA, 133
  persistence of, 200-201, 257

Sphincter external
  dilatation of, 126

Stab wound, 152-153

Status epilepticus, 96

Statutory declaration, 76-77

Steroids
  anabolic, 167

Stillbirth, 215

Stipendiary magistrates, 26

Straddle injury, 134

Substance misuse and mental illness, 184

Suicide risk, 185

Summary cases, 26-27

Summary complaint, 28

Supervising pathologist, 302

Suspicious death, 161, 244

Swab, 30, 46, 124-125
  of anus, 206
  endocervical, 204
  high vaginal, 204
  for lubricants, 257
  moistened, 68
  of mouth, 40, 200
  of penis, 205
  saliva, 46, 200, 291
  sterile untreated, 265
  vaginal, 203
    examination of, 257, 265
  vulval, 203

Symptom led medication, 95, 97

Syphilis, 133

T

Tachycardia, 107, 167, 177-178, 312

Tampons, 123, 200, 204

Tanner growth charts, 123

Tanner Stages, 203

Temazepam, 96

Temporary mortuary plan, 300

Tetanus, 317

Threadworms, 135

Tokyo Declaration, 160

Tone
  anal, 126

Torture, 19, 160-161

Traffic wardens, 313

Trial
  order of, 13

Tramline bruising, 69, 148

Treasure trove, 276

Treatment plans, 93

Triage at disaster site, 299

Trichomonas vaginalis, 133, 213

U

Ultraviolet light, 68, 72, 206

Ultraviolet photography, 250, 292

Urethra
prolapse of, 134

Urine for alcohol & drugs, 268

V

Vagina
foreign bodies in, 135, 204

Vaginal
discharge, 135
lacerations, 210

Valproate, 96

Verdict
not proven, 26

Victims
dental charting of, 294

Volatile substance
inhalation of, 168

Vulnerable persons
representation of, 51

Vulva in children, 125

Vulvitis, 130, 135, 146

W

Ward of Court, 121

Warts
ano-genital, 127, 133

Weapons
ballistic testing of, 252
rifled, 156
smooth bore, 155

Withdrawal
alcohol, 177-178
benzodiazepine, 168
heroin, 168-169

Witness(es)
child, 12-13, 122
competent, 12
expert, 4, 30, 76
fees for, 88
of fact, 75 84
professional, 1, 4, 75, 84, 87
payment of, 88

Witness summons, 83

Wood's light, 206

Wound
age of, 144
description of, 143
firearm, 155-160
location of, 145
penetrating, 70
self-inflicted, 72, 154
shape of, 145